FRONTIERS IN NEUROENDOCRINOLOGY
VOLUME 5

Frontiers in Neuroendocrinology

Volume 5

Edited by

William F. Ganong, M.D.
Professor of Physiology
Chairman, Department of Physiology
University of California
San Francisco, California

Luciano Martini, M.D.
Professor and Chairman
Institute of Endocrinology
University of Milan
Milan, Italy

Raven Press ▪ New York

Raven Press, 1140 Avenue of the Americas, New York, New York 10036

Made in the United States of America

International Standard Book Number 0–89004–1350
Library of Congress Catalog Card Number: 77–82030

Preface

This book is the fifth in a series of volumes surveying the frontiers of the new and rapidly expanding science of neuroendocrinology. Neuroendocrinologists are concerned not only with neural control of endocrine secretion, but also with the effects of hormones on the brain and behavior, and with the broader problems of the interactions between the brain and the internal environment. The field was reviewed in a comprehensive two volume survey published twelve years ago (*Neuroendocrinology,* L. Martini and W. F. Ganong, eds., Academic Press, New York, Volume I, 1966; Volume II, 1967). The present series is designed to update the initial survey by publishing, at intervals of approximately two years, a collection of papers reviewing the areas of neuroendocrinology in which there have been advances, innovations, and controversies. The first three volumes in the *Frontiers in Neuroendocrinology* series were published by Oxford University Press; one in 1969, one in 1971, and one in 1973. Volume 4 was published by Raven Press in 1976. The present volume, Volume 5, again focusses on particularly active, exciting areas in neuroendocrinology.

Since the appearance of *Frontiers in Neuroendocrinology,* Volume 4, there has been immense progress in our knowledge of the nature, distribution and function of peptides in the brain. Enkephalins and endorphins, the brain peptides that act on opiate receptors, have been isolated and characterized, and a precursor molecule from which these peptides are formed has been found in the pituitary gland. Somatostatin, the growth hormone inhibiting hormone first isolated from the hypothalamus, has also been found in the gastrointestinal tract, and several other peptides have been shown to be common to the brain and gastrointestinal system. There has been continuing rapid progress in the immunocytochemical localization of peptides that are putative synaptic transmitters in the nervous system, including the enkephalins. The "brain renin-angiotensin system" continues to be a subject for active research and spirited debate. Important advances have been made in our knowledge of the interactions between catecholamines and steroids in various parts of the body. The suprachiasmatic nuclei have been shown to regulate many circadian rhythms and the entrainment of these rhythms by light. These and other subjects are covered in the present volume. Rapid publication has made it possible to combine the features of review monographs and journal articles. The contributors are experts in their fields, and they have been encouraged to include not only published data, but also, where pertinent, the results of their own current research. This should make the book of particular value to investigators engaged in research in neuroendocrinology and other aspects of neurobiology. It should also be of interest to endocrinologists, neurochemists, psychologists, psychiatrists, neurologists, biochemists, and all those concerned with any of the multiple facets of the interactions between the brain and the endocrine glands.

William F. Ganong, M.D.
Luciano Martini, M.D.

Contents

Contributors

Howard W. Blume
Division of Neurology
The Montreal General Hospital and
  McGill University
1650 Cedar Avenue
Montreal, Quebec H3G 1A4 Canada

Steven R. Childers
Departments of Pharmacology and
  Experimental Therapeutics
Johns Hopkins University
School of Medicine
Baltimore, Maryland 21205

Emilio del Pozo
Department of Experimental Thera-
  peutics
Medical and Biological Research Di-
  vision
Sandoz Ltd.
CH-4002 Basel, Switzerland

Robert Elde
Department of Anatomy
University of Minnesota
321 Church Street, SE
Minneapolis, Minnesota 55455

Alan N. Epstein
Department of Biology
University of Pennsylvania
326 Leidy Lab G-7
Philadelphia, Pennsylvania 19174

Kjell Fuxe
Department of Histology
Karolinska Institute
Stockholm 60 Sweden

Detlev Ganten
University of Heidelberg
Im Neuenheimer Feld 366
6900 Heidelberg, Germany

Ursula Ganten
University of Heidelberg
Im Neuenheimer Feld 366
6900 Heidelberg, Germany

John E. Gerich
Diabetes and Metabolism Research
  Laboratory
Mayo Medical School and Mayo Clinic
Rochester, Minnesota 55901

Tomas Hökfelt
Department of Histology
Karolinska Institute
Stockholm 60 Sweden

E. Knobil
Department of Physiology
University of Pittsburgh
School of Medicine
Pittsburgh, Pennsylvania 15261

Ioana Lancranjan
Department of Experimental Thera-
  peutics
Medical and Biological Research Di-
  vision
Sandoz Ltd.
CH-4002 Basel, Switzerland

Mara Lorenzi
Metabolic Research Unit
University of California
San Francisco, California 94143

Johannes F. E. Mann
University of Heidelberg
Im Neuenheimer Feld 366
6900 Heidelberg, Germany

Neville Marks
New York Institute for Neurochemis-
  try and Drug Addiction
Rockland Research Institute
Wards Island, New York 10035

Robert Y. Moore
Department of Neurosciences M-008
University of California at San Diego
La Jolla, California 92093

U. Otten

Department of Pharmacology
Biocenter of the University
Klingelbergstr. 70
CH-4056 Basel, Switzerland

M. Ian Phillips

University of Heidelberg
Im Neuenheimer Feld 366
6900 Heidelberg, Germany

Quentin J. Pittman

Division of Neurology
The Montreal General Hospital and
  McGill University
1650 Cedar Avenue
Montreal, Quebec H3G 1A4 Canada

T. M. Plant

Department of Physiology
University of Pittsburgh
School of Medicine
Pittsburgh, Pennsylvania 15261

Leo P. Renaud

Division of Neurology
The Montreal General Hospital and
  McGill University
1650 Cedar Avenue
Montreal, Quebec H3G 1A4 Canada

Alan G. Robinson

Department of Medicine
University of Pittsburgh
School of Medicine
Pittsburgh, Pennsylvania 15261

Solomon H. Snyder

Departments of Pharmacology and
  Experimental Therapeutics
Johns Hopkins University
School of Medicine
Baltimore, Maryland 21205

H. Thoenen

Department of Pharmacology
Biocenter of the University
Klingelbergstr. 70
CH-4056 Basel, Switzerland

George R. Uhl

Departments of Pharmacology and
  Experimental Therapeutics
Johns Hopkins University
School of Medicine
Baltimore, Maryland 21205

Frontiers in Neuroendocrinology, Vol. 5,
edited by W. F. Ganong and L. Martini.
Raven Press, New York © 1978.

Chapter 1

Distribution of Hypothalamic Hormones and Other Peptides in the Brain

*Robert Elde and Tomas Hökfelt

Karolinska Institute, Department of Histology, S–104 01 Stockholm, Sweden

In the previous volume in this series, Zimmerman (193) reviewed advances in immunohistochemical mapping of neuropeptides, focusing especially on posterior pituitary hormones and luteinizing hormone releasing hormone (LRH). Since then, a number of studies have provided many more details of the organization of neuroendocrine systems. In addition, widely distributed peptidergic neuronal systems have now been localized throughout the central and peripheral nervous systems (85). The functional implications of prominent peptide-containing neuronal systems are largely unknown, but these matters are currently under intensive investigation. These findings have added new aspects to the discussions of differences and similarities of the concepts of neurosecretion and neurotransmission (25,165).

The study of peptidergic neurons clearly has its roots in neuroendocrinology. Perhaps the first biologically active peptide to be isolated in crude form from the central nervous system was the neurohormone vasopressin (100,137). Half a century later the sequence and synthesis of oxytocin and vasopressin (50,51) served to mark the beginning of the era of neuropeptide research. The characterization of three hypothalamic regulatory hormones has been another milestone in this field (73,164). The present rate of progress in neuropeptide research can be illustrated by the recent but now voluminous account of the morphinomimetic peptides. Evidence that such factors existed was first offered in the early seventies (152,173,177). By 1975 the first of these peptides was isolated, characterized, and its sequence was determined and confirmed by chemical synthesis (101). Within weeks of this report other laboratories isolated, sequenced, and synthesized other members of the family of morphinomimetic peptides. The availability of the synthetic peptides has enabled a large number of laboratories to investigate their manifold activities (see 72,73,176) and to produce antibodies so that the distribution of these substances could be established by immunohistochemistry (55,84,88,172).

* Present address: Department of Anatomy, University of Minnesota, Minneapolis, Minnesota 55455.

In this report we summarize results obtained to date on the distribution of neuropeptides, especially within the hypothalamus. Brief mention is made of the distribution of these peptides within the other areas of the nervous system. For a more thorough account of the latter we refer to recent review articles (54,85). The studies we report rely on immunohistochemical techniques which are inherently qualitative tools; at certain points in this chapter we attempt to relate our findings to quantitative studies from other laboratories.

IMMUNOHISTOCHEMICAL METHODS

Much of what is currently known about the cellular distribution of peptides rests on the achievements of neuroendocrine physiologists and peptide chemists who have extracted and chromatographed extremely small quantities of biologically active materials, making possible the determination of their primary structure. Subsequently, synthetic peptides have been coupled to large carrier proteins and used as immunogens to elicit the production of specific antibodies.

Antibodies

We have used primary antibodies generated in our own laboratories as well as those generously provided by other investigators (Table 1). In all cases the peptide was coupled to a larger carrier protein in order to render the peptide more antigenic. For example, several of our antibodies have been raised in response to peptides coupled to keyhole limpet hemocyanin or thyroglobulin (somatostatin, vasopressin, oxytocin, luteinizing hormone releasing hormone, enkephalins; see 174). In many cases these antibodies have also been characterized and used in radioimmunoassays. The characterization of several of these antisera in such competitive peptide binding studies has served as an independent test of the specificity of the antigen-antibody interaction. In all cases the specificity of the antisera was verified within the immunohistochemical method by the use of antibodies whose combining sites had been blocked by treatment of the serum with an excess of the antigen. The secondary, fluorescein-labeled antibodies were obtained from commercial sources (Statens Bakteriologiska Laboratorium, Stockholm; Antibodies Incorporated, Davis, California).

Tissue Preparation

Tissues to be studied using the light microscopic, immunofluoresence procedure were fixed by transcardiac perfusion of ice cold, phosphate-buffered 4% paraformaldehyde (145). After perfusion for 30 min, the brain was removed and placed in the above fixative for an additional 90 min. In prepa-

TABLE 1–1. Peptides and sources of antisera

Peptide	Abbreviation[a]	Structural characterization	Carrier protein	Antisera Code[b]	Antisera Source
Vasopressin	VP	duVigneaud (50)	Thyroglobulin	GP24a	Elde (52)
Oxytocin	OXY	duVigneaud et al. (51)	Hemocyanin	R111g	Elde[e]
Neurophysins	NP	Hope (99)	—	RNF9[c]	Seybold and Elde[e]
		Walter et al. (185)		R81a[d]	Elde[e]
Thyrotropin releasing hormone	TRH	Burgus et al. (36)	Albumin	R79	Jeffcoate et al. (103)
		Nair et al. (132)			
Luteinizing hormone releasing hormone	LRH	Amoss et al. (3)	Albumin	R-N	Jeffcoate et al. (104)
		Schally et al. (163)	Hemocyanin	R122a	Elde[e]
Somatostatin	SOM	Brazeau et al. (26)	Thyroglobulin	GP2d	Elde and Parsons (56)
			Hemocyanin	R141c	Elde et al. (56)
Substance P	SP	Chang et al. (38)	Albumin	R16	Nilsson et al. (134)
Leucine-enkephalin	ENK	Hughes et al. (101)	Thyroglobulin	GP14b	Elde et al. (55)
Methionine-enkephalin	ENK	Hughes et al. (101)	Hemocyanin	R6c	Elde et al. (55)

[a] Refers to immunoreactivity identified by antibodies to the named peptide.
[b] GP, antisera raised in guinea pigs; R, antisera raised in rabbits.
[c] Antisera specific for bovine neurophysin II.
[d] Antisera directed against all porcine neurophysins.
[e] Unpublished observations.

ration for sectioning, the tissue was transferred to 5% sucrose in phosphate buffer. The tissue was sectioned at 10 μm in a cryostat (Dittes, Heidelberg) at $-20°$C.

Immunohistochemical Reactions

The indirect immunofluorescence technique of Coons and collaborators (40) formed the basis for the studies reported. Tissues sections were exposed to a dilution (range 1:10 to 1:100) of the primary antiserum in phosphate-buffered saline (PBS) for 30 min in a humid atmosphere at 37°C. After rinsing to remove unbound serum proteins, the fluorescein-labeled second antibody (diluted 1:4) was applied and incubated in a similar manner. After rinsing, a coverslip was mounted with glycerin:PBS (3:1). Both primary and secondary antisera were diluted so as to contain 0.3% Triton X-100 (77). In all cases, the primary antiserum was pretreated with an excess of the carrier protein, in order to remove antibodies directed against this portion of the immunogen. The tissues were examined in a Zeiss fluorescence microscope.

Experimental Animals

Tissues studied were obtained from normal male rats and guinea pigs. To enhance the staining of certain peptides within neuronal perikarya, we administered colchicine (30 to 150 μg/kg) intraventricularly or intracisternally 24 to 48 hr prior to sacrifice (88). Some rats were treated with stereotaxically placed electrolytic lesions 5 days prior to sacrifice in order to study the connectivity of certain cell bodies and terminals. Hypothalamic deafferentations (75) were also performed in order to study peptidergic pathways projecting to the hypothalamus.

VASOPRESSIN, OXYTOCIN, AND NEUROPHYSINS

Since the discussion in the previous volume of this series (193), it has become even more clear that each of the posterior pituitary nonapeptides has a unique cellular distribution, and that the differential distribution of the neurophysins parallels that of the peptides (5,169,181,182,184). Thus, a specific neurophysin seems to be associated with vasopressin and another

$\longrightarrow$

FIG. 1–1. Immunofluorescence micrograph (mount) of a coronal section of the rat hypothalamus after incubation with an antiserum to bovine neurophysin II. Note the numerous axons of paraventricular nucleus origin which are approaching the supraoptic nucleus (*) and optic chiasm (CO). These beaded, varicose fibers join with axons originating from the supraoptic nucleus and project to the median eminence and posterior lobe of the pituitary. The neurophysin-positive cell bodies have been intentionally overexposed in order to record the details of the varicose nerve fibers. +, intrachiasmatic portion, supraoptic nucleus. Magnification 120$\times$.

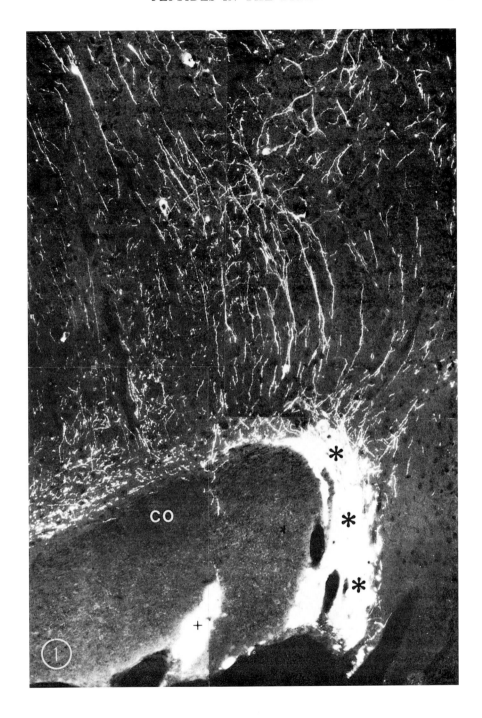

with oxytocin. Neuronal perikarya detectable by immunohistochemical methods for vasopressin and oxytocin are found primarily in the magnocellular neurosecretory nuclei of the hypothalamus—the supraoptic and paraventricular nuclei (181,186,193). Small groups of vasopressin- and oxytocin-positive neurons, often closely associated with blood vessels, are found scattered between the boundaries of the supraoptic and paraventricular nuclei. The retrochiasmatic division of the supraoptic nucleus also contains these peptides. In addition, the suprachiasmatic nucleus contains a number of small, densely packed, vasopressin-positive neuronal perikarya (183). In all regions studied, the distribution of a specific neurophysin is essentially parallel to that of its respective peptide. Recently, Weindl and Sofroniew (187) described a previously unrecognized group of neurophysin-containing neuronal perikarya within the triangular nucleus of the septum.

The axons projecting from the vasopressin and oxytocinergic neurons are readily observed using immunohistochemical techniques. The arching projections of axons laterally and then ventrally from the paraventricular nucleus toward the supraoptic nucleus are especially striking (Fig. 1–1). Brownfield and Kozlowski (27) have recently traced a group of neurophysin-containing fibers from the paraventricular nucleus which diverge from the ventrally arching fibers, and instead pass dorsally toward the lateral ventricles where they appear to terminate within the choroid plexus. The response of the choroid plexus to exogenously administered vasopressin suggests a possible functional role for a vasopressin/neurophysin projection to the choroid plexus (166).

Using classic staining techniques for neurosecretory material or immunohistochemical techniques, several investigators have noted the presence of terminals containing vasopressin in the external layer of the median eminence [Fig. 1–2; reviewed by Zimmerman (193)]. The quantity of vasopressin and neurophysin within these terminals increases following adrenalectomy. Thus, the possibility that vasopressin might be present in high concentrations in hypophyseal portal blood has been discussed, and the suggestion that vasopressin may act to release ACTH from the pituitary under certain conditions has been revived (193). Vandesande et al. (180,183) proposed on the basis of axonal morphology that the vasopressin present in the external layer of the median eminence might originate from the vasopressin-containing

→

FIGS. 1–2, 1–3, 1–4. Immunofluorescence micrographs of coronal sections of the ventral aspect of the normal (Fig. 1–2) and experimentally altered (Figs. 1–3 and 1–4) rat hypothalamus after incubation with antiserum to bovine neurophysin II. The internal layer (IL) of the normal rat median eminence displays the massive neurophysin projection to the posterior pituitary, whereas the external layer (EL) contains a more delicate array of neurophysin-positive nerve terminals adjacent to portal capillaries. Neurophysin immunoactivity is greatly reduced in the external layer of the median eminence from animals sacrificed 5 days after bilateral thermal lesions that include the paraventricular nucleus (Fig. 1–3). Similarly, the amount of neurophysin immunoreactivity in the external layer is greatly reduced in animals sacrificed 24 hr after injection of reserpine (10 mg/kg, i.p.) (Fig. 1–4). *, third ventricle. Magnification 120× (Figs. 1–2, 1–4); 300× (Fig. 1–3).

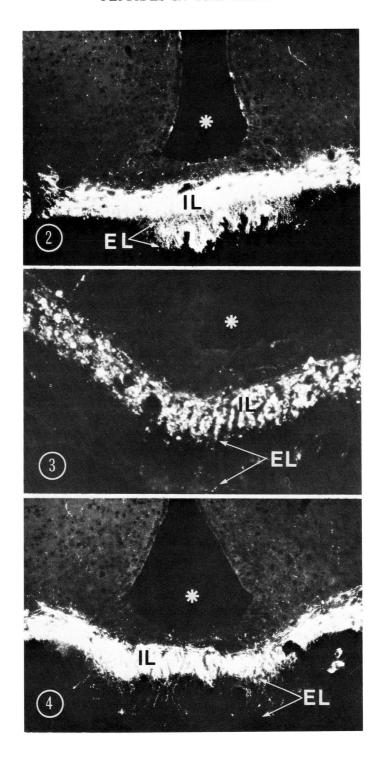

neurons of the suprachiasmatic nucleus. However, lesion studies have not
supported this notion. Immunohistochemical staining for vasopressin and
neurophysin on sections of the median eminence of rats sacrificed 5 days
after stereotactically placed bilateral electrolytic lesions confined to the
suprachiasmatic nucleus revealed no decrease in the amount of vasopressin
or neurophysin in the external layer of the median eminence (R. Elde and
T. Hökfelt, *unpublished observations*). Recently, Antunes et al. (4) reported that lesions of the paraventricular nucleus in the monkey selectively
remove stainable vasopressin and neurophysin from the external layer of
the median eminence. We have studied this projection in the rat and have
also found the paraventricular nucleus to project to the external layer of
the median eminence (R. Elde and T. Hökfelt, *unpublished observations;*
Fig. 1–3).

We have found that storage of the neurosecretory products of this subsystem of vasopressinergic neurons is extremely sensitive to reserpine, an
agent which is known to deplete monoamines. Vasopressin and neurophysin
disappear from the external layer of the median eminence 24 hr after administration of reserpine (10 mg/kg, i.p.) (Fig. 1–4). Administration of
reserpine did not induce changes in the vasopressin and neurophysin staining
pattern in the posterior lobe of the pituitary. The sensitivity of the paraventricular nucleus–external layer vasopressinergic system to reserpine is interesting in light of the findings of Bhattacharya and Marks (23) who reported
the disappearance of bioassayable corticotropin releasing hormone (CRF)
activity from the median eminence 24 hr after reserpine. Although the reserpine effect may not be mediated by an aminergic mechanism (24), there is
a striking parallel in the time course of the depletion of CRF and immuno-
histochemically stainable vasopressin/neurophysin. In summary, these findings add weight to the possibility that this vasopressin/neurophysin subsystem might act to specifically release ACTH from the pituitary under certain
physiological conditions.

The recent findings of vasopressinergic projections to extrahypothalamic
sites (27) and what may be an entirely separate vasopressinergic system in
the septal area (187) suggest a greater functional role for vasopressin than
previously considered. Schultz and collaborators (166) have suggested that
innervation of the choroid plexus by vasopressinergic fibers may serve to
control fluid and electrolyte balance of the cerebrospinal fluid by acting on
choroid receptors whose function may be similar to those in the distal tubule

$\longrightarrow$

FIG. 1–5. Immunofluorescence micrographs of longitudinal sections of the rat spinal cord after incubation
with antisera to bovine neurophysin II, substance P, and methionine-enkephalin, respectively. A very few
brightly fluorescent descending neurophysin-containing nerve fibers are seen in the dorsal horn (A). A
rather dense network of substance P-containing fibers and terminals is localized in the vicinity of the intermediolateral cell column (B). Fibers containing enkephalin are found in the dorsal horn (C) as well as in
the area around the central canal. Arrow indicates rostrocaudal axis of spinal cord. Magnification 300×.

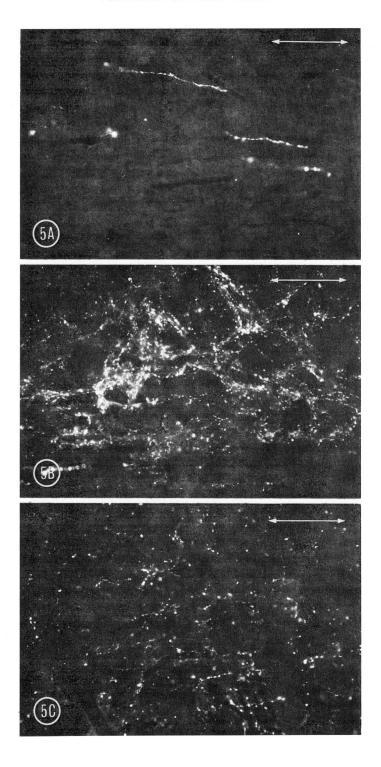

of the kidney. Immunohistochemical evidence for vasopressin in the septal area strengthens the proposed role of vasopressin in certain aspects of behavior (187,190). We have recently demonstrated the presence of a small number of intensely fluorescent nerve fibers in the spinal cord which often run transversely from the region of the central canal toward the dorsolateral aspect of the intermediate gray matter (Fig. 1–5A). These fibers disappear below a total transection of the cord. Such a projection from the paraventricular nucleus has been suggested from autoradiographic studies (39,162).

THYROTROPIN RELEASING HORMONE

The tripeptide thyrotropin releasing hormone (TRH) was isolated from hypothalamic extracts and characterized by Burgus et al. (36) and by Nair et al. (132). Although this peptide was identified because of its ability to induce the release of thyroid stimulating hormone from the pituitary, its extrahypothalamic distribution signaled a broader functional role than regulation of pituitary function (12,33,102,115,116,136,191).

Although a number of laboratories have successfully generated antibodies to this peptide that are useful for radioimmunoassay, its immunohistochemical localization has proven to be extremely difficult. It may be that a tripeptide is close to the lower limit of peptides which can be chemically stabilized *in situ* by a histological fixative and still present the complete antigenic determinant necessary for binding of the specific antibody. Using one of the several TRH antisera raised by Jeffcoate et al. (103), investigators have localized TRH in a number of hypothalamic and extrahypothalamic structures by immunofluorescence procedures (89,90). The medial portion of the external layer of the median eminence contains a high density of TRH-positive terminals that appear to abut on the capillary loops of the portal plexus (Fig. 1–6). Nerve terminals containing TRH immunoreactivity are found in several hypothalamic nuclei including the dorsomedial nucleus, the paraventricular nucleus, and the perifornical region. Less prominent TRH fibers are found in the medial aspect of the ventromedial nucleus, the zona incerta, and the periventricular area. Occasional fibers are encountered in the suprachiasmatic nucleus, the ventral preoptic area, the magnocellular paraventricular nucleus, and the medial forebrain bundle. The organum vasculosum of the lamina terminalis (OVLT) contains only a few TRH-positive fibers. Outside of the hypothalamus, TRH terminals are seen in nucleus ac-

→

FIGS. 1–6, 1–7, 1–8. Immunofluorescence micrographs of coronal sections of the ventral aspect of the normal (Fig. 1–6) and experimentally altered (Figs. 1–7 and 1–8) rat hypothalamus after incubation with antiserum to TRH. Fibers and terminals containing TRH are seen, especially in the medial aspects of the median eminence (Fig. 1–6). The TRH-containing terminals are greatly reduced in the median eminence of rats sacrificed 5 days after bilateral electrolytic lesions of the hypothalamic periventricular nucleus (Fig. 1–7). However, thermal lesions of the paraventricular and dorsomedial nuclei had no effect on the TRH-containing elements of the median eminence (Fig. 1–8). *, third ventricle. Magnification 120× (Figs. 1–6 and 1–8); 300× (Fig. 1–7).

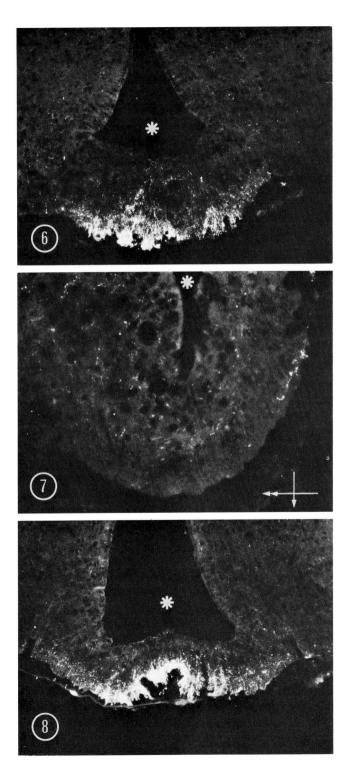

cumbens, nucleus interstitialis stria terminalis, and the lateral septal nucleus. In addition, a number of brainstem nuclei, the ventral horn, and the intermediolateral cell column of the spinal cord contain TRH-positive terminals.

Cell bodies containing TRH immunoreactivity have been found in the lateral hypothalamus, dorsomedial nucleus, paraventricular nucleus, perifornical region, and periventricular nucleus. Bilateral electrolytic lesions that include the latter area result in the disappearance of TRH from the external layer of the median eminence (Fig. 1–7). A limited rostral deafferentation of the medial basal hypothalamus at the caudal border of the optic chiasm also leads to disappearance of TRH from the external layer. However, neither the lesion nor the deafferentation reduces the number of terminals containing TRH in the dorsomedial nucleus. Furthermore, lesions that include the paraventricular and dorsomedial nuclei do not diminish the amount of stainable TRH in the median eminence (Fig. 1–8). Our interpretation of these findings is that the TRH neuroendocrine system has its cell bodies in the periventricular region dorsal to the optic chiasm and that these neurons project to the external layer of the median eminence. The location of these cell bodies coincides closely with the so-called thyrotropic area described using other techniques (61,69,75,113,156).

LUTEINIZING HORMONE RELEASING HORMONE

The decapeptide LRH was isolated, characterized, and synthesized in 1971 (3,163). A number of laboratories succeeded in producing antibodies to this peptide, and its distribution was established by radioimmunoassays of extracts of specific brain regions (32,34,142,189) and by immunohistochemistry (22,37,125). Since then, numerous immunohistochemical studies of this peptide have been published and several lines of controversy have emerged. There is little dispute concerning the distribution of LRH in the median eminence (13,44,111,193).

In the rostral portions of the median eminence LRH terminals are rather evenly distributed across the extent of the external layer. Caudal to this region, LRH terminals are found in extremely high numbers in the lateral lips of the median eminence at the tuberoinfundibular sulcus. A large number of LRH terminals are also found abutting on the capillaries of the OVLT.

There is controversy over the localization of LRH cell bodies using immunohistochemical techniques. A number of investigators (using peroxidase immunohistochemical techniques) have exhaustively searched the hypothalamus and other regions of the central nervous system for LRH-positive cell bodies and have found none (8,9,104,108,109,112). Barry and collaborators (13–22,168,170) have for several years reported scattered LRH-positive cell bodies in the preoptic and suprachiasmatic regions of a number of animals. In some cases they have manipulated the state of the LRH neurons with colchicine, methanol, melatonin, and barbiturates in order to increase the intensity of immunofluorescent staining. Most of the positive cell bodies they have localized lie outside of the hypophysiotrophic area. However, Zimmerman and co-workers (193,194) reported LRH-positive cell bodies in the arcuate nucleus of the mouse, and Naik (130,131) reported similar findings in the arcuate nucleus of the rat. Recently, Hoffman et al. (80) reported their study of LRH positivity in arcuate neurons using different antisera, each of which recognized a unique determinant site on the LRH molecule. One of these antisera localized LRH-containing arcuate neurons; the other demonstrated preoptic neurons, but all antisera could stain LRH terminals in the median eminence and OVLT. These findings may account for the disparate results of the several laboratories involved.

SOMATOSTATIN

The biological activity of a peptide with growth hormone release inhibiting activity was first described by Krulich and colleagues (115). This peptide was completely characterized, sequenced, and synthesized by Brazeau et al. (26). Studies on the distribution of the tetradecapeptide by bioassay (178) and radioimmunoassay (29,57,114,141; R. Elde, S. Efendić, T. Hökfelt, O. Johansson, R. Luft, J. Parsons, A. Roovete and R. Sorenson, submitted for publication) have indicated that this peptide, like TRH, is widely distributed throughout the central nervous system. Numerous immunohistochemical studies have added to our understanding of the details of the somatostatin-containing systems within the brain (for reviews see 82,83,85, 143). These localizations have revealed somatostatin-containing elements in the median eminence (10,42,45,53,81,82,107,143,146,148,149,167), and hypothalamic cell bodies in the periventricular area (1,46,56,82). In addition, somatostatin-containing nerve fibers have been found in the peripheral nervous system in the gut (91) and in small-caliber primary afferent neurons which terminate in the substantia gelatinosa of the dorsal horn of the spinal cord (86,87). Somatostatin has also been localized to cellular elements of the gastroentero-pancreatic endocrine system (43,47,48,58,67,78,82,122, 127,138,139,147,153,158,159). In addition, somatostatin-containing cells are found in the thyroid (82).

Somatostatin-containing neuronal cell bodies can be found in several areas of the CNS. A prominent group of such neurons can be found in the hypothalamic periventricular area at caudal levels of the optic chiasm. Under optimal immunohistochemical staining conditions, the axons of these neurons can be seen to arch laterally and ventrally toward the optic chiasm. They then turn caudally, merge medially with fibers from the contralateral side, and project to the external layer of the median eminence where a large portion terminate across the extent of the median eminence in the vicinity of portal capillaries (Fig. 1–9). The pathway of these cell bodies has been confirmed in lesion studies in which the periventricular area was destroyed by bilateral

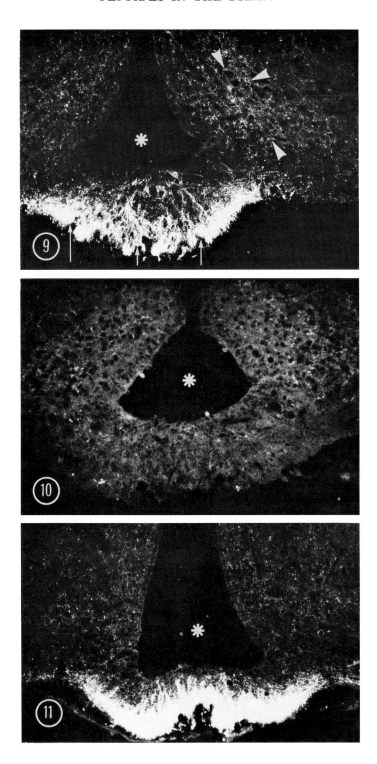

electrolytic lesions (Fig. 1–10) or, alternatively, the axons were severed caudal to the chiasm with a Halász knife (see also 28). Interestingly, the somatostatin-containing terminals in the ventromedial and arcuate nuclei (see below) were unaffected by such lesions, indicating that other (possibly extrahypothalamic) neuronal perikarya may project to these hypothalamic nuclei. Lesions of the paraventricular and dorsomedial nuclei are without effect on somatostatin-containing elements in the median eminence (Fig. 1–11). Thus, among the several somatostatin systems, one appears to be uniquely neuroendocrine in nature, whereas the other systems probably mediate other modalities of neuronal function.

High concentrations of somatostatin-containing nerve terminals are found in the ventromedial-arcuate complex, and great numbers of somatostatin-containing terminals are also found in the suprachiasmatic and ventral premammillary nuclei, as well as in the OVLT. Outside of the hypothalamus, fibers are found in the stria terminalis, the nucleus accumbens, the medial portion of the caudate nucleus, the olfactory tubercle, the amygdaloid complex, and certain cortical areas. In addition, somatostatin fibers and terminals are found in the parabrachial nucleus of the brainstem and in the substantia gelatinosa of the spinal nucleus of the trigeminal nerve. This column of somatostatin terminals continues the length of the substantia gelatinosa of the dorsal horn of the spinal cord. The terminals in the substantia gelatinosa of the spinal cord and medulla have their cell bodies in the dorsal root and trigeminal ganglia, respectively. The sites of neuronal cell bodies which give rise to most of the other previously mentioned terminals are presently unknown, although somatostatin-containing cell bodies have also been localized in the zona incerta, bed nucleus of the stria terminalis; the cortical amygdaloid nucleus, the dentate gyrus, and the piriform, entorhinal, and neocortex. Lesion studies of these cell bodies should provide insight into the nature of the connectivity of these peptidergic systems.

SUBSTANCE P

Substance P was discovered in equine hypothalamic and gut extracts by von Euler and Gaddum (59). This factor was more completely characterized in Leeman's laboratory (38,123).

←

FIGS. 1–9, 1–10, 1–11. Immunofluorescence micrographs of coronal sections of the ventral aspect of the normal (Fig. 1–9) and experimentally altered (Figs. 1–10 and 1–11) rat hypothalamus after incubation with antiserum to somatostatin. Note the high density of somatostatin-containing nerve terminals adjacent to the portal capillaries (Fig. 1–9, *arrows*). The neuropil of the arcuate nucleus also has a striking component of somatostatin-containing fibers and terminals (Fig. 1–9, *arrowheads*). The somatostatin-containing nerve terminals are virtually absent from the median eminence of rats sacrificed 5 days after bilateral electrolytic lesions of the hypothalamus periventricular nucleus (Fig. 1–10). Note, however, that the arcuate nucleus still contains somatostatin-positive elements. Bilateral thermal lesions that include the paraventricular and dorsomedial nuclei have no effect on the SOM-containing fibers and terminals in either the median eminence or the arcuate nucleus (Fig. 1–11). *, third ventricle. Magnification 120×.

Preliminary mappings of the distribution of substance P bioactivity determined that this factor was concentrated in certain regions of the CNS (2,38, 124,140,150,192). The availability of relatively large quantities of the synthetic peptide has enabled the production of antibodies to it (135,154). Immunochemical techniques are generally much more sensitive detectors of peptides and have enabled detailed studies on the occurrence of substance P neuronal systems. Several groups have reported the distribution of substance P on the basis of radioimmunoassay studies (30,31,49,105). The cellular nature of substance P immunoreactivity has been determined using immunohistochemistry (84,87,92–96,133,134,144).

The above immunohistochemical studies have revealed extensive systems of neuronal cell bodies, processes, and their terminals that contain substance P. When viewed as a whole, they rival the extent of the catecholaminergic systems. Within the hypothalamus, substance P-positive cell bodies are found in the dorsomedial, ventromedial, premammillary, and, to a lesser extent, lateral preoptic areas. Their projections are presently unknown. Terminals containing substance P immunoreactivity are also found in most hypothalamic nuclei. The most striking terminal areas are found in the medial preoptic nucleus. Somewhat lower concentrations of substance P-positive terminals are found in the periventricular area, the anterior hypothalamic nucleus, the lateral hypothalamus, the dorsomedial nucleus, the ventrolateral part of the ventromedial nucleus, and the arcuate nucleus. Substance P fibers are encountered in other hypothalamic nuclei but are conspicuously absent from the external layer of the median eminence. Thus, in the rodent hypothalamus, there does not appear to be a neuroendocrine terminal system containing substance P that is capable of affecting anterior pituitary function via the portal vessels.

Except for neocortical areas and the cerebellum, substance P neurons and their fibers are found in varying numbers in the brain. Extrahypothalamic cell bodies have been found in the amygdala, nucleus interstitialis stria terminalis, the medial habenular nucleus, the interpeduncular nucleus, the periaqueductal central gray, the dorsal tegmental nucleus, the commissural nucleus, and the nuclei raphe magnus and pallidus.

Many fluorescent terminals are seen in the following regions after immunofluorescence histochemistry with antibodies to substance P: the amygdala, nucleus interstitialis stria terminalis, the lateral septal nucleus, zona reticulata of the substantia nigra, the interpeduncular nucleus (lateral aspects), the periaqueductal central gray, nucleus parabrachialis dorsalis, the marginal zone of the caudal portion of the nucleus of the spinal trigeminal tract, the nucleus of the solitary tract, and the commissural nucleus.

A few pathways that contain substance P (perhaps among other neurotransmitter systems) include the habenulointerpeduncular tract (84,92,97, 128), a striatonigral pathway (31,98,106), and a descending projection from the raphe nuclei to the spinal cord (T. Hökfelt, Å. Ljungdahl, L. Terenius, R. Elde and G. Nilsson, submitted for publication).

In addition, substance P is found within a subpopulation of primary afferent neurons which have small cell bodies in the dorsal root ganglia and terminals in the marginal laminae (I and II) of the dorsal horn of the spinal cord (87,94,95). Supraspinal and possibly propriospinal substance P systems have terminals in other regions of the spinal cord gray matter (Fig. 1–5B).

ENKEPHALINS

The peptides methionine-enkephalin and leucine-enkephalin were characterized by Hughes and collaborators (101). The existence of endogenous ligands for the opiate receptor was suggested from the work of several groups. More recently, a number of other morphinomimetic peptides, the endorphins, have been characterized (68,74,176).

In preliminary studies, an antiserum raised to leucine-enkephalin was used to localize enkephalin-containing nerve terminals within the nervous system (55). This antiserum was later found to cross-react about 20% with methionine-enkephalin, so it is likely that these findings represented localizations of both enkephalins. More recently an antiserum raised to methionine-enkephalin has been used to localize enkephalin immunoreactivity in terminals and cell bodies within the nervous system (88). This antiserum cross-reacts with leucine-enkephalin, but only at a level of 10%. Since the ratio of methionine- to leucine-enkephalin in the rat brain is approximately 3:1 (175), it is likely that the latter studies primarily represent localizations of methionine enkephalin. However, no major discrepancies have been found between localizations with either antiserum. Neither antiserum has greater than 0.1% cross-reactivity with the endorphins (α, β, γ), somatostatin, or substance P (L. Terenius, *unpublished observations*). The distribution of enkephalins has also been studied in Snyder's laboratory, using a radioreceptor assay (171) and immunohistochemistry (172). In all cases, the distribution of the morphinomimetic peptides has shown a striking parallel to the distribution of opiate receptors (6,7,79,117,118,151).

Groups of enkephalin-containing neuronal cell bodies are found throughout most of the neuraxis. Many hypothalamic nuclei contain groups of enkephalin cell bodies, including the preoptic periventricular nucleus, the medial preoptic nucleus, the paraventricular nucleus, the ventromedial nucleus, the dorsal and ventral premammillary nuclei, the perifornical area, and the arcuate nucleus. Enkephalin-positive neuronal cell bodies are found in nearly 20 other nuclei or regions outside of the hypothalamus (88).

Nerve terminals containing enkephalin immunoreactivity are also found discretely distributed throughout the nervous system. Within the hypothalamus, immunofluorescence localizations reveal enkephalin-positive nerve terminals within the external layer of the median eminence. No enkephalin immunoreactivity could be detected in the pituitary stalk or in any portions of the pituitary. However, nearly all hypothalamic nuclei appear to have moderate to high concentrations of enkephalin fibers and terminals. Outside of the hypothalamus, enkephalin terminals are found in numerous areas, including densely packed terminals in the globus pallidus, patches of terminals within nucleus accumbens, in the lateral septal nucleus, the amygdaloid complex, several brainstem nuclei, and the dorsal and ventral horn of the spinal cord (Fig. 1–5C). Furthermore, enkephalin-immunoreactive terminals are found in the wall of the gut, especially surrounding the ganglion cells in the myenteric (Auerbach's) plexus.

The connections of enkephalin cell bodies and terminals have not been determined. Within the hypothalamus, the localization of enkephalin in the external layer of the median eminence suggests the peptide has a neuroendocrine role. The enkephalin-positive cell bodies in many hypothalamic nuclei could be the origin of this newly discovered neuroendocrine system.

GASTRIN

Gastrin has been shown to exist in several forms, including 17- and 34-amino acid peptides (70,71). Recently, Vanderhaeghen et al. (179) reported that brain extracts contained a peptide that could compete with labeled gastrin for the antibody used in a gastrin radioimmunoassay. The material, however, did not appear to be authentic gastrin since it did not displace labeled gastrin in a manner parallel to that of authentic gastrin. This peptide was found to be distributed in a heterogenous manner within the nervous system.

Using a gastrin antibody generated by Rehfeld et al. (155), investigators could detect gastrin immunoreactivity using fluorescence immunohistochemical techniques. Within the hypothalamus, gastrin-immunoreactive nerve terminals were found in the periventricular area, the dorso- and ventromedial nuclei, and in the medial portion of the external layer of the median eminence. Terminals also occurred in other areas including the cerebral cortex. Nerve cell bodies were found in the hippocampal formation. Dockray (41), Rehfeld (*personal communication*), and Vanderhaeghen (*personal communication*) have recently found that the brain peptide that reacts with the gastrin antibody is smaller than gastrin. It may be an octapeptide related to cholecystokinin.

ANGIOTENSIN II

The brain contains an isorenin-angiotensin system (60; Chapter 3). Recently, angiotensin II immunoreactivity has been demonstrated in the nervous system, using an immunohistochemical approach (62,63). Cell bodies in the paraventricular nucleus and perifornical area contain angiotensin II immunoreactivity (83,85). Within the hypothalamus, angiotensin II terminals are found in the external layer of the median eminence, the dorsomedial nucleus, and the ventral portions of the hypothalamus. Other hypothalamic regions contain only scattered fibers. Outside of the hypothalamus a rather dense network of terminals containing angiotensin II immunoreactivity has been observed in the marginal layers of the dorsal horn of the spinal cord and the substantia gelatinosa of the spinal trigeminal nucleus. The sympathetic intermediolateral cell column as well as the amygdaloid nuclei also receive afferent fibers containing angiotensin II immunoreactivity. The angiotensin II immunoreactivity in the brain is discussed in greater detail in Chapter 3.

VASOACTIVE INTESTINAL POLYPEPTIDE

Mutt and Said (129) have described a 28-amino acid peptide which they isolated from porcine gut. Radioimmunoassay studies have established that this peptide is widely distributed in the periphery (160) as well as in the central nervous system (66,161). Immunohistochemical localizations have demonstrated vasoactive intestinal polypeptide (VIP) immunoreactivity in neurons and their processes in the CNS. Larsson and collaborators (119,120) localized VIP nerve terminals closely associated with cerebrovascular nerves and found cell bodies in the mouse hypothalamus. They also found VIP-containing elements in the peripheral nervous system of the gut, as did Bryant et al. (35). Fuxe et al. (63,64) have localized similar neuronal structures, except that they were unable to confirm the localization of VIP cell bodies in the hypothalamus. However, they found a striking array of VIP-positive neocortical neurons. Terminals containing VIPs were also found in the anterior hypothalamus, the amygdaloid complex, and the neostriatum.

DISCUSSION

Most of our present knowledge of the distribution of peptides within the nervous system has been established with immunochemical techniques. However, neither radioimmunoassay nor immunohistochemical studies are able to describe the distribution of the biological activity of a peptide. Thus, the description by both of the immunological techniques of a neuronal system containing a peptide is necessarily a description of a peptide(s) with immunoreactivity similar to that of the native peptide. Radioimmunoassay of extracts of a certain brain region at several dilutions enables one to determine if the immunoreactivity present in the extract parallels dilutions of the peptide used as a standard. Parallelism of dilutions of the standard and the sample is a necessary although not sufficient criterion to establish identity of sample and unknown (157).

To a certain extent, the specificity of the immunohistochemical reaction can be established if staining is abolished after pretreatment of the primary antiserum with an excess of the antigen. In a similar manner, one can pre-treat the primary antiserum with an excess of another peptide to see if the staining is in any way diminished, thereby indicating cross-reactivity. Therefore, an immunohistochemical localization of a peptide is said to be "specific" if the antibody can bind the desired antigen and is unable to bind known, unrelated peptides. At the same time, it is presently impossible to establish that all immunohistochemical localizations represent only the native peptide and not precursor molecules, peptide fragments, or uncharacterized peptides bearing a partial amino acid sequence homology.

It must also be emphasized that negative results with the immunohistochemical technique do not necessarily indicate the absence of the peptide being studied. This may simply reflect the lack of adequate fixation of the tissue or a low-affinity antibody which is unable to bind the antigen in areas of low concentrations of the peptide.

In spite of these limitations, immunohistochemical and radioimmunoassay techniques are powerful tools which can be judiciously used to uncover the distribution and nature of peptidergic neuronal systems. In terms of sensitivity, both of these techniques are orders of magnitude more sensitive than conventional bioassay procedures. Furthermore, immunohistochemical localizations at the light and electron microscopic levels are able to provide insight into the relationship of specifically identified neuronal elements.

Neuroendocrine Systems

There now seems to be an emerging pattern with respect to the distribution of neuronal perikarya whose axons project to the external layer of the median eminence. With several of these neuroendocrine systems, the nerve cell bodies have been found in the preoptic area and the hypothalamic gray matter dorsal to the optic chiasm. Thus, somatostatin, neurophysin, vasopressin, TRH, and LRH cell bodies projecting to the external layer of the median eminence are for the most part rostral to the caudal border of the optic chiasm (Fig. 1–12). These projections have been established after anterior deafferentation of the medial basal hypothalamus and the consequent disappearance of the specific peptidergic terminals in the external layer of the median eminence (53).

The concept of a hypophysiotrophic area in the medial basal hypothalamus (76) has emphasized the important role of this region in neuroendocrine regulation. It now appears as if more rostrally located structures also play a significant role.

Although LRH-positive cell bodies have been reported in the arcuate nucleus (80,194), they may not send axons to the external layer of the median eminence. Recently, Lechan et al. (121) produced glutamate-induced lesions of the arcuate nucleus and such lesions did not diminish the quantity of LRH terminals in the median eminence. On the other hand, anterior deafferentation of the median eminence (141,188) significantly diminished

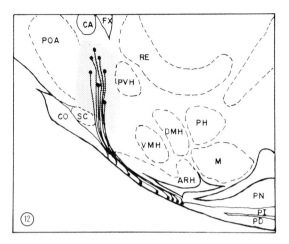

FIG. 1–12. Schematic parasagittal diagram indicating the location of neuronal perikarya (*stippled area*) which project to the external layer of the median eminence in the rat. The suprachiasmatic localization of these perikarya has been determined by immunohistochemistry and their projections have been established by lesions and transection of their axons. The perikarya illustrated represent those of the neuroendocrine somatostatin system that projects to the median eminence. ARH, nucleus arcuatus hypothalami; CA, commissura anterior; CO, chiasma opticum; DMH, nucleus dorsomedialis hypothalami; FX, fornix; M, nucleus mammillaris; PD, pars distalis hypophysis; PH, nucleus posterior hypothalami; PI, pars intermedia hypophysis; PN, pars nervosa hypophysis; POA, area preoptica; PVH, nucleus paraventricularis hypothalami; RE, nucleus reuniens thalami; SC, nucleus suprachiasmaticus; VMH, nucleus ventromedialis hypothalami.

the quantity of LRH in the median eminence. Thus, it seems likely that this system also arises from cell bodies in the rostral hypothalamus, in agreement with Barry's findings (13). The occurrence of somatostatin and TRH cell bodies in the anterior periventricular region, and the disappearance of somatostatin and TRH nerve terminals from the median eminence after lesions of this area, also point to the importance of rostral hypothalamic structures in neuroendocrine regulation.

The vasopressin/neurophysin projection from the paraventricular nucleus to the external layer of the median eminence (4; R. Elde and T. Hökfelt, *unpublished observations*) indicates that these terminals are not random collaterals of the massive hypothalamo-neurohypophyseal projection to the posterior pituitary. In addition to being morphologically separate from the larger vasopressin hypothalamo-neurohypophyseal pathway, a functional separation also is suggested by these findings. This notion is further supported by the sensitivity of the vasopressin/neurophysin paraventricular-median eminence pathway to reserpine. The vasopressin/neurophysin terminals in the posterior pituitary were not depleted of vasopressin/neurophysin after such treatment. Since the time course of the disappearance of these peptides from the external layer of the median eminence paralleled the reduction of bioassayable CRF from the median eminence (23), it is tempting to speculate that this vasopressin/neurophysin subsystem may in some way be related to at least part of the CRF activity. Further evidence regarding the role of vasopressin as a CRF has been reviewed by Zimmerman (193). However, it should be cautioned that there may be several peptidergic neuroendocrine systems that regulate ACTH secretion, and they are also likely to be influenced by neurotransmitters such as the monoamines (65).

The localization of newly discovered peptidergic systems with terminals in the external layer of the median eminence suggests a neuroendocrine role for these peptides (83). The function of neuroendocrine systems containing gastrin and angiotensin II immunoreactivity is not known, but the enkephalin-containing terminals in the median eminence may regulate prolactin release. Lien et al. (126) found exogenous enkephalin increased circulating prolactin levels.

Peptides in Other Neural Systems

The occurrence of biologically active peptides in diverse neuronal networks suggests they may have a regulatory role in these systems. This suggestion is further supported by the morphological similarity of peptidergic neuronal perikarya, axons, and terminals with those of established neurotransmitters such as the monoamines. Using immunofluorescence microscopy, the intense dot- and fiber-like appearance of peptidergic nerve terminals is strikingly similar to monoaminergic terminals as revealed by either formaldehyde- or glyoxylic acid-induced fluorescence, or by immunofluorescence localization of the catecholamine-synthesizing enzymes (see 83). In some terminal regions, peptidergic endings are sparse and somewhat randomly scattered. In other areas, however, peptidergic terminals are dense and may be organized as dense "baskets" of endings surrounding individual neurons. In regions such as the septal, amygdaloid, and parabrachial nuclei, several peptidergic systems seem to converge. In spite of such convergence, each of these terminal systems presents a somewhat unique arrangement and/or density of terminals within these nuclei. In many other regions of the brain, only a single peptide presently studied projects to a certain nucleus. These observations, in addition to the methodological controls, point to the uniqueness of the individual peptidergic pathways.

Peptidergic neurons resemble other neuronal systems in that the nerve terminal is dependent on axonal transport for replenishment of the peptide. Thus, 24 hr after axon transection or ligation, marked accumulations of peptides can be localized immediately proximal to the site of transection (53,87). In favorable planes of sections, this blockade of axonal transport allows visualization of the entire axon back to the cell body. Further evidence for axonal transport of neuropeptides is derived from experiments in which colchicine was administered 24 to 48 hr prior to sacrifice (88). In this case, nerve terminals seem to be partially depleted of their stores of peptides, whereas proximal axons and neural perikarya appear to contain increased quantities of the peptides.

In spite of this evidence, it is not yet clear if peptides function as neurotransmitters (see Chapter 5). Barker and Smith (11) have recently suggested that peptides may act within the neuropil as neurohormones and are therefore a category of biologically active substances distinct from the classic neurotransmitters. Much of their evidence for this distinction is based on morphological and physiological findings from invertebrate systems. One tenet of their hypothesis is that the action of peptides does not occur via a synaptic specialization. Whereas this may be true for the invertebrate systems they have studied, recent evidence suggests that at least some terminals containing substance P in the dorsal horn of the rat spinal cord synapse on substantia gelatinosa dendrites (85; O. Johansson and T. Hökfelt, *unpublished observations*). However, it must be stressed that these ultrastructural immunocytochemical localizations are preliminary in nature, and that much further work is clearly required to determine if synaptic specializations are a common feature of peptidergic terminals within the neuropil.

Immunohistochemistry at the ultrastructural level may also provide answers to two other important questions regarding the role of peptidergic terminals within the neuropil. Firstly, the nature of the subcellular organelle(s) responsible for storage of neuropeptides must be determined. Although a large body of evidence suggests that peptides in classic neuroendocrine systems are stored within large "neurosecretory" granules (see 5,146,149), such organelles have not been frequently described in the neuropil where peptides are now being localized. Therefore, thorough ultrastructural immunohistochemical studies of these regions are necessary.

Finally, immunohistochemical techniques may be useful in revealing whether peptides are the only biologically active occupants of their nerve terminals, or if other classic neurotransmitters or other substances are localized within and possibly released from the same nerve terminals.

ACKNOWLEDGMENTS

Robert Elde was supported by a National Research Service Award (NS 05047-01) from the National Institute of Neurological, Communicative Disorders and Stroke (U.S.A.). This work was supported by grants from the Minnesota Medical Foundation, the University of Minnesota Graduate School, Minnesota Affiliate of the American Diabetes Association, the Swedish Medical Research Council (04X-2887, 19X-3412, 04X-4495, 04X-2886), Magnus Bergwalls Stiftelse, Knut och Alice Wallenbergs Stiftelse, and Harald och Greta Jeanssons Stiftelse. Portions of this work were made possible by the generous gifts of antisera from the laboratories of Drs. S. L. Jeffcoate, G. Nilsson, and G. Seybold. The technical assistance of A. Nygards and K. Rivers is gratefully acknowledged.

REFERENCES

1. Alpert, L. C., Brawer, J. R., Patel, Y. C., and Reichlin, S. (1976): Somato-statinergic neurons in anterior hypothalamus: Immunohistochemical localization. *Endocrinology*, 98:255–258.
2. Amin, A. H., Crawford, T. B. B., and Gaddum, J. H. (1954): The distribution of substance P and 5-hydroxytryptamine in the central nervous system of the dog. *J. Physiol.*, 126:596–618.
3. Amoss, M., Burgus, R., Blackwell, R., Vale, W., Fellows, R., and Guillemin, R. (1971): Purification, amino acid composition and N-terminus of the hypothalamic luteinizing hormone releasing factor (LRF) of ovine origin. *Biochem. Biophys. Res. Commun.*, 44:205–210.
4. Antunes, J. L., Carmel, P. W., and Zimmerman, E. A. (1977): Projections from the paraventricular nucleus to the zona externa of the median eminence of the rhesus monkey: An immunohistochemical study. *Brain Res. (in press)*.
5. Aspelagh, M.-R., Vandesande, F., and Dierickx, K. (1976): Electron microscopic immunocytochemical demonstration of separate neurophysin-vasopressinergic and neurophysin-oxytocinergic nerve fibers in the neural lobe of the rat hypophysis. *Cell Tissue Res.*, 171:31–37.
6. Atweh, S. F., and Kuhar, M. J. (1977): Autoradiographic localization of opiate receptors in rat brain. I. Spinal cord and lower medulla. *Brain Res.*, 124:53–67.
7. Atweh, S. F., and Kuhar, M. J. (1977): Autoradiographic localization of opiate receptors in rat brain. II. The brainstem. *Brain Res.*, 129:1–12.
8. Baker, B. L., Dermody, W. C., and Reel, J. R. (1974): Localization of luteinizing hormone-releasing hormone in the mammalian hypothalamus. *Am. J. Anat.*, 139: 129–134.
9. Baker, B. L., Dermody, W. C., and Reel, J. R. (1975): Distribution of gonado-tropin-releasing hormone in the rat brain as observed with immunocytochemistry. *Endocrinology*, 97:125–135.
10. Baker, B. L., and Yen, Y.-Y. (1976): The influence of hypophysectomy on the stores of somatostatin in the hypothalamus and pituitary stem. *Proc. Soc. Exp. Biol. Med.*, 151:599–602.
11. Barker, J. L., and Smith, T. G., Jr. (1977): Peptides as neurohormones. In: *Neuroscience Symposia, Vol. II*. Society for Neuroscience, Bethesda *(in press)*.
12. Barnea, A., Ben-Jonathan, N., Colston, C., Johnston, J. M., and Porter, J. C. (1975): Differential sub-cellular compartmentalization of thyrotropin releasing hormone (TRH) and gonadotropin releasing hormone (LRH) in hypothalamic tissue. *Proc. Natl. Acad. Sci. USA*, 72:3153–3157.
13. Barry, J. (1976): Immunohistochemical localization of hypothalamic hormones (especially LRF) at the light microscopy level. In: *Hypothalamus and Endocrine Functions*, edited by F. Labrie, J. Meites, and G. Pelletier, pp. 451–474. Plenum Press, New York.
14. Barry, J., and Carette, B. (1975): Etude en immunofluorescence des neurones elaborateurs de LRF chez les Cebides. *C. R. Acad. Sci. [D] (Paris)*, 281:735–738.
15. Barry, J., and Carette, B. (1975): Immunofluorescence study of LRF neurons in primates. *Cell Tissue Res.*, 164:163–178.
16. Barry, J., and Dubois, M.-P. (1973): Etude en immunofluorescence des structures hypothalamiques a competence gonadotrope. *Ann. Endocrinol. (Paris)*, 34:735–742.
17. Barry, J., and Dubois, M.-P. (1974): Etude en immunofluorescence de la differenci-ation prenatale des cellules hypothalamiques elaboratrices de LH-RF et de la maturation de la voie neurosecretrice preoptico-infundibulaire chez le cobaye. *Brain Res.*, 67:103–113.
18. Barry, J., and Dubois, M.-P. (1974): Immunofluorescence study of the preoptico-infundibular LH-RH neurosecretory pathway of the guinea pig during the estrous cycle. *Neuroendocrinology*, 15:200–208.
19. Barry, J., and Dubois, M.-P. (1975): Immunofluorescence study of LRF-producing neurons in the cat and the dog. *Neuroendocrinology*, 18:290–298.
20. Barry, J., and Dubois, M.-P. (1976): Immunoreactive LRF neurosecretory path-ways in mammals. *Acta. Anat.*, 94:497–503.

21. Barry, J., Dubois, M.-P., and Carette, B. (1974): Immunofluorescence study of the preoptic-infundibular LRF neurosecretory pathway in the normal, castrated or testosterone-treated male guinea pig. *Endocrinology,* 95:1416–1423.
22. Barry, J., Dubois, M.-P., and Poulain, P. (1973): LRF producing cells of the mammalian hypothalamus. A fluorescent antibody study. *Z. Zellforsch.,* 146:351–366.
23. Bhattacharya, A. N., and Marks, B. H. (1969): Reserpine- and chlorpromazine-induced changes in hypothalamo-hypophyseal-adrenal system in rats in the presence and absence of hypothermia. *J. Pharmacol. Exp. Ther.,* 165:108–116.
24. Bhattacharya, A. N., and Marks, B. H. (1970): Effects of alpha methyl tyrosine and p-chlorophenylalanine on the regulation of ACTH secretion. *Neuroendocrinology,* 6:49–55.
25. Bern, H. A., and Knowles, F. G. W. (1966): Neurosecretion. In: *Neuroendocrinology,* edited by L. Martini and W. F. Ganong, pp. 139–186. Academic Press, New York.
26. Brazeau, P., Vale, W., Burgus, R., Ling, N., Butcher, M., Rivier, J., and Guillemin, R. (1973): Hypothalamic polypeptide that inhibits the secretion of immunoreactive pituitary growth hormone. *Science,* 179:77–79.
27. Brownfield, M. S., and Kozlowski, G. P. (1977): The hypothalamo-choroidal tract I. Immunohistochemical demonstration of neurophysin pathways to telencephalic choroidal plexuses and cerebrospinal fluid. *Cell Tissue Res.,* 178:111–127.
28. Brownstein, M. J., Arimura, A., Fernandez-Durango, R., Schally, A. V., Palkovits, M., and Kizer, J. S. (1977): The effect of hypothalamic deafferentation on somatostatin-like activity in the rat brain. *Endocrinology,* 100:246–249.
29. Brownstein, M., Arimura, A., Sato, H., Schally, A. V., and Kizer, J. S. (1975): The regional distribution of somatostatin in the rat brain. *Endocrinology,* 96:1456–1461.
30. Brownstein, M. J., Mroz, E. A., Kizer, J. S., Palkovits, M., and Leeman, S. E. (1976): Regional distribution of substance P in the brain of the rat. *Brain Res.,* 116:299–305.
31. Brownstein, M. J., Mroz, E. A., Tappaz, M. L., and Leeman, S. E. (1977): On the origin of substance P and glutamic acid decarboxylase (GAD) in the substantia nigra. *Brain Res. (in press).*
32. Brownstein, M., Palkovits, M., and Kizer, J. S. (1975): On the origin of luteinizing hormone-releasing hormone (LH-RH) in the supraoptic crest. *Life Sci.,* 17:679–682.
33. Brownstein, M., Palkovits, M., Saavedra, J. M., Bassiri, R., and Utiger, R. D. (1974): Thyrotropin-releasing hormone in specific nuclei of rat brain. *Science,* 185:267–269.
34. Brownstein, M. J., Palkovits, M., Saavedra, J. M., and Kizer, J. S. (1976): Distribution of hypothalamic hormones and neurotransmitters within the diencephalon. In: *Frontiers in Neuroendocrinology, Vol. 4,* edited by L. Martini and W. F. Ganong, pp. 1–23. Raven Press, New York.
35. Bryant, M. G., Polak, J. M., Modlin, I., Bloom, S. R., Albuquerque, R. H., and Pearse, A. G. E. (1976): Possible dual role for vasoactive intestinal peptide as gastrointestinal hormone and neurotransmitter substance. *Lancet,* 1:991–993.
36. Burgus, R., Dunn, T. F., Desiderion, D., Ward, D. N., Vale, W., and Guillemin, R. (1970): Characterization of ovine hypothalamic hypophysiotropic TSH-releasing factor. *Nature,* 226:321–325.
37. Calas, A., Kerdelhue, B., Assenmacher, I., and Jutisz, M. (1973): Les axones a LH-RH de l'eminence mediane. Mise en evidence chez le canard par une technique immunocytochimique. *C. R. Acad. Sci. [D] (Paris),* 277:2765–2768.
38. Chang, M. M., Leeman, S. E., and Niall, H. D. (1971): Amino acid sequence of substance P. *Nature [New Biol.],* 232:86–87.
39. Conrad, L. C. A., and Pfaff, D. W. (1976): Efferents from medial basal forebrain and hypothalamus in the rat. II. An autoradiographic study of the anterior hypothalamus. *J. Comp. Neurol.,* 169:221–261.
40. Coons, A. H. (1958): Fluorescent antibody methods. In: *General Cytochemical Methods,* edited by J. F. Danielli, pp. 399–422. Academic Press, New York.

41. Dockray, G. J. (1976): Immunohistochemical evidence of cholecystokinin-like peptides in brain. *Nature,* 264:568–570.
42. Dube, D., Leclerc, R., Pelletier, G., Arimura, A., and Schally, A. V. (1975): Immunohistochemical detection of growth hormone-release inhibiting hormone (somatostatin) in the guinea-pig brain. *Cell Tissue Res.,* 161:385–392.
43. Dubois, M. P. (1975): Immunoreactive somatostatin is present in discrete cells of the endocrine pancreas. *Proc. Natl. Acad. Sci. USA,* 72:1340–1343.
44. Dubois, M. P. (1976): Immunocytological evidence of LH-RF in hypothalamus and median eminence. A review. *Ann. Biol. Anim. Biochim. Biophys.,* 16:177–194.
45. Dubois, M. P., Barry, J., and Leonardelli, J. (1974): Mise en evidence par immunofluorescence et repartition de la somatostatine (SRIF) dans l'eminence mediale des Vertebres (Mammiferes, Oiseaux, Amphibiens, Poissons). *C. R. Acad. Sci. [D] (Paris),* 279:1899–1902.
46. Dubois, M. P., and Kolodziejczyk, E. (1975): Centres hypothalamiques du rat secretant la somatostatine: repartition des pericaryons en 2 systemes magno et parvocellulaires (edute immunocytologique). *C. R. Acad. Sci. [D]* (Paris), 281: 1737–1740.
47. Dubois, M. P., and Paulin, C. (1976): Gastrointestinal somatostatin cells in the human fetus. *Cell Tissue Res.,* 166:179–184.
48. Dubois, M. P., Paulin, C., Assan, R., and Dubois, M. P. (1975): Evidence for immunoreactive somatostatin in the endocrine cells of human foetal pancreas. *Nature,* 26:731–732.
49. Duffy, M. J., Mulhall, D., and Powell, D. (1975): Subcellular distribution of substance P in bovine hypothalamus and substantia nigra. *J. Neurochem.,* 25:305–307.
50. duVigneaud, V. (1954): Hormones of the posterior pituitary gland: Oxytocin and vasopressin. *Harvey Lect.,* Series L, pp. 1–26.
51. duVigneaud, V., Ressler, C., Swann, J. M., Roberts, C. W., Katsoyannis, P. G., and Gordon, S. (1953): The synthesis of an octapeptide amide with the hormone activity of oxytocin. *J. Am. Chem. Soc.,* 75:4879–4880.
52. Elde, R. P. (1974): The production and characterization of anti-vasopressin antibodies and their use in the immunoenzyme histochemical localization of vasopressins in the hypothalamo-neurohypophysial neurosecretory system of several mammals. Ph.D. thesis, University of Minnesota, Minneapolis.
53. Elde, R. P., Hökfelt, T., Johansson, O., Efendic, S., and Luft, R. (1976): Somatostatin containing pathways in the nervous system. *Neurosci. Abstr.,* II:759.
54. Elde, R. P., Hökfelt, T., Johansson, O., Ljungdahl, A., Nilsson, G., and Jeffcoate, S. L. (1977): Immunohistochemical localization of peptides in the nervous system. In: *Centrally Acting Peptides,* edited by John Hughes. Macmillan, Hampshire, England *(in press).*
55. Elde, R. P., Hökfelt, T., Johansson, O., and Terenius, L. (1976): Immunohistochemical studies using antibodies to leucine-enkephalin: Initial observations on the nervous system of the rat. *Neuroscience,* 1:349–351.
56. Elde, R. P., and Parsons, J. A. (1975): Immunocytochemical localization of somatostatin in cell bodies of the rat hypothalamus. *Am. J. Anat.,* 144:541–548.
57. Epelbaum, J., Brazeau, P., Tsang, D., Brawer, J., and Martin, J. (1977): Subcellular distribution of radioimmunoassayable somatostatin in rat brain. *Brain Res.,* 126:309–323.
58. Erlandsen, S. L., Hegre, O. D., Parsons, J. A., McEvoy, R. C., and Elde, R. P. (1976): Pancreatic islet cell hormones. Distribution of cell types in the islet and evidence for the presence of somatostatin and gastrin within the D cell. *J. Histochem. Cytochem.,* 24:883–897.
59. Euler, U. S. von, and Gaddum, J. H. (1931): An unidentified depressor substance in certain tissue extracts. *J. Physiol.,* 72:74–87.
60. Fischer-Ferraro, C., Nahmod, V. E., Goldstein, D. J., and Finkielman, S. (1971): Angiotensin and renin in rat and dog brain. *J. Exp. Med.,* 133:353–361.
61. Flament-Durand, J., and Desclin, L. (1968): A topographical study of a hypothalamic region with a thyrotrophic action. *J. Endocrinol.,* 41:531–539.
62. Fuxe, K., Ganten, D., Hökfelt, T., and Bolme, P. (1976): Immunohistochemical

evidence for the existence of angiotensin II-containing nerve terminals in the brain and spinal cord in the rat. *Neurosci. Lett.,* 2:229–234.

63. Fuxe, K., Hökfelt, T., Johansson, O., Ganten, D., Goldstein, M., Perez de la Mora, M., Possani, L., Tapia, R., Teran, L., Palacios, R., Said, S., and Mutt, V. (1976): Monoamine neuron systems in the hypothalamus and their relation to the GABA and peptide containing neurons. In: *Colloque de Synthese des Actions Thematiques 22 et 35. Neuromediateurs et Polypeptides Hypothalamiques a Action Relachante ou Inhibitrice,* edited by R. Mornex and J. Barry. Institut National de la Sante et de la Recherche Medicale, Paris (*in press*).

64. Fuxe, K., Hökfelt, T., Said, S., and Mutt, V. (1977): Evidence for the existence of VIP containing nerve terminals in the rat brain. *Neurosci. Lett.* (*in press*).

65. Ganong, W. F. (1973): Catecholamines and the secretion of renin, ACTH and growth hormone. In: *Frontiers in Catecholamine Research,* edited by E. Usdin and S. Snyder, pp. 819–824. Pergamon Press, New York.

66. Giachetti, A., Rosenberg, R. N., and Said, S. I. (1976): Vasoactive intestinal polypeptide in brain synaptosomes. *Lancet,* II:741–742.

67. Goldsmith, P. C., Rose, J. C., Arimura, A., and Ganong, W. F. (1975): Ultrastructural localization of somatostatin in pancreatic islets of the rat. *Endocrinology,* 97:1061–1064.

68. Goldstein, A. (1976): Opioid peptides (endorphins) in pituitary and brain. *Science,* 193:1081–1086.

69. Greer, M. A. (1951): Evidence of hypothalamic control of pituitary release of thyrotrophin. *Proc. Soc. Exp. Biol. Med.,* 77:603–608.

70. Gregory, R. A., and Tracy, H. J. (1964): The constitution and properties of two gastrins extracted from hog antral mucosa. *Gut,* 5:103–114.

71. Gregory, R. A., and Tracy, H. J. (1972): Isolation of two "big gastrins" from Zollinger-Ellison tumor tissue. *Lancet,* ii:797–799.

72. Guillemin, R. (1977): Endorphins, brain peptides that act like opiates. *N. Engl. J. Med.,* 296:226–228.

73. Guillemin, R. (1977): Chemistry of brain peptides. In: *The Hypothalamus. Association for Research in Nervous and Mental Diseases Publication, Vol. 56,* edited by S. Reichlin. Raven Press, New York (*in press*).

74. Guillemin, R., Ling, N., and Burgus, R. (1976): Endorphines, peptides, d'origine hypothalamique et neurohypophysaire a activite morphinomimetique. Isolement et structure moleculaire de l'd-endorphine. *C. R. Acad. Sci. [D] (Paris),* 282:783–785.

75. Halász, B., Florsheim, W. H., Coreorran, N. L., and Gorski, R. A. (1967): Thyrotrophic hormone secretion in rats after partial or total interruption of neural afferents to the medial basal hypothalamus. *Endocrinology,* 80:1075–1082.

76. Halász, B., Pupp, L., and Uhlarik, S. (1962): Hypophysiotrophic area in the hypothalamus. *J. Endocrinol.,* 25:147–154.

77. Hartman, B. K. (1973): Immunofluorescence of dopamine-B-hydroxylase. Application of improved methodology to the localization of the peripheral and central noradrenergic nervous system. *J. Histochem. Cytochem.,* 21:312–332.

78. l'Hermite, A., Lefranc, G., Pradal, G., Andre, J.-J., and Dubois, M. P. (1976): Identification ultrastructurale et etude immunocytochimique des cellules a somatostatine de la muqueuse antrale du lapin et de la souris. *Histochemistry,* 47:31–41.

79. Hiller, J. M., Pearson, J., and Simon, E. J. (1973): Distribution of stereospecific binding of the potent narcotic analgesic etorphine in the human brain: Predominance in the limbic system. *Res. Commun. Chem. Pathol. Pharmacol.,* 6:1052–1062.

80. Hoffman, G. E., Moynihan, J. A., and Knigge, K. M. (1976): Immunocytochemical localization of luteinizing hormone-releasing hormone (LH-RH). Differences with different antisera. *Neurosci. Abstr.,* II:673.

81. Hökfelt, T., Efendić, S., Johansson, O., Luft, R., and Arimura, A. (1974): Immunohistochemical localization of somatostatin (growth hormone release-inhibiting factor) in the guinea pig brain. *Brain Res.,* 80:165–169.

82. Hökfelt, T., Efendić, S., Hellerström, C., Johansson, O., Luft, R., and Arimura, A. (1975): Cellular localization of somatostatin in endocrine like cells and neurons of the rat with special references to the A_1 cells of the pancreatic islets and to the hypothalamus. *Acta Endocrinol. [Suppl.] (Kbh.),* 200:5–41.

83. Hökfelt, T., Elde, R., Fuxe, K., Johansson, O., Ljungdahl, Å., Goldstein, M., Luft, R., Nilsson, G., Said, S., Fraser, H., Jeffcoate, S. L., White, N., Ganten, D., and Rehfeld, J. (1977): Aminergic and peptidergic pathways in the nervous system with special reference to the hypothalamus. In: *The Hypothalamus. Association for Research in Nervous and Mental Disease Publication, Vol. 56,* edited by S. Reichlin. Raven Press, New York (*in press*).
84. Hökfelt, T., Elde, R. P., Johansson, O., Kellerth, J.-O., Ljungdahl, Å., Nilsson, G., Pernow, B., and Terenius, L. (1977): Substance P and enkephalin: Distribution in the nervous system as revealed with immunohistochemistry. In: *Proc. CINP,* edited by S. Radouco-Thomas (*in press*).
85. Hökfelt, T., Elde, R. P., Johansson, O., Ljungdahl, Å., Schultzberg, M., Fuxe, K., Goldstein, M., Nilsson, G., Pernow, B., Terenius, L., Ganten, D., Jeffcoate, S. L., Rehfeld, J., and Said, S. (1977): The distribution of peptide containing neurons in the nervous system. In: *Psychopharmacology: A Generation of Progress,* edited by K. Killam, M. Linton, and A. DiMascio. Raven Press, New York (*in press*).
86. Hökfelt, T., Elde, R. P., Johansson, O., Luft, R., and Arimura, A. (1975): Immuno-histochemical evidence for the presence of somatostatin, a powerful inhibitory peptide in some primary sensory neurons. *Neurosci. Lett.,* 1:231–235.
87. Hökfelt, T., Elde, R., Johansson, O., Luft, R., Nilsson, G., and Arimura, A. (1976): Immunohistochemical evidence for separate populations of somatostatin-containing and substance P-containing primary afferent neurons in the rat. *Neuroscience,* 1:131–136.
88. Hökfelt, T., Elde, R. P., Johansson, O., Terenius, L., and Stein, L. (1977): Distri-bution of enkephalin-like immunoreactivity in the rat central nervous system. I. Cell bodies. *Neurosci. Lett.,* 5:25–31.
89. Hökfelt, T., Fuxe, K., Johansson, O., Jeffcoate, S. L., and White, N. (1975): Dis-tribution of thyrotropin-releasing hormone (TRH) in the central nervous system as revealed with immunohistochemistry. *Eur. J. Pharmacol.,* 34:389–392.
90. Hökfelt, T., Fuxe, K., Johansson, O., Jeffcoate, S., and White, N. (1975): Thy-rotropin releasing hormone (TRH)-containing nerve terminals in certain brain stem nuclei and in the spinal cord. *Neurosci. Lett.,* 1:133–139.
91. Hökfelt, T., Johansson, O., Efendic, S., Luft, R., and Arimura, A. (1975): Are there somatostatin-containing nerves in the rat gut? Immunohistochemical evidence for a new type of peripheral nerves. *Experientia,* 31:852–854.
92. Hökfelt, T., Johansson, O., Kellerth, J.-O., Ljungdahl, Å., Nilsson, G., Nygards, A., and Pernow, B. (1977): Immunohistochemical distribution of substance P. In: *Substance P Nobel Symposium, Vol. 37,* edited by U. S. von Euler and B. Pernow. Raven Press, New York (*in press*).
93. Hökfelt, T., Kellerth, J.-O., Ljungdahl, Å., Nilsson, G., Nygards, A., and Pernow, B. (1976): Immunohistochemical localization of substance P in the central and peripheral nervous system. In: *Neuroregulators and Hypotheses of Psychiatric Disorders,* edited by J. Barchas, E. Costa, and E. Usdin. Oxford University Press, Oxford (*in press*).
94. Hökfelt, T., Kellerth, J.-O., Nilsson, G., and Pernow, B. (1975): Experimental immunohistochemical studies on the localization and distribution of substance P in cat primary sensory neurons. *Brain Res.,* 100:235–252.
95. Hökfelt, T., Kellerth, J.-O., Nilsson, G., and Pernow, B. (1975): Substance P: Localization in the central nervous system and in some primary sensory neurons. *Science,* 190:889–890.
96. Hökfelt, T., Meyerson, B., Nilsson, G., Pernow, B., and Sachs, Ch. (1976): Im-munohistochemical evidence for substance P-containing nerve endings in the human cortex. *Brain Res.,* 104:181–186.
97. Hong, J. S., Costa, E., and Yang, H.-Y. T. (1976): Effects of habenular lesions on the substance P content of various brain regions. *Brain Res.,* 118:523–525.
98. Hong, J. S., Yang, H.-Y. T., Racagni, G., and Costa, E. (1977): Projections of substance P containing neurons from neostriatum to substantia nigra. *Brain Res.,* 122:541–544.
99. Hope, D. B. (1968): Neurophysin, oxytocin and vasopressin in neurosecretory

granules and in crystalline complexes. Pharmacology of hormonal polypeptides and proteins. *Adv. Exp. Med. Biol.,* 2:73–83.

100. Howell, W. H. (1898): The physiological effects of extracts of the hypophysis cerebri and infundibular body. *J. Exp. Med.,* 3:245–258.

101. Hughes, I., Smith, T. W., Kosterlitz, H. W., Fothergill, L. H., Morgan, B. A., and Morris, H. R. (1975): Identification of two related pentapeptides from the brain with potent opiate agonist activity. *Nature,* 258:577–579.

102. Jackson, I. M. D., and Reichlin, S. (1974): Thyrotropin-releasing hormone (TRH): Distribution in hypothalamic and extrahypothalamic brain tissue of mammalian and submammalian chordates. *Endocrinology,* 95:854–862.

103. Jeffcoate, S. L., Fraser, H. M., Gunn, A., and White, N. (1973): Radioimmuno-assay of thyrotrophin releasing hormone. *J. Endocrinol.,* 59:191–192.

104. Jeffcoate, S. L., Hollan, D. T., Fraser, H. M., and Gunn, A. (1974): Preparation and specificity of antibodies to the decapeptide, luteinizing hormone-releasing hormone (LH-RH). *Immunochemistry,* 11:75–77.

105. Kanazawa, I., and Jessell, T. (1976): Post mortem changes and regional distribution of substance P in the rat and mouse nervous system. *Brain Res.,* 117:362–367.

106. Kanazawa, I., Emson, P. C., and Cuello, A. C. (1977): Evidence for the existence of substance P-containing fibres in striato-nigral and pallido-nigral pathways in rat brain. *Brain Res.,* 119:447–453.

107. King, J. C., Arimura, A., Gerall, A. G., Fishback, J. B., and Elking, K. E. (1975): Growth hormone-release inhibiting hormone (GH-RIH) pathway of the rat hypo-thalamus revealed by the unlabeled antibody peroxidase-antiperoxidase method. *Cell Tissue Res.,* 160:423–430.

108. King, J. C., and Gerall, A. A. (1976): Localization of luteinizing hormone-releasing hormone. *J. Histochem. Cytochem.,* 24:829–845.

109. King, J. C., Parsons, J. A., Erlandsen, S. L., and Williams, T. H. (1974): Lutein-izing hormone-releasing hormone (LH-RH) pathway of the rat hypothalamus revealed by the unlabeled peroxidase-anti-peroxidase method. *Cell Tissue Res.,* 153:211–217.

110. King, J. C., Williams, T. H., and Arimura, A. (1975): Localization of luteinizing hormone-releasing hormone in rat hypothalamus using radioimmunoassay. *J. Anat.,* 120:275–288.

111. Knigge, K. M. (1977): Anatomy of the endocrine hypothalamus. In: *The Hypo-thalamus. Association for Research in Nervous and Mental Disease Publication, Vol. 56,* edited by S. Reichlin. Raven Press, New York (*in press*).

112. Kordon, C., Kerdelhue, B., Pattou, E., and Jutisz, M. (1974): Immunocyto-chemical localization of LH-RH in axons and nerve terminals of the rat median eminence. *Proc. Soc. Exp. Biol. Med.,* 147:122–127.

113. Koves, K., and Magyar, A. (1975): On the location of TRH producing neurons: Thyroid response to PTU treatment after stereotaxic interventions in hypothala-mus. *Endocrinol. Exp.,* 9:247–257.

114. Kronheim, S., Berelowitz, M., and Pimstone, B. L. (1976): A radioimmunoassay for growth hormone release-inhibiting hormone; Method and quantitative tissue distribution. *Clin. Endocrinol.,* 5:619–630.

115. Krulich, L., Dhariwal, A. P. S., and McCann, S. M. (1968): Stimulatory and inhibitory effects of purified hypothalamic extracts on growth hormone release from rat pituitary *in vitro. Endocrinology,* 83:783–790.

116. Krulich, L., Quijda, M., Hefco, E., and Sundberg, D. K. (1974): Localization of thyrotropin-releasing factor (TRF) in the hypothalamus of the rat. *Endocrinology,* 95:9–17.

117. Kuhar, M. J., Pert, C. B., and Snyder, S. H. (1973): Regional distribution of opiate receptor binding in monkey and human brain. *Nature,* 245:447–450.

118. Lamotte, C., Pert, C. B., and Snyder, S. H. (1976): Opiate receptor binding in primate spinal cord: Distribution and changes after dorsal root section. *Brain Res.,* 112:407–412.

119. Larsson, L.-I., Edvinsson, L., Fahrenkrug, J., Håkanson, R., Owman, Ch., Schaffalitzky de Muckadell, O., and Sundler, F. (1976): Immunohistochemical

localization of a vasodilatory polypeptide (VIP) in cerebrovascular nerves. *Brain Res.*, 113:400–404.

120. Larsson, L.-I., Fahrenkrug, J., Schaffalitzky de Muckadell, O., Sundler, F., Håkanson, R., and Rehfeld, J. F. (1976): Localization of vasoactive intestinal polypeptide (VIP) to central and peripheral neurons. *Proc. Natl. Acad. Sci. U.S.A.*, 73:3197–3200.

121. Lechan, R. M., Alpert, L. C., and Jackson, I. M. D. (1976): Synthesis of luteinizing hormone releasing factor and thyrotropin-releasing factor in glutamate lesioned mice. *Nature*, 264:463–465.

122. Leclerc, R., Pelletier, G., Puviani, R., Arimura, A., and Schally, A. V. (1976): Immunohistochemical localization of somatostatin in endocrine cells of the rat stomach. *Mol. Cell. Endocrinol.*, 4:257–261.

123. Leeman, S. E., and Mroz, E. A. (1975): Substance P. *Life Sci.*, 15:2033–2044.

124. Lembeck, F., and Zetler, G. (1962): Substance P: A polypeptide of possible physiological significance, especially within the nervous system. *Int. Rev. Neurobiol.*, 4:159–215.

125. Leonardelli, J., Barry, J., and Dubois, M. P. (1973): Mise en evidence par immunofluorescence d'un constituant immunologiquement apparente au LH-RH dans l'hypothalamus et l'eminence mediane chez les Mammiferes. *C. R. Acad. Sci [D] (Paris)*, 276:2043–2046.

126. Lien, E. L., Fenichel, R. L., Garsky, V., Sarantakis, D., and Grant, N. H. (1976): Enkephalin-stimulated prolactin release. *Life Sci.*, 19:837–840.

127. Luft, R., Efendić, S., Hökfelt, T., Johansson, O., and Arimura, A. (1974): Immunohistochemical evidence for the localization of somatostatin-like immunoreactivity in a cell population of the pancreatic islets. *Med. Biol.*, 52:428–430.

128. Mroz, E. A., Brownstein, M. J., and Lemman, S. E. (1976): Evidence for substance P in the habenulo-interpeduncular tract. *Brain Res.*, 113:597–599.

129. Mutt, V., and Said, S. I. (1974): Structure of the porcine vasoactive intestinal octacosapeptide. The amino-acid sequence. Use of kallikrein in its determination. *Eur. J. Biochem.*, 42:581–589.

130. Naik, D. V. (1975): Immunoreactive LH-RH neurons in the hypothalamus identified by light and fluorescent microscopy. *Cell Tissue Res.*, 157:423–436.

131. Naik, D. V. (1976): Immunohistochemical localization of LH-RH during different phases of estrus cycle of rat, with reference to the preoptic and arcuate neurons, and the ependymal cells. *Cell Tissue Res.*, 173:143–166.

132. Nair, R. M. G., Barrett, J. F., Bower, C. Y., and Schally, A. V. (1970): Structure of porcine thyrotropin releasing hormone. *Biochemistry*, 9:1103–1106.

133. Nilsson, G., Hökfelt, T., and Pernow, B. (1974): Distribution of substance P-like immunoreactivity in the rat central nervous system as revealed by immunohistochemistry. *Med. Biol.*, 52:424–427.

134. Nilsson, G., Larsson, L. I., Håkansson, R., Brodin, E., Sundler, F., and Pernow, B. (1975): Localization of substance P-like immunoreactivity in mouse gut. *Histochemistry*, 43:97–99.

135. Nilsson, G., Pernow, B., Fischer, G. H., and Folkers, K. (1975): Presence of substance P-like immunoreactivity in plasma from man and dog. *Acta Physiol. Scand.*, 94:542–544.

136. Oliver, C., Eskay, R. L., Ben-Jonathan, N., and Porter, J. C. (1974): Distribution and concentration of TRH in the rat brain. *Endocrinology*, 96:540–546.

137. Oliver, G., and Schafer, E. A. (1895): On the physiological action of extracts of pituitary body and certain other glandular organs. *J. Physiol.*, 18:277–279.

138. Orci, L., Baetens, D., Dubois, M. P., and Rufener, C. (1975): Evidence for the D-cell of the pancreas secreting somatostatin. *Horm. Metab. Res.*, 7:400–402.

139. Orci, M. L., Baetens, D., Rufener, C., Amherdt, M., Ravazzola, M., Studer, P., Malaisse-Lagae, F., and Unger, R. H. (1975): Reactivite de la cellule a somatostatine de l'ilot de Langerhans dans le diabete experimental. *C. R. Acad. Sci. [D] (Paris)*, 281:1883–1885.

140. Paasonen, M. K., and Vogt, M. (1956): The effect of drugs on the amounts of substance P and 5-hydroxytryptamine in mammalian brain. *J. Physiol.*, 131:617–626.

141. Palkovits, M., Brownstein, M., and Kizer, S. J. (1976): Effect of total hypothalamic deafferentation on releasing hormone and neurotransmitter concentrations of the mediobasal hypothalamus in rat. In: *International Symposium on Cellular and Molecular Bases of Neuroendocrine Processes,* edited by E. Endroczy, pp. 575–599. Akademiai Kiado, Budapest.

142. Palkovits, M., Brownstein, M., Saavedra, J. M., and Axelrod, J. (1974): Luteinizing hormone releasing hormone (LH-RH) content of the hypothalamic nuclei in rat. *Endocrinology,* 96:554–558.

143. Parsons, J. A., Erlandsen, S. L., Hegre, O., McEvoy, R., and Elde, R. P. (1976): Central and peripheral localization of somatostatin. Immunoenzyme immunocytochemical studies. *J. Histochem. Cytochem.,* 24:872–882.

144. Pearse, A. G. E., and Polak, J. (1975): Immunocytochemical localization of substance P in mammalian intestine. *Histochemistry,* 41:373–375.

145. Pease, D. C. (1962): Buffered formaldehyde as a killing agent and primary fixative for electron microscopy. *Anat. Rec.,* 142:342.

146. Pelletier, G., Labrie, F., Arimura, A., and Schally, A. V. (1974): Electron microscopic immunohistochemical localization of growth hormone release inhibiting hormone (somatostatin) in the rat median eminence. *Am. J. Anat.,* 140:445–450.

147. Pelletier, G., Leclerc, R., Arimura, A., and Schally, A. V. (1975): Immunohistochemical localization of somatostatin in the rat pancreas. *J. Histochem. Cytochem.,* 23:699–701.

148. Pelletier, G., Leclerc, R., Dube, D., Labrie, F., Puviani, R., Arimura, A., and Schally, A. V. (1975): Localization of growth hormone-release inhibiting hormone (somatostatin) in the rat brain. *Am. J. Anat.,* 142:397–401.

149. Pelletier, G., Leclerc, R., and Dube, D. (1976): Immunohistochemical localization of hypothalamic hormones. *J. Histochem. Cytochem.,* 24:864–871.

150. Pernow, B. (1953): Studies on substance P. Purification, occurrence and biological actions. *Acta. Physiol. Scand. [Suppl.],* 105 29:1–90.

151. Pert, C. B., Kuhar, M. J., and Snyder, S. H. (1976): Opiate receptor: Autoradiographic localization in rat brain. *Proc. Natl. Acad. Sci. U.S.A.,* 73:3729–3733.

152. Pert, C. B., and Snyder, S. H. (1973): Opiate receptor: Demonstration in nervous tissue. *Science,* 179:1001–1014.

153. Polak, J. M., Grimelius, L., Pearse, A. G. E., Bloom, S. R., and Arimura, A. (1975): Growth-hormone release-inhibiting hormone in gastrointestinal and pancreatic D-cells. *Lancet,* 1:1220–1222.

154. Powell, D., Leeman, S. E., Tregear, G. W., Niall, H. D., and Potts, J. T. (1973): Radioimmunoassay for substance P. *Nature [New Biol.],* 241:252–254.

155. Rehfeld, J. F., Stadil, F., and Rubin, B. (1972): Production and evaluation of antibodies for the radioimmunoassay of gastrin. *Scand. J. Clin. Lab. Invest,* 30:221–232.

156. Reichlin, S. (1960): Thyroid function, body temperature regulation and growth in rats with hypothalamic lesions. *Endocrinology,* 66:340–354.

157. Rodbard, D. (1974): Statistical quality control and routine data processing for radioimmunoassays and immunoradiometric assays. *Clin. Chem.,* 20:1255–1273.

158. Rufener, C., Amherdt, M., Dubois, M. P., and Orci, L. (1975): Ultrastructural immunocytochemical localization of somatostatin in rat pancreatic monolayer culture. *J. Histochem. Cytochem.,* 23:866–869.

159. Rufener, C., Dubois, M. P., Malaisse-Lagae, F., and Orci, L. (1975): Immunofluorescent reactivity to anti-somatostatin in the gastrointestinal mucosa of the dog. *Diabetologia,* 11:321–324.

160. Said, S. I., and Faloona, G. R. (1975): A radioimmunoassay of vasoactive intestinal polypeptide. *N. Engl. J. Med.,* 293:155.

161. Said, S. I., and Rosenberg, R. M. (1976): Vasoactive intestinal polypeptide: Abundant immunoreactivity in neural cell lines and normal nervous tissue. *Science,* 192:907–908.

162. Saper, C. B., Loewy, A. L., Swanson, L. W., and Cowan, W. M. (1976): Direct hypothalamo-autonomic connections. *Brain Res.,* 117:305–312.

163. Schally, A. V., Arimura, A., Baba, Y., Nair, R. M. G., Matsuo, J., Redding, T. W., Debeljuk, L., and White, W. F. (1971): Isolation and properties of the

FSH- and LH-releasing hormone. *Biochem. Biophys. Res. Commun.,* 43:393–399.
164. Schally, A. V., and Kastin, A. J. (1976): Les hormones de l'hypothalamus. *La Recherche,* 7:36–45.
165. Scharrer, E., and Scharrer, B. (1954): Hormones produced by neurosecretory cells. *Recent Prog. Horm. Res.,* 10:183–240.
166. Schultz, W. J., Brownfield, M. S., and Kozlowski, G. P. (1977): The hypothalamo-choroidal tract. II. Ultrastructural response of the choroid plexus to vasopressin. *Cell Tissue Res.,* 178:129–141.
167. Setalo, G., Vigh, S., Schally, A. V., Arimura, A., and Flerko, B. (1975): GH-RIH containing neural elements in the hypothalamus. *Brain Res.,* 90:352–356.
168. Setalo, G., Vigh, S., Schally, A. V., Arimura, A., and Flerko, B. (1976): Immuno-histological study of the origin of LH-RH-containing nerve fibers of the rat hypothalamus. *Brain Res.,* 103:597–602.
169. Silverman, A. J. (1975): The hypothalamic magnocellular neurosecretory system of the guinea pig. I. Immunohistochemical localization of neurophysin in the adult. *Am. J. Anat.,* 144:433–444.
170. Silverman, A. J. (1976): Distribution of luteinizing hormone-releasing hormone (LH-RH) in the guinea pig brain. *Endocrinology,* 99:30–41.
171. Simantov, R., Kuhar, M. J., Pasternak, G. W., and Snyder, S. H. (1976): The regional distribution of a morphine-like factor enkephalin in monkey brain. *Brain Res.,* 106:189–197.
172. Simantov, R., Kuhar, M. J., Uhl, G. R., and Snyder, S. H. (1977): Opioid peptide enkephalin: Immunohistochemical mapping in the rat central nervous system. *Proc. Natl. Acad. Sci. USA,* 74:2167–2171.
173. Simon, E. J., Hiller, J. M., and Fidelman, I. (1973): Stereospecific binding of the potent narcotic analgesic [³H] etorphine to rat brain homogenate. *Proc. Natl. Acad. Sci. U.S.A.,* 70:1947–1949.
174. Skowsky, W. R., and Fisher, D. A. (1972): The use of thyroglobulin to induce antigenicity to small molecules. *J. Lab. Clin. Med.,* 80:134–144.
175. Smith, T. W., Hughes, J., Kosterlitz, H. W. and Sosa, R. P. (1976): Enkephalins: Isolation, distribution and function. In: *Opiates and Endogenous Opioid Peptides,* pp. 57–62. North Holland, Amsterdam.
176. Snyder, S. H. and Simantov, R. (1977): The opiate receptor and opioid peptides. *J. Neurochem.,* 28:13–20.
177. Terenius, L. (1973): Characteristics of the receptor for narcotic analgesics in synaptic membrane fractions from rat brain. *Acta Pharmacol. (Kbh.),* 33:377–384.
178. Vale, W., Brazeau, P., Rivier, C., Brown, M., Boss, B., Rivier, J., Burgus, R., Ling, N., and Guillemin, R. (1975): Somatostatin. *Recent Prog. Horm. Res.,* 31:365.
179. Vanderhaeghen, J. J., Signeau, J. C., and Gepts, W. (1975): New peptide in the vertebrate CNS reacting with antigastrin antibodies. *Nature,* 257:604–605.
180. Vandesande, F., DeMey, J., and Dierickx, K. (1974): Identification of neuro-physin producing cells. I. The origin of the neurophysin-like substance-containing nerve fibers of the external region of the median eminence of the rat. *Cell Tissue Res.,* 151:187–200.
181. Vandesande, F., and Dierickx, K. (1975): Identification of the vasopressin pro-ducing and of the oxytocin producing neurons in the hypothalamic magnocellular neurosecretory system of the rat. *Cell Tissue Res.,* 164:153–162.
182. Vandesande, F., Dierickx, K., and DeMey, J. (1975): Identification of the vaso-pressin-neurophysin II and the oxytocin-neurophysin I producing neurons in the bovine hypothalamus. *Cell Tissue Res.,* 156:189–200.
183. Vandesande, F., Dierickx, K., and DeMey, J. (1975): Identification of the vaso-pressin-neurophysin producing neurons of the rat suprachiasmatic nuclei. *Cell Tissue Res.,* 156:377–380.
184. Vandesande, F., Dierickx, K., and DeMey, J. (1975): Identification of separate vasopressin-neurophysin II and oxytocin-neurophysin I containing nerve fibers in the external region of the bovine median eminence. *Cell Tissue Res.,* 158:509–516.
185. Walter, R., Schlesinger, D. H., Schwartz, I. L., and Capra, J. D. (1971): Com-

plete amino acid sequence of bovine neurophysin II. *Biochem. Biophys. Res. Commun.*, 44:293–298.

186. Watkins, W. B. (1975): Immunohistochemical demonstration of neurophysin in the hypothalamo-neurohypophysial system. *Int. Rev. Cytol.*, 41:241–284.

187. Weindl, A., and Sofroniew, M. V. (1976): Demonstration of extrahypothalamic peptide secreting neurons. A morphologic contribution to the investigation of psychotropic effects of neurohormones. *Pharmakopsych.*, 9:226–234.

188. Weiner, R. I., Pattou, E., Kerdelhue, B., and Kordon, C. (1975): Differential effects of hypothalamic deafferentation upon luteinizing hormone-releasing hormone in the median eminence and organum vasculosum of the lamina terminalis. *Endocrinology*, 97:1597–1600.

189. Wheaton, J. E., Krulich, L., and McCann, S. M. (1975): Localization of luteinizing hormone-releasing hormone in the preoptic area and hypothalamus of the rat using radioimmunoassay. *Endocrinology,* 97:30–38.

190. Wimersma Greidanus, T. B. van, Bohus, B., and Wied, D. de (1975): CNS sites of action of ACTH, MSH and vasopressin in relation to avoidance behavior. In: *Anatomical Neuroendocrinology,* edited by W. E. Stumpf and L. D. Grant, pp. 284–289. S. Karger, Basel.

191. Winokur, A., and Utiger, R. D. (1974): Thyrotropin-releasing hormone: Regional distribution in rat brain. *Science,* 185:265–267.

192. Zetler, G. (1970): Distribution of peptidergic neurons in mammalian brain. In: *Aspects of Neuroendocrinology,* edited by W. Bargmann and B. Scharrer, pp. 287–295. Springer-Verlag, Berlin.

193. Zimmerman, E. A. (1976): Localization of hypothalamic hormones by immunocytochemical techniques. In: *Frontiers in Neuroendocrinology, Vol. 4,* edited by L. Martini and W. R. Ganong, pp. 25–62. Raven Press, New York.

194. Zimmerman, E. A., Hsu, K. G., Ferin, M., and Kozlowski, G. P. (1974): Localization of gonadotropin-releasing hormone (Gn-RH) in the hypothalamus of mouse by immunoperoxidase technique. *Endocrinology,* 95:1–8.

Frontiers in Neuroendocrinology, Vol. 5,
edited by W. F. Ganong and L. Martini.
Raven Press, New York © 1978.

Chapter 2

Neurophysins, an Aid to Understanding the Structure and Function of the Neurohypophysis

Alan G. Robinson

Department of Medicine, University of Pittsburgh School of Medicine, Pittsburgh, Pennsylvania 15261

Before neurophysins were isolated and recognized biochemically, they had already provided the means of detailed study of the neurohypophysis (33,69) because Bargmann and his collaborators (6,71) found that the chromalum-hematoxylin stain, which had been developed by Gomori to stain the beta cells of the pancreas (70), selectively stained the neurosecretory material of the neurohypophysis (5). It is now known that this dye and aldehyde fuchsin have a special affinity for sulfhydryl groups and that the high cysteine content of neurophysins results in a dense concentration of sulfhydryl groups in neurosecretory granules of the neurohypophysis (98). Because neurosecretory granules are present throughout the neurons of the neurohypophysis, it was possible to study the entire system by staining granules (71,76). It was shown that the secretory material of the posterior pituitary was synthesized in clusters of cells in the hypothalamus and that the terminals of the long axons of these neurons ended on blood vessels rather than in synapses with other neurons [a finding which provided the most definitive anatomic evidence for the concept of neurosecretion—see review of Berta Scharrer (69)]. It is also of interest that Bargmann and Scharrer (6) described and diagrammed a close connection between the supraoptico-hypophyseal tract and the long portal vessels which drained to the adenohypophysis (Fig. 2–1). Studies with the Gomori stain led these workers to conclude that the supraoptico-hypophyseal tract had minor projections to the zona externa of the median eminence and to the third ventricle (6,71). Recent technical advances in immunohistology provide additional evidence that neurohypophyseal peptides are secreted into cerebrospinal fluid (CSF) and into the long portal vessels of the median eminence (98).

At about the same time that the anatomic pathways of the neurohypophysis were being defined, other workers were identifying the secretory peptides of the neurohypophysis (33). The early work of Van Dyke (86) showed that the biologic activities of the posterior pituitary could be precipitated from

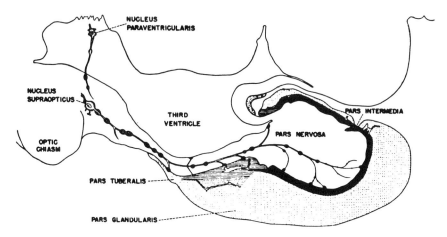

FIG. 2–1. Supraoptico-hypophyseal tract as drawn by Bargmann and Scharrer in 1951. Note the projections to the third ventricle and to the external zone of the median eminence in addition to the major pathway to the posterior lobe. Reprinted with permission from (6).

aqueous extracts of the pituitary gland by the addition of salt. Extracts of neural lobe were shown to have vasopressor, antidiuretic, galactogenic, and uterotonic properties in test animals, and it was eventually demonstrated that the biologic activity resided in two separate hormones, vasopressin and oxytocin (25,82). When the purified hormones became available it was not possible to precipitate the biologic activity with salt, and the protein in the aqueous extract which combined with the hormone and allowed salt to induce precipitation was neurophysin (36). Acher et al. showed that the two biologically active hormones were loosely combined by noncovalent binding to the larger peptide, neurophysin (1,2). As neurophysins were not demonstrated to have biologic activity, they were assigned the role of intraneuronal carrier proteins for the biologically active hormones oxytocin and vasopressin. Neurophysins were relatively unstudied during the next decade, but interest in neurophysins emerged recently for two reasons: the demonstration that in many species there is a specific neurophysin for oxytocin and a different and specific neurophysin for vasopressin; and the demonstration that the neurophysins are not confined to the hypothalamic neurons but are secreted into the general circulation.

NUMBER OF NEUROPHYSINS

The number of neurophysins in the posterior lobe has been a matter of some disagreement. With the original sulfuric acid extraction of Du Vigneaud (25), numerous neurophysin-like peptides were isolated from bovine and porcine posterior pituitaries. As many as seven hormone binding fractions with similar amino acid composition were described (34). It was subsequently shown that degradative enzymes in the neurohypophyseal extracts were active after sulfuric acid extraction but inactive in 0.1 N HCl (35). Extraction of the posterior pituitary of bovine species with 0.1 N HCl yielded predominantly two major peptide bands, and it was believed that any neurophysins in excess of two which were present in extracts of the posterior lobe were due to catabolic degradation of the two natural neurophysins. The concept of two neurophysins was appealing because of the presence of two hormones in the posterior lobe. Isolation of neurosecretory granules indicated the association of a specific neurophysin with oxytocin, bovine neurophysin I, and a different neurophysin with vasopressin, bovine neurophysin II (18). The concept of oxytocin-neurophysin and vasopressin-neurophysin has persisted in spite of the isolation of a third neurophysin from cow (20) and pig (14,83,94) and the suggestion of only a single neurophysin in sheep (12) and guinea pig (64).

Neurophysins have also been grouped into two main classes based on their amino acid composition (11). Amino acid sequences of neurophysins show a large area of homology among the various neurophysins from individual species and the neurophysins from various species. The central amino acid sequence of the neurophysins appears to be most stable in comparing various species of neurophysins (10,11,91). Alanine is consistently the N terminal amino acid in all neurophysins so far sequenced, which suggests that the N terminus forms the peptide bond with any putative precursor molecule (10). Chauvet and co-workers (11) have proposed that the amino acid positions 2, 3, 6, and 7 from the N terminus can be used to divide neurophysins into two groups of neurophysins called MSEL (Met, Ser, Glu, Leu) and VLDV (Val, Leu, Asp, Val) based on the amino acids present in these positions. However, the human neurophysin isolated by Foss et al. (29) and the work of Capra, et al. (9) with the human neurophysin I isolated by Cheng and Friesen (15) have both shown that the N terminus contains an alanine-alanine sequence which does not fit into either of the two groups proposed by Chauvet et al. Fresh dog neurophysin isolated by Walter et al. (91) also contains a similar alanine-alanine sequence. The more variable portions of the neurophysin molecule are the nine N terminal residues and the approximately twenty C terminal residues (10). Within the central core of the neurophysin molecule is the only tyrosine in the molecule, and this highly charged area may be important in binding (10).

Extraction of neurophysin in 0.1 N HCl eliminates catheptic activity, and the results of hydrochloric acid extraction led to the conclusion that the numerous neurophysins of bovine posterior pituitary were in fact only two natural neurophysins (35). Further studies with hydrochloric acid extractions, however, have proven that even with this method there may be at least a third neurophysin present in the cow (20), pig (14,83,94), rat (74), and man (54). One might explain the extra neurophysin as an artifact of the separation technique and assume that the extra neurophysin represents an *in vitro* degradation product of one of the two major neurophysins thought to be present in most species. Indeed, radioimmunoassay studies have indicated that the extra neurophysins in cow (20) and man (54) react with complete identity with one of the two major neurophysins. Amino acid analysis of the third porcine neurophysin has shown that it is just three amino acids longer than porcine neurophysin I (94) and, therefore, that porcine neurophysin I may have been derived from porcine neurophysin III by proteolysis. Furthermore, the work of North and associates (51) has demonstrated that there are enzymes present in hypothalamic extracts which will convert one neurophysin to a different neurophysin by proteolysis. Thus, there is considerable evidence that extracted neurophysins can be further broken down by proteolytic enzymes, but even rapid extraction of the freshest tissue has identified more than two neurophysins in the dog and the cow (91,90). Burford and Pickering (8) used the rat to study *in vivo* synthesis of neurophysins. From the turnover times of three rat neurophysins, called A, B, and C, they determined that A and B were synthesized first and that C was derived from B by enzymatic conversion by a proteinase "within the granule." Enzymes which can cause the catabolic proteolysis of neurophysins may then exist within neurosecretory granules and the "extra" neurophysins may be formed *in vivo*. It is reasonable to assume that catabolic enzymes in the neurosecretory granules have some biologic function. As we have no evidence that it is biologically important to degrade the neurophysins from their two major components to the minor derivatives, it might be assumed that the enzymes are present to cleave neurophysins from some larger precursor molecule.

NEUROPHYSIN SYNTHESIS

A precursor molecule has been postulated to be the parent molecule for neurophysin and its companion hormone, oxytocin or vasopressin. The concept stems from the work of Sachs in the 1960s and 1970s (63,65,66). From Sach's studies it is well known that ^{35}S-cysteine injected into the third ventricle is incorporated into vasopressin and neurophysin. Inhibition of protein synthesis inhibited simultaneously the incorporation of cysteine into vasopressin and neurophysin suggesting that the biosynthesis of these two peptides was linked. If the label was introduced into CSF as a pulse for 1.5 to 3 hr *in vivo* and then incubated *in vitro* under conditions in which further protein synthesis was blocked by the presence of puromycin and label incorporation was blocked by a large pool of unlabeled amino acid, there was still a further production of radioactive vasopressin and neurophysin *in vitro*. Because *de novo* protein synthesis was blocked, the data were interpreted to indicate formation of a labeled precursor *in vivo* during the initial infusion period and subsequent formation of vasopressin and neurophysin from the prelabeled precursor during *in vitro* incubation (65,66). Gainer, Sarne, and Brownstein

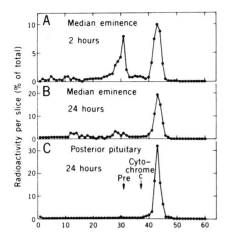

FIG. 2–2. Pattern of labeled protein transported to the median eminence at (A) 2 hr and (B) 24 hr; and to the posterior pituitary at (C) 24 hr after injection of the SON with ^{35}S-cysteine. Proteins were run on 15% acid urea polyacrylamide gel. The putative precursor of neurophysin is the peak at tube #30 which is present in the median eminence 2 hr after injection but absent 24 hr after injection. Reprinted with permission from (30).

(30) used a similar technique in the rat. One to six hours after pulse labeling with cysteine, a sulfhydryl-labeled peptide of about 20,000 molecular weight (MW) which was thought to represent a precursor for neurophysin was isolated from the supraoptic nucleus (SON). By 24 hr after injection all of the label in the SON resided in the 10,000 MW neurophysin fraction. The putative precursor was also present in the neurohypophyseal axons in the median eminence 2 hr after injection, but absent 24 hr after injection of label (Fig. 2–2). The presence of precursor in axons in the median eminence indicates that the precursor is present in the neurosecretory granules because all the neurophysin in axons of the median eminence is within granules. Packaging of precursor into neurosecretory granules is a logical explanation for the presence of proteolytic enzymes within the granules. The enzymes may be necessary to split neurophysin (and hormone?) from the precursor molecule. These proteolytic enzymes may explain the further degradation of neurophysins into the various minor neurophysins which have been isolated from the posterior lobe.

NEUROPHYSINS AND HORMONE RELEASE

There is some evidence that precursor neurophysin may be membrane bound. In the studies of Swann and Pickering (80) most of the ^{35}S-labeled neurophysin which was synthesized in the rat and packaged in neurosecretory granules could be released by treatment of the rat with 2% saline. A small but significant proportion of the neurosecretory granule neurophysin, however, could be sedimented with the granule membrane after exhaustion of the neurosecretory contents. This was thought to represent membrane-bound neurophysin. A similar finding was obtained by Norstrom and Hansson in 1972 (48,50). It is uncertain whether the membrane-bound neurophysin is part of a lipid-neurophysin complex (47) and whether membrane-bound neurophysin plays a role in release of neurosecretory granules. McKelvy (46) has summarized the evidence for a possible role of cyclic AMP-stimulated protein kinase in the release of neurohypophyseal peptides and has suggested that neurosecretory granule membranes can be phosphorylated by activated cyclic AMP. However, bovine neurophysin was not found to possess any protein kinase activity, nor to serve as a substrate for the protein kinase activity in neurosecretory granules. The results would indicate that a membrane-associated neurophysin was not involved in phosphorylation and in extrusion of the neurosecretory contents into the perivascular space, if cAMP plays any role.

Similarly, the methanol-forming enzyme described by Axelrod and Daly (4) and Edgar and Hope (26) has been postulated to play some role in regulating release of posterior pituitary hormones. The postulate was based on the observation that neurophysins are a particularly active substrate for the protein-carboxyl methyltransferase enzyme. However, as with the studies of membrane-bound neurophysin, subcellular fractionation of fresh bovine posterior pituitary glands indicated that the methyltransferase activity was not associated with the particulate fractions which contained neurosecretory granules (26). Thus, the enzyme is compartmentalized away from neurophysins and the neurophysins are unlikely to serve as a natural substrate in the intact neuron. There are no data at the present time to indicate that neurophysins play an active role in the process of neurosecretion.

NEUROPHYSIN PATHWAYS

Histologic studies of the neurohypophysis have been greatly aided by the advent of immunohistochemistry, and in fact the immunohistologic study of neurophysins has provided a prototype for location of peptides in nerve cells by immunohistologic techniques (95). In general, the observations have confirmed the concept of hormone and neurophysin being synthesized in specific cells of the supraoptic and paraventricular nuclei and transported down the long axons to the posterior lobe. Some interesting new observations which have been reviewed elsewhere (98) are discussed here briefly. Because of the greater sensitivity of the immunohistochemical technique as compared to the previous Gomori stain, it has been noted that magnocellular neurons reside outside the strict confines of the supraoptic and the paraventricular nuclei. Magnocellular neurons are located between the supraoptic and paraventricular (PVN) nuclei indicating a greater overlap in these two nuclei than was previously appreciated, and accessory cells containing neurophysin lie scattered beyond the anterior hypothalamus. Staining with antisera for individual neurophysins (which are thought to be hormone specific) and staining with antisera for vasopressin and oxytocin have clearly demonstrated that both hormones are formed in both nuclei (98). However, they are probably formed within separate neurons (21). There may be geographic separation of vasopressin neurons and oxytocin neurons within the nuclei. Studies of the Brattleboro rat homozygous for diabetes insipidus (as compared with the normal rat) indicate that vasopressin and its neurophysin are synthesized in the ventral portion of the SON and the more medial portion of the PVN (77). Oxytocin and its neurophysin are retained as a dorsal cap of the SON and a lateral group of cells in the PVN in the Brattleboro rat and in the same position in the normal rat (Fig. 2–3). A similar geographic separation of oxytocin and vasopressin neurons has been described in the human (97,98). It should be noted that at least two groups of workers have reported the presence of vasopressin in what would otherwise be presumed to be oxytocin-secreting neurons in the normal rat (40,77). Thus, it cannot be completely excluded that some cells can synthesize both hormones [see review of Zimmerman and Robinson (98)].

Early studies of Bargmann and Scharrer (6) based on comparative anatomy studies with the Gomori stain led them to conclude that axons of the supraoptico-hypophyseal tract projected to the zona externa of the median eminence where there might be secretion into the long portal vessels which drain to the adenohypophysis (see Fig. 2–1). This observation was lost for

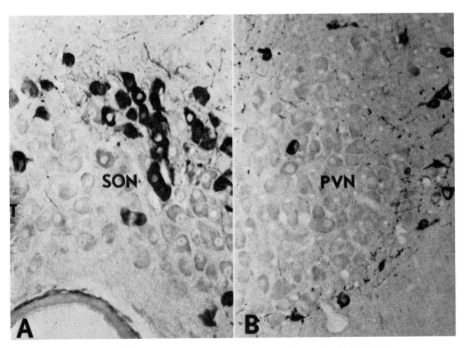

FIG. 2–3. Neurophysin stained by immunoperoxidase technique shown as the dark color in neurosecretory neurons of homozygous Brattleboro rat with diabetes insipidus. (A): Supraoptic nucleus (SON) with neurophysin-containing cells in the dorsal region. (B): Paraventricular nucleus (PVN) with neurophysin-containing cells in the periphery. Neurophysin in the Brattleboro rat identifies the position of the oxytocin-containing cells. Reprinted with permission from (77).

nearly 20 years until the neurohypophysis was re-examined using immuno-histochemical techniques. Several laboratories have confirmed an intense staining of neurophysin in the external zone of the monkey (96), rat (77,84), and cow (19,99). The concurrence of the observation in several animals would indicate that neurophysin in the external zone is both real and physio-logically significant. This comparative approach was used with great success by Bargmann and Scharrer (6), Scharrer and Scharrer [see review of Berta Scharrer (69)], Sawyer (68), and others. The origin of the neurophysin-containing axons of the external zone is not certain. Antunes et al. (3) per-formed unilateral lesion of the paraventricular nucleus in the monkey and showed a depletion of the immunoreactive neurophysin (and vasopressin) in the zona externa of the ipsilateral median eminence. Therefore, the axons in the external zone probably arrive from the supraoptico-hypophyseal tract. Still unknown is whether there are separate neurons within the paraventricular nucleus with single axons which extend only to the external zone or if the fibers to the external zone are collaterals of axons projecting to the posterior lobe.

It is probable that both oxytocin and vasopressin are present in the external zone of the median eminence as both hormones have been demonstrated there by specific immunohistochemistry (98) and both bovine neurophysin I and bovine neurophysin II have been localized in the external zone of the cow (21). Also, the observation of neurophysin-containing fibers in the ex-ternal zone of the median eminence of the Brattleboro rat homozygous for diabetes insipidus (77) indicates that oxytocin fibers reach the external zone.

When neurophysins were first recognized in the external zone of the mon-key (96), there was an associated heavy staining of neurophysin in tanycytes of the median eminence. These "stretch cells" which reach from the third ventricle to the external zone of the median eminence have been postulated to have a transport function for the transfer of peptides from the CSF to the portal vessels. The heavy staining in the tanycytes, the presence of neuro-physin around portal vessels, and the presence of neurophysin in CSF led to the suggestion that tanycytes might be one source of neurophysin in the external zone. Investigation of other animals has shown that neurophysins are not present in tanycytes of all species, and importantly tanycyte staining is lacking in some animals when there is obvious staining in the external zone (98). Furthermore, the studies of Antunes et al. (3) demonstrating that in-terruption of the paraventricular tract decreases the staining in the external zone indicates a supraoptico-hypophyseal origin for the fibers in the external zone. Vandesande et al. (85) observed that bovine neurophysin I and bovine neurophysin II are present in separate cells around portal vessels and that there was an appropriate association of neurophysin I with oxytocin and neu-rophysin II with vasopressin. They made the cogent argument that if neuro-physins were first secreted into CSF and then taken up again by cells for transport to the portal vessels, it would be likely that both neurophysins and both hormones would be present in the same cells. It would be unlikely that transport cells would selectively take up one neurophysin and one hormone from CSF. Thus, it is most consistent with the recently developed data that the neurohypophyseal peptides in the external zone arise from the supra-optico-hypophyseal tract.

The presence of neurophysins in CSF in concentrations in excess of plasma and the demonstration that neurophysins do not cross from plasma into CSF have provided firm support for the previous suggestion that vasopressin, and probably oxytocin, are secreted into CSF (59). The source of secretion of vasopressin and neurophysin into CSF is not fully established. Some free nerve endings have been described in the floor of the third ventricle (73), and some of these endings contain large granules typical of the magnocellular system. Possibly axons of the supraoptico-hypophyseal tract secrete into the ventricular system, but the physiological role of neurohypophyseal peptides in CSF is undetermined. Interesting work by Van Wimersma et al. (87–89) suggests that vasopressin may play a role in memory consolidation in rats, and other workers have postulated that peptides in CSF may influence thirst (28). At present, it can be stated that should a physiologic function of neu-rohypophyseal peptides in CSF be discovered, the anatomic groundwork on which to build a physiologic principle is established.

Thus, neurophysins and the hormones vasopressin and oxytocin are syn-thesized within the magnocellular system, which is primarily localized in two groups of cells in the supraoptic and paraventricular nuclei but which has cells scattered in other areas of the hypothalamus. The axons project by long axons to the posterior lobe and by somewhat shorter axons (which may be branches) to the external zone of the median eminence and to the third ventricle. Based on immunohistology, neurohypophyseal peptide secretion from the posterior lobe would appear to be quantitatively the most important, but lesser quantities of peptides secreted into the alternate pathways may be found to subserve major physiologic functions.

MEDIAN EMINENCE NEUROPHYSIN AND ADRENALECTOMY

Although it is known that neurohypophyseal peptides are present in the external zone of the median eminence, it is not known: (a) if the secretion of neurohypophyseal peptides into the portal system varies in a physiologically significant way; (b) whether this is a quantitatively important pathway for the release of neurohypophyseal peptides after injury to the posterior lobe; or (c) if the neurohypophyseal peptides which are secreted into the portal vessels influence the secretory activity of the anterior pituitary. In the studies of Zimmerman and co-workers (96) in the monkey and of Oliver et al. (52) in the rat, vasopressin was present in high concentrations in the portal blood draining to the anterior pituitary, $> 10,000$ pg/ml. The concentrations in the portal blood were of a quantity close to the predicted values of Goldman and

Lindner (31), which would stimulate ACTH release. Several workers have confirmed in the rat an increase in neurosecretory material in the median eminence after adrenalectomy (23,72,84,93). Stillman et al. (78) showed that the neurophysin in the external zone after adrenalectomy was accompanied by a similar increase in vasopressin without a concomitant increase in oxytocin and that the increased vasopressin appeared to be due specifically to the lack of glucocorticoids. Increased vasopressin was not found in the zona externa of severely dehydrated rats, but was present in adrenalectomized rats maintained on sodium chloride replacement, and was absent in adrenalectomized rats replaced with prednisone (Fig. 2–4). The presence of neurophysin and vasopressin in the external zone and the secretion of vasopressin into portal vessels place vasopressin in a position to act as a releasing factor but do not prove that vasopressin is the corticotrophin releasing factor. Certainly there are substances in the hypothalamus which are not vasopressin but which have been shown to release ACTH (39). Nonetheless, vasopressin secretion into the portal blood and the increased content of vasopressin and neurophysin in the external zone after adrenalectomy raise the possibility that

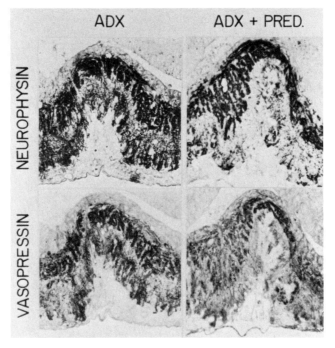

FIG. 2–4. Comparison of neurophysin and vasopressin in the median eminence 2 weeks after adrenalectomy in a rat maintained on 0.9% NaCl volume replacement (*left*) and in a rat treated with prednisone (*right*). Increased staining is demonstrated in the zona interna and in the zona externa, with both vasopressin and neurophysin. Prednisone administration suppresses the increase of both neurophysin and vasopressin. Coronal section, ×250. Figure courtesy of Stillman et al. (78).

vasopressin may serve as one of the ACTH releasing factors in certain situations.

AXON TRANSPORT

Neurophysin and hormone are packaged together in neurosecretory granules, and the granules are carried down the axons by rapid transport (63). In the rat, radioactive cysteine injected into the hypothalamus appears in the posterior lobe as neurophysin and vasopressin in 2 to 3 hr. Allowing an approximate 1.5-hr delay for incorporation of ^{35}S-cysteine into neurophysin, Norstrom (49) calculated a transport rate of 190 mm/day. Similar results were obtained by Jones and Pickering (38) and Burford and Pickering (8). It is debatable if any neurophysin and vasopressin exist outside granules and if any neurophysin and hormone are transported by slow axon transport (see 49).

When secretion of neurohypophyseal hormones is stimulated by hemorrhage, suckling, or hypertonic saline administration, there is a decrease in the absolute neurophysin content of the posterior lobe but an increase in turnover of labeled neurosecretory material indicating an initial release of stored hormone and a more rapid release of newly synthesized hormone. Studies of axon transport during periods of stimulated release do not demonstrate an increased transport time from the nuclei of synthesis to the posterior lobe (49,63). Under such conditions there is believed to be increased synthesis in the perikaryon on one end of the long axon and increased secretion from the axon terminal on the other end of the axon. If the transport rate is fixed, then there should be an increase in neurosecretory material transported per unit axon. One might anticipate that increased neurosecretory material could be demonstrated in the axons by specific immunohistochemical stains of the hypothalamus. A recent study of neurohypophyseal axons in rats after adrenalectomy supports this concept (78). In adrenalectomized rats there is an increase in circulating plasma vasopressin with a decrease in posterior lobe content of vasopressin, data consistent with increased secretion (75). In the median eminence, the axons of the supraoptico-hypophyseal tract were shown by specific immunohistochemistry to contain neurophysin and vasopressin in amounts which greatly exceeded the contents of these peptides in the normal rat (see above Fig. 1–4; 78).

In the posterior pituitary heterogeneity of storage of neurophysin and vasopressin has been found. As summarized by Douglas (24), the evidence indicates that newly arrived neurosecretory granules are the first to be secreted. It was hypothesized that the newly arrived neurosecretory granules are closer to the membrane surface and that this anatomic location allows for a rapid release when secretion is stimulated. When vasopressin and neurophysin are tagged *in vivo* by incorporation of ^{35}S-labeled cysteine, some label may remain in the posterior pituitary for greater than 3 weeks (65). The slow release of label from the posterior lobe has been variously interpreted to represent: (a) slow transport of neurohypophyseal peptides over a period of days; (b) existence of a precursor peptide which is slowly transformed into neurophysin and vasopressin in the neurosecretory granules; and (c) movement of mature neurosecretory granules into a less readily releasable pool.

NEUROPHYSIN SECRETION

With the knowledge that hormone secretion in a number of glands occurred by exocytosis of granules and with the data of Douglas that exocytosis was the method of secretion of neurohypophyseal peptides (24), it was reasonable to assume that the entire contents of neurosecretory granules would be secreted into the perivascular space. Neurophysins are a major component of the peptides in neurosecretory granules, and the studies of Fawcett, Powell, and Sachs (27) were the first to demonstrate secretion of neurophysins into the bloodstream. A dog model which has been discussed above was used to study synthesis and secretion of vasopressin by the injection of ^{35}S-cysteine into the third ventricle. After time was allowed for labeling of neurohypophyseal peptides, the dogs were hemorrhaged and a ^{35}S-cysteine labeled peptide which had the molecular weight of neurophysin was secreted into the bloodstream. This marked the beginning of the investigation of neurophysin secretion. Subsequent progress was accelerated by the development of radioimmunoassays for neurophysins. Neurophysin was detected in the blood of pregnant women using a radioimmunoassay of bovine neurophysin by Legros et al. in 1969 (43), and this observation was followed shortly by reports of Cheng and Friesen (13) and Robinson et al. (60,61) on the measurement of plasma neurophysin in the rat, pig, and ox. The secretion of neurophysin in plasma in response to physiologic stimulation of the neurohypophysis was quickly established in a variety of animals (56). Studies of bovine neurophysins were of special interest because the cow was the first species in which the two major neurophysins, bovine neurophysin I and bovine neurophysin II, could be separately measured by specific radioimmunoassays (60,61). With these assays it was found that the two neurophysins were independently secreted in the cow, consistent with bioassay data suggesting independent secretion of vasopressin and oxytocin. Subsequently, other specific bovine neurophysin assays (44) demonstrated a clear-cut increase in bovine neurophysin I with milking, with values in the range of 1.8 to 2.7 ng/ml before milking and in the range of 2.2 to 6.1 ng/ml after milking. Bovine neurophysin II values were unchanged by milking. An opposite effect on bovine neurophysins was found with hemorrhage where there was an increase in bovine neurophysin II from values less than 1 ng/ml to peak values of greater than 30 ng/ml while bovine neurophysin I showed only a slight increase in some animals (45). Consistent with the earlier studies of isolated granules (18), there was an association of bovine neurophysin I with oxytocin and bovine neurophysin II with vasopressin. The supraoptic and paraventricular nuclei of the cow were dissected and extracted for radioimmunoassay of neurophysins and bioassay of oxytocin and vasopressin, and again neurophysin I was associated with oxytocin and neurophysin II with vasopressin (99). De Mey and co-workers (21) have now shown the same association by immunohistology of individual neurons (21). In the cow, the relationships of neurophysins and hormones are sufficiently established that one might speak of bovine neurophysin I as oxytocin-neurophysin and bovine neurophysin II as vasopressin-neurophysin.

Data in the rat also support the concept of oxytocin-neurophysin and vasopressin-neurophysin. By analytic disc gel electrophoresis, investigators identified three bands of neurophysin peptides in the normal rat, whereas in the Brattleboro rat homozygous for diabetes insipidus (DI) one of the neurophysin bands was lacking. It has been suggested that the absent neurophysin in the DI rat was the neurophysin which in the normal rat was associated with vasopressin (7,79). In the hypothalamus of the DI rat only some neurons show a positive stain for neurophysin, and all of these neurons contain oxytocin. The unstained cells in the DI rat are in the position of cells which in the normal rat contain vasopressin and neurophysin (77). Although specific rat neurophysins have not been identified by amino acid composition nor by specific antisera, the anatomic evidence indicates there is a vasopressin-neurophysin in the rat.

Seif et al. (74) have recently developed a homologous radioimmunoassay for rat neurophysin, but unfortunately the assay does not distinguish between the various neurophysins of the rat. Basal neurophysin values were somewhat higher in the rat than in other animals, 3.7 ± 0.2 ng/ml in unrestrained and unanesthetized rats on *ad libitum* water and food. The assay appears to be especially good for measurement of vasopressin-related neurophysin because plasma neurophysin was suppressed to 2.8 ± 0.1 ng/ml after water loading and stimulated to 10.4 ± 2.1 ng/ml after hypertonic saline injection intraperitoneally. A similar brisk response of neurophysin to hemorrhage was noted in five rats which had 1 ml of blood removed from a carotid cannula every 5 min for 40 min (Fig. 2–5). When the red cells resuspended in saline were reinjected there was a fall of neurophysin to base line, but a second and massive hemorrhage at 155 min resulted in a further outpouring of neurophysin. The assay may also measure a neurophysin associated with oxytocin. In Fig. 2–6 periodic plasma neurophysin levels in 10 pregnant rats were compared with plasma neurophysin in 10 age-matched nonpregnant controls. In the pregnant rats plasma neurophysin showed a statistically significant increase by day 14, rose steadily to greater than 13 ng/ml by day 21, and fell dramatically toward normal by 2 days postpartum. Sixteen blood samples collected from four rats during parturition showed significantly higher values than before parturition with a mean of 40 ± 5.3 ng/ml (74). This homologous assay must measure vasopressin-neurophysin and oxytocin-neurophysin in the rat.

In the human in spite of methods of extraction of neurophysins which are

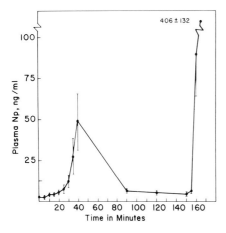

FIG. 2–5. Changes in plasma neurophysin (Np) in 5 rats subjected to hemorrhage. Mean ± SEM are indicated. One milliliter blood was removed every 5 min from 0 to 40 min and the volume was replaced at 40 min. Rats were subjected to massive hemorrhage at 155 min. Reprinted with permission from (74).

reported to minimize enzymatic degradation, more than two neurophysins were found in extracts of human posterior pituitary (54,92). Antisera raised in response to injection of the various human neurophysin peptides have, however, detected only two distinct antigenic sites in the various neurophysin peptides from human posterior pituitary (15,54). Considerable confusion exists about the comparison of human neurophysins isolated in different laboratories. Numbering of individual neurophysins has been proposed as a method of identification giving the number 1 to the peptide with the fastest mobility. Unfortunately, if some fast-migrating neurophysin peptides are recognized in one laboratory but not in another, the neurophysin assigned number 1 in the second laboratory may be assigned the number 3 in the first laboratory (54). It is desirable to refer to the neurophysins based on their

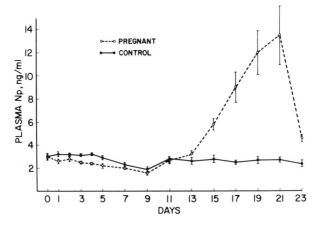

FIG. 2–6. Plasma neurophysin (Np) during pregnancy in 10 pregnant rats compared to 10 age-matched controls. Blood samples were obtained by tail vein. None of the samples was obtained during parturition. Mean ± SEM are indicated. Reprinted with permission from (74).

associated hormone so that we refer to vasopressin-neurophysin and oxytocin-neurophysin in any species. Proof that neurophysin is associated with a specific hormone would best be obtained by absolute separation of neurosecretory granules which contained oxytocin and one neurophysin from another type of granule which contained vasopressin and a different neurophysin. Evidence might also be obtained by specific immunohistochemical stain of the hypothalamus which would demonstrate the association of one neurophysin with oxytocin and another neurophysin with vasopressin within separate neurons or by the associated release of hormone and specific neurophysin into the bloodstream in response to stimuli which independently stimulate oxytocin or vasopressin. Further evidence might be obtained from pathologic situations in which vasopressin or oxytocin is known to be either chronically stimulated or regularly absent, as was done in the Brattleboro rat with congenital lack of vasopressin. Some "proof" of a vasopressin-neurophysin and an oxytocin-neurophysin has been accumulated in humans. We have determined that for the two different neurophysins assayed in our laboratory there are pharmacologic stimuli which specifically cause the secretion of individual neurophysins into the plasma of normal humans. The characteristic response to pharmacologic stimuli can be used to compare human neurophysins in different laboratories. The two neurophysins isolated from human posterior pituitary (54) have been identified as nicotine-stimulated neurophysin (NSN) and estrogen-stimulated neurophysin (ESN) (Figs. 2–7, 2–8).

There is considerable evidence that nicotine-stimulated neurophysin is associated with vasopressin release. Nicotine inhalation is an accepted stimulus

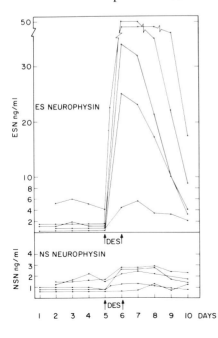

FIG. 2–7. Changes in plasma ESN (*top*) and NSN (*bottom*) in 5 normal male subjects given 5 mg diethystilbestrol (DES) on days 5 and 6. Reprinted with permission from (54).

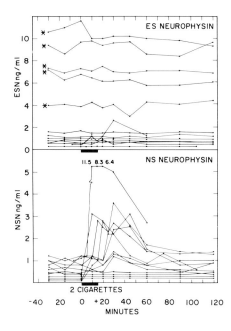

FIG. 2–8. Changes in plasma ESN (*top*) and NSN (*bottom*) in 13 normal subjects who smoked two cigarettes from 0 to 12 min. The asterisk indicates women who were not taking estrogen-containing oral contraceptives. The one subject with a rise in plasma ESN to 2.6 ng/ml was the subject whose NSN rose to 11.5 ng/ml. Reprinted with permission from (54).

for release of vasopressin in humans, and Husain et al. (37) assayed NSN and vasopressin in plasma samples collected after inhalation of the smoke from two cigarettes in 21 tests in 14 volunteers. Vasopressin and neurophysin showed similar secretion curves in all individuals tested (Fig. 2–9), and there was a close correlation between neurophysin and vasopressin concentrations using correlations of the peak value, the area under the curve, or the individual plasma values. When alcohol was administered prior to nicotine stimulation, both NSN secretion and vasopressin secretion were inhibited. Nicotine did not stimulate the secretion of ESN in any subjects. Hypertonic saline infusion in four subjects also caused an increase in NSN, whereas no subjects had a rise in ESN, demonstrating the response of NSN to an osmolar stimulus (57). Tilt table testing produced postural hypotension and a brisk rise of NSN with no change of ESN, demonstrating the response of NSN to a volume stimulus (57). Therefore, physiologic maneuvers which are thought to stimulate osmolar receptors or volume receptors and pharmacologic maneuvers which stimulate vasopressin secretion all caused a secretion of NSN independent of any secretion of ESN.

It was also demonstrated that the secretion of ESN was independent of NSN (see Fig. 2–7), but it has been difficult to prove the association of ESN with oxytocin. Stimuli for the release of oxytocin in humans have not been reliably proved by specific assay of hormone in the bloodstream. Elevated neurophysin has been found in pregnant women by all investigators who measured neurophysin with heterologous assays, and we have demonstrated that the neurophysin elevated in pregnancy is a specific neurophysin which

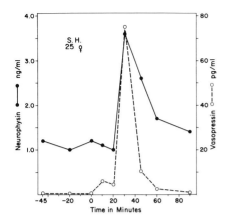

FIG. 2–9. Plasma vasopressin and NSN in response to two cigarettes smoked from 0 to 12 mins. Reprinted with permission from (37).

has been called estrogen-stimulated neurophysin. Estrogen in pharmacologic doses stimulated the secretion of ESN in humans (54) and monkeys (60,61) without any change in NSN. The physiologic rise of estrogen at midcycle in monkeys is associated with a rise of ESN (60,61), and this has been found in some women (42). It is most consistent with the previous animal work to assume that human ESN is associated with oxytocin, but this assumption does not explain the response of ESN (and oxytocin) to changes in estrogen, and any role for the neurohypophysis in reproductive function is at present obscure.

Immunohistochemical studies provide some support for the association of NSN with vasopressin and ESN with oxytocin. Defendini et al. (95,97) used the antisera for ESN and NSN to stain human hypothalamus. In the human SON and PVN there was a geographic distribution of vasopressin and oxytocin similar to that reported in the rat (77) and cow (21). Oxytocin in the human tends to form a superior cap of the SON and a lateral group of cells in the PVN. ESN was most heavily stained in a group of cells in the superior cap of the SON and the lateral part of the PVN whereas NSN was stained predominantly in cells in the inferior portion of the SON and the medial portion of the PVN (95,97). Studies of pathologic situations also support the association of NSN with vasopressin. Patients with the syndrome of inappropriate secretion of antidiuretic hormone had a mean NSN value of 3.2 ± 0.8, significantly above normal, $p < 0.01$, and greater than 2 standard deviations from normal in 8 of 13 patients tested. Mean ESN was not significantly different from the normal, 1.3 ± 0.5, and was elevated in only 2 of the 13 patients, both of whom also had an elevation of NSN (57). In central diabetes insipidus where vasopressin secretion is lacking, NSN was less than 1 ng/ml in 7 of 7 patients tested. Orthostatic hypotension produced no response in 3 of 3 patients tested, and cigarette smoking produced an elevation of plasma NSN in 1 of 5 patients tested with a rise in NSN from 0.8 to 1.8 ng/ml. Interestingly, this patient had only partial diabetes insipidus by de-

TABLE 2–1. *ESN response to estrogen in diabetes insipidus*

	ESN	
Diagnosis	Base line	After estrogen
Idiopathic	< 0.5	6.7
Traumatic	< 0.5	7.6
CNS leukemia	0.9	46.0
Traumatic	1.1	2.0
Postoperative	1.2	9.5
Idiopathic	1.7	24.6
Postoperative	2.9	> 50.0
Postoperative	3.7[a]	> 50.0
Idiopathic	4.5[a]	44.5
Postoperative	15.4[a]	> 50.0

[a] Taking oral contraceptives.

hydration testing and subsequently the diabetes insipidus resolved after irradiation of a hypothalamic tumor. Therefore, syndromes of excess vasopressin secretion were accompanied by elevated plasma NSN, and absence of vasopressin was accompanied by absence of NSN (57).

ESN secretion was remarkably intact in patients with diabetes insipidus (55). Nine of ten patients with diabetes insipidus given a single oral dose of estrogen responded with a marked increase in ESN and no change in NSN (Table 2–1). Included in the series were patients with idiopathic diabetes insipidus, diabetes insipidus due to tumor, and traumatically induced diabetes insipidus. Only a single patient (diabetes insipidus induced by an auto accident) failed to respond to estrogen. The reason ESN remained intact when the neurohypophysis was damaged is unknown, but the data confirm that ESN is not associated with vasopressin, and ESN may therefore be associated with oxytocin.

BIOLOGIC ACTIVITY

Various biologic activities such as lipolytic activity (62,81), hypocalcemic activity (81), and natriuretic activity (17,58) have been found in neurophysins extracted from the neurohypophysis. Although it seems possible that some neurophysins may possess some biologic activity, no physiologic function of neurophysins after secretion from the posterior lobe has been established.

ECTOPIC PRODUCTION OF NEUROPHYSIN

Elevated levels of NSN have been found in the plasma of patients with the syndrome of inappropriate antidiuretic hormone secretion. In some of these cases, vasopressin was believed to be produced ectopically by a carcinoma. Hamilton et al. (32) and Legros (41) have studied extracts of carcinoma of the lung and demonstrated that some of the tumors which contained vasopressin also contained a human neurophysin. Presumably the neurophysin was made by the tumor, and this observation has been quoted to prove that neurophysin synthesis is necessary for vasopressin synthesis. On the other hand, Pettengill et al. (53) have grown an oat cell tumor of the lung in tissue culture and have demonstrated that the tumor produced vasopressin in the absence of any synthesis of neurophysin. There is no evidence that hypothalamic neurons ever synthesize hormone without neurophysin. The mouse hypothalamic cells maintained in tissue culture by De Vitry (22) synthesize both vasopressin and neurophysin, but some tumor cells, as shown by Pettengill et al. (53), must have the ability to synthesize vasopressin alone.

Ciarochi et al. (16) reported the interesting observation of high levels of neurophysins in the uterus and kidney of the rat. When neurophysin isolated from rat posterior pituitary was injected intravenously into intact rats, it was taken up by the kidney but not by the uterus. The data were interpreted to indicate that the neurophysin in the uterus might be the product of local synthesis. Estrogen administration caused a marked increase in the neurophysin concentration of the uterus without a concomitant increase in plasma neurophysin, whereas with pregnancy there was an even greater increase of neurophysin in the rat uterus accompanied by an increase in neurophysin in plasma. The material isolated from the rat uterus has been identified as neurophysin by radioimmunoassay; in a standard radioimmunoassay there was a parallel displacement with pituitary neurophysins. The material from the rat uterus has a molecular weight identical to rat pituitary neurophysin and moves in a position on analytic disc gel electrophoresis which is characteristic of the neurophysin in the rat which has been thought to be associated with oxytocin. Characteristic binding of vasopressin and oxytocin by this neurophysin-like material has not been demonstrated as yet, and sufficient quantities have not been isolated for amino acid sequencing. Further studies of rat uterus neurophysin are progressing in our laboratory. The peptide is likely to offer some unique insights into the synthesis of neurophysin and possibly the synthesis and mode of action of oxytocin.

CONCLUSIONS

The demonstration (in some species) of a specific neurophysin for oxytocin and a different and specific neurophysin for vasopressin, along with the demonstration that the neurophysins are secreted into the general circulation, prompted a renewed interest in these neuronal peptides. Although more than two neurophysin peptides have been isolated from a number of animals, the concept that every species synthesizes a vasopressin-neurophysin and an oxytocin-neurophysin is the most generally accepted hypothesis. Extra (more than two) neurophysins in any species probably represent degradation products of the two major neurophysins. Some of this degradation may occur during extraction, but neurophysins may also be broken down enzymatically within neurosecretory granules. Intragranular proteolysis of neurophysins may represent progression of normal proteolytic cleavage of neurophysin (and hormone) from a precursor protein containing neurophysin and hormone, but the exact role of neurophysins in hormone biosynthesis is yet to be established. At least one tumor tissue has been reported to synthesize vasopressin without neurophysin. Neurophysins accompany neurohypophyseal hormones throughout the magnocellular system and have provided markers to study neurohypophyseal peptide secretion from the posterior lobe. They have additionally been used to show neurohypophyseal pathways to the long portal vessels of the median eminence and to the third ventricle. In the cow there is good evidence of specific release into the general circulation of an oxytocin-neurophysin and a vasopressin-neurophysin. In the human independent secretion of two separate neurophysins has also been proven. The human "nicotine-stimulated neurophysin" qualifies as a vasopressin-neurophysin based on its association with vasopressin in hypothalamic neurons, its release with vasopressin during pharmacologic testing and physiologic stimulation, and its elevation in plasma during pathologic states of vasopressin excess. The alternate human neurophysin "estrogen-stimulated neurophysin" is associated with oxytocin within neurons of the human hypothalamus, but has not been proven to be secreted in tandem with oxytocin in human plasma. Estrogen-stimulated neurophysin is elevated in pregnant women and in monkeys at mid-menstrual cycle, but whether oxytocin is increased at these times is unknown. After release from the posterior pituitary, neurophysins have not been shown to have biologic function. Thus, neurophysins have provided the means of detailed study of the anatomy of the neurohypophysis and have provided a new measure of posterior pituitary function. The major discovery with neurophysin assays has been that estrogen stimulates secretion of one neurophysin in humans. The physiologic significance of this stimulation is obscure and is the subject of continued research. Recent research has also focused on the role of neurophysins in hormone synthesis and on the investigation of "ectopic" neurophysin synthesis.

ACKNOWLEDGMENTS

This work was supported by NIH Grant AM16166; Clinical Research Unit Grant of the University of Pittsburgh, FR-56; Population Council Grant, M7432; and the Health Research and Services Foundation of Pittsburgh. Dr. Robinson is the recipient of an NIH Research Career Development Award, AM00093. I wish to thank co-workers mentioned in the text for allowing me to quote their work and to publish their ideas. Ms. Catherine Haluszczak and Ms. Julie Wilkins are acknowledged for their assistance in the laboratory, and Ms. Karen Bodnar for her secretarial assistance.

REFERENCES

1. Acher, R. (1968): Neurophysin and neurohypophysial hormones. *Proc. Roy. Soc. [Biol.]*, 170:7–16.
2. Acher, R., Chauvet, J., and Olivry, G. (1956): Sur l'existence d'une hormone unique neurohypophysaire: Relation entre l'oxytocin, la vasopressine, et la protein de Van Dyke extradites de la neurohypophyse du boeuf. *Biochem. Biophys. Acta*, 22:428–433.
3. Antunes, J. L., Carmel, P. W., Ferin, M., and Zimmerman, E. A. (1977): Paraventricular nucleus: The origin of vasopressin secreting terminals on hypophysial portal vessels in the monkey (abstract). *Endocrinology (in press)*.
4. Axelrod, J., and Daly, J. (1965): Pituitary gland: Enzymic formation of methanol from S-adenosylmethionine. *Science*, 150:892–893.
5. Bargmann, W. (1949): Uber die neurosekretorische verknupfung von hypothalamus und neurohypophyse. *Z. Zellforsch.*, 34:610–634.
6. Bargmann, W., and Scharrer, E. (1951): The site of origin of the hormones of the posterior pituitary. *Am. Sci.*, 39:255–259.
7. Burford, G. D., Jones, C. W., and Pickering, B. T. (1971): Tentative identification of a vasopressin-neurophysin and an oxytocin-neurophysin in the rat. *Biochem. J.*, 124:809–813.
8. Burford, G. D., and Pickering, B. T. (1973): Intra-axonal transport and turnover of neurophysin in the rat: A proposal for a possible origin of the minor neurophysin component. *Biochem. J.*, 136:1047–1052.
9. Capra, J. D., Cheng, K. W., Friesen, H. G., North, W. G., and Walter, R. (1974): Evolution of neurophysin proteins: The partial sequence of human neurophysin-I. *FEBS Lett.*, 46:71–75.
10. Capra, J. D., and Walter, R. (1975): Primary structure and evolution of neurophysins. *Ann. N.Y. Acad. Sci.*, 248:397–407.
11. Chauvet, M., Chauvet, J., and Acher, R. (1975): Phylogeny of neurophysins: Partial amino acid sequence of a sheep neurophysin. *FEBS Lett.*, 52:212–215.
12. Chauvet, M., Coffe, G., Chauvet, J., and Acher, R. (1975): On the biological significance of neurophysins: Presence of a major neurophysin in sheep. *FEBS Lett.*, 53:331–333.
13. Cheng, K. W., and Friesen, H. G. (1970): Physiological factors regulating secretion of neurophysin. *Metabolism*, 19:876–890.
14. Cheng, K. W., and Friesen, H. G. (1971): Isolation and characterization of a third component of porcine neurophysin. *J. Biol. Chem.*, 246:7656–7665.
15. Cheng, K. W., and Friesen, H. G. (1972): Studies of human neurophysin by radioimmunoassay. *J. Clin. Endocrinol. Metab.*, 34:165–176.
16. Ciarochi, F. F., Haluszczak, C., and Robinson, A. G. (1976): Neurophysin activity and dynamics in the rat. The Endocrine Society, Abstract 356.
17. Cort, J. H., Sedlakova, E., and Kluh, I. (1975): Neurophysin binding and natriuretic peptides from the posterior pituitary. *Ann. N.Y. Acad. Sci.*, 248:336–344.
18. Dean, C. R., Hope, D. B., and Kazic, T. (1968): Evidence for a storage of oxytocin with neurophysin-I and of vasopressin with neurophysin-II in separate neurosecretory granules. *Br. J. Pharmacol.*, 34:192P–193P.
19. De Mey, J., Dierickx, K., and Vandesande, F. (1975): Immunohistochemical demonstration of neurophysin I- and neurophysin II-containing nerve fibres in the external region of the bovine median eminence. *Cell Tissue Res.*, 157:517–519.
20. De Mey, J., and Vandesande, F. (1976): Bovine neurophysins I, II and C: New methods for their purification and for the production of specific antibodies. *Eur. J. Biochem.*, 69:153–162.
21. De Mey, J., Vandesande, F., and Dierickx, K. (1975): Immunohistochemical identification of the neurophysin I and of the neurophysin II producing neurons in the bovine hypothalamus. *Ann. Endocrinol. (Paris)*, 36:377–378.
22. De Vitry, F., Camier, M., Czernichow, P., Benda, P., Cohen, P., and Tixier-Vidal, A. (1974): Establishment of a clone of mouse hypothalamic neurosecretory cells synthesizing neurophysin and vasopressin. *Proc. Natl. Acad. Sci. USA*, 71:3575–3579.

23. Dierickx, K., Vandesande, F., and De Mey, J. (1975): Identification and origin of the vasopressin-neurophysin containing nerve fibres of the external region of the rat median eminence. *Ann. Endocrinol. (Paris)*, 36:383–384.
24. Douglas, W. W. (1974): Mechanism of release of neurohypophysial hormones: Stimulus-secretion coupling. In: *Handbook of Physiology, Vol. 4*, edited by E. Knobil and W. H. Sawyer, pp. 191–224. American Physiological Society, Washington, D.C.
25. Du Vigneaud, V. (1956): Hormones of the posterior pituitary gland: Oxytocin and vasopressin. *Harvey Lect.*, L:1–26.
26. Edgar, D. H., and Hope, D. B. (1976): Protein-carboxyl methyltransferase of the bovine posterior pituitary gland: Neurophysin as a potential endogenous substrate. *J. Neurochem.*, 27:949–955.
27. Fawcett, C. P., Powell, A. E., and Sachs, H. (1968): Biosynthesis and release of neurophysin. *Endocrinology*, 83:1299–1310.
28. Fitzsimmons, J. T. (1969): The effect on drinking of peptide precursors and of shorter-chain peptide fragments of angiotensin II injected into the rats dicenplalon. *J. Physiol.*, 201:349–368.
29. Foss, I., Sletten, K., and Trygstad, O. (1973): Studies on the primary structure and biological activity of a human neurophysin. *FEBS Lett.*, 30:151–156.
30. Gainer, H., Sarne, Y., and Brownstein, M. J. (1977): Neurophysin biosynthesis: Conversion of a putative precursor during axonal transport. *Science*, 195:1354–1356.
31. Goldman, H., and Lindner, L. (1962): Antidiuretic hormone concentration in blood perfusing the adenohypophysis. *Experientia*, 18:279–281.
32. Hamilton, B. P. M., Upton, G. V., and Amatruda, T. T., Jr. (1972): Evidence for the presence of neurophysin in tumors producing the syndrome of inappropriate antidiuresis. *J. Clin. Endocrinol. Metab.*, 35:764–767.
33. Heller, H. (1974): History of neurohypophysial research. In: *Handbook of Physiology, Vol. 4*, edited by E. Knobil and W. H. Sawyer, pp. 103–126. American Physiological Society, Washington, D.C.
34. Hollenberg, M. D., and Hope, D. B. (1967): Fractionation of neurophysin by molecular-sieve and ion-exchange chromatography. *Biochem. J.*, 104:122–127.
35. Hollenberg, M. D., and Hope, D. B. (1968): The isolation of the native hormone-binding proteins from bovine pituitary posterior lobes. *Biochem. J.*, 106:557–564.
36. Hope, D. B. (1975): The neurophysin proteins: Historical aspects. *Ann. N.Y. Acad. Sci.*, 248:6–14.
37. Husain, M. K., Frantz, A. G., Ciarochi, F. F., and Robinson, A. G. (1975): Nicotine stimulated release of neurophysin and vasopressin in humans. *J. Clin. Endocrinol. Metab.*, 41:1113–1117.
38. Jones, C. W., and Pickering, B. T. (1972): Intra-axonal transport and turnover of neurohypophysial hormones in the rat. *J. Physiol. (Lond.)*, 227:553–561.
39. Krieger, D. T., and Zimmerman, E. A. (1977): The nature of CRF and its relationship to vasopressin. In: *Clinical Neuroendocrinology*, edited by G. M. Besser and L. Martini. Academic Press, New York *(in press)*.
40. Le Clerc, R., and Pelletier, G. (1974): Electron microscope immunohistochemical localization of vasopressin in the hypothalamus and neurohypophysis of the normal and Brattleboro rat. *Am. J. Anat.*, 140:583–588.
41. Legros, J. J. (1975): The radioimmunoassay of human neurophysins: Contribution to the understanding of the physiopathology of neurohypophyseal function. *Ann. N.Y. Acad. Sci.*, 248:281–303.
42. Legros, J. J., Franchimont, P., and Burfer, H. (1975): Variations in neurohypophyseal function in normally cycling women. *J. Clin. Endocrinol. Metab.*, 41:54–59.
43. Legros, J. J., Franchimont, P., and Hendrick, J. C. (1970): Dosage radioimmunologique de la neurophysine dans le serum des femmes normales et des femmes enceintes. *C. R. Soc. Biol. [D] (Paris)*, 163:2773–2777.
44. Legros, J. J., Reynaert, R., and Peeters, G. (1974): Specific release of bovine neurophysin I during milking and suckling in the cow. *J. Endocrinol.*, 60:327–332.
45. Legros, J. J., Reynaert, R., and Peeters, G. (1975): Specific release of bovine neurophysin II during arterial or venous haemorrhage in the cow. *J. Endocrinol.*, 67:297–302.

46. McKelvy, J. F. (1975): Phosphorylation of neurosecretory granules by cAMP-stimulated protein kinase and its implication for transport and release of neurophysin proteins. *Ann. N.Y. Acad. Sci.,* 248:80–91.
47. Meyer-Grass, M., and Pliska, V. (1974): Properties of neurophysin from neurosecretory granules ('native' neurophysin). *Experientia,* 30:689–694.
48. Norstrom, A. (1974): Biosynthesis of neurohypophysial proteins in rats with hereditary hypothalamic diabetes insipidus (Brattleboro strain). *Brain Res.,* 68:309–317.
49. Norstrom, A. (1975): Axonal transport and turnover of neurohypophyseal peptides in the rat. *Ann. N.Y. Acad. Sci.,* 248:46–63.
50. Norstrom, A., and Hansson, H. A. (1972): Isolation and characterization of neurosecretory granules of the rat posterior pituitary gland. *Z. Zellforsch.,* 129:92–113.
51. North, W. G., Morris, J. F., La Rochelle, T. F., and Valtin, H. (1977): Enzymatic interconversions of neurophysins. In: *Proceedings of the Conference on the Neurohypophysis,* edited by A. Moses. S. Karger, Basel *(in press).*
52. Oliver, C., Mical, R. S., and Porter, J. C. (1977): Hypothalamic-pituitary vasculature: Evidence for retrograde blood flow in the pituitary stalk. *Endocrinology,* 101:598–604.
53. Pettengill, O. S., Faulkner, C. S., Wurster-Hill, D. H., Maurer, L. H., Sorenson, G. D., Robinson, A. G., and Zimmerman, E. A. (1977): Isolation and characterization of a hormone producing cell line from human small cell anaplastic carcinoma of the lung. *J. Natl. Cancer Inst.,* 58:511–518.
54. Robinson, A. G. (1975): Isolation, assay and secretion of individual human neurophysins. *J. Clin. Invest.,* 55:360–367.
55. Robinson, A. G. (1977): The neurophysins—health and disease. *Clin. Endocrinol. Metabol.,* 6:261–275.
56. Robinson, A. G., and Frantz, A. G. (1973): Radioimmunoassay of posterior pituitary peptides—a review. *Metabolism,* 22:1047–1057.
57. Robinson, A. G., Haluszczak, C., Wilkins, J. A., Huellmantel, A. B., and Watson, C. G. (1977): Physiologic control of two neurophysins in humans. *J. Clin. Endocrinol. Metab.,* 44:330–339.
58. Robinson, A. G., Michelis, M. F., Warms, P. C., and Davis, B. B. (1974): Natriuretic effect of posterior pituitary neurophysin. *J. Clin. Endocrinol. Metab.,* 39:913–918.
59. Robinson, A. G., and Zimmerman, E. A. (1973): Cerebrospinal fluid and ependymal neurophysin. *J. Clin. Invest.,* 52:1260–1267.
60. Robinson, A. G., Zimmerman, E. A., Engleman, E. A., and Frantz, A. G. (1971): Radioimmunoassay of bovine neurophysin: Specificity of neurophysin I and II. *Metabolism,* 20:1138–1147.
61. Robinson, A. G., Zimmerman, E. A., and Frantz, A. G. (1971): Physiologic investigation of the posterior pituitary binding proteins neurophysin I and neurophysin II. *Metabolism,* 20:1148–1155.
62. Rudman, D., Chawla, R. K., Khatra, B. S., and Yodaiken, R. E. (1975): Observations on the lipolytic and melanotropic properties of neurophysin proteins. *Ann. N.Y. Acad. Sci.,* 248:324–335.
63. Sachs, H., Fawcett, P., and Takabatake, Y. (1975): Biosynthesis and release of vasopressin and neurophysin. *Recent Prog. Horm. Res.,* 25:46–63.
64. Sachs, H., Pearson, D., and Nureddin, A. (1975): Guinea pig neurophysin: Isolation, developmental aspects, biosynthesis in organ culture. *Ann. N.Y. Acad. Sci.,* 248:36–45.
65. Sachs, H., Pearson, D., Shainbetg, A., Shin, S., Bryce, G., Malamed, S., and Mowles, T. (1974): Studies on the hypothalamo-neurohypophysial complex in organ culture. In: *Recent Studies of Hypothalamic Function, International Symposium, Calgary 1973,* pp. 50–66. S. Karger, Basel.
66. Sachs, H., Saito, S., and Sunde, D. (1970): Biochemical studies on the neurosecretory and neuroglial cells of the hypothalamo-neurohypophysial complex. In: *Memoirs of the Society for Endocrinology, No. 19,* edited by H. Heller and K. Lederis, p. 325. Cambridge University Press, Cambridge.
67. Sachs, H., and Takabatake, Y. (1964): Evidence for a precursor in vasopressin biosynthesis. *Endocrinology,* 75:939–948.

68. Sawyer, W. H. (1967): Evolution of antidiuretic hormones and their functions. *Am. J. Med.,* 42:678–691.

69. Scharrer, B. (1974): The concept of neurosecretion past and present. In: *Recent Studies of Hypothalamic Function International Symposium, Calgary 1973,* pp. 1–7. S. Karger, Basel.

70. Scharrer, B. (1975): Neurosecretion and its role in neuroendocrine regulation. In: *Pioneers in Neuroendocrinology,* edited by J. Meites, B. T. Donovan, and S. M. McCann, p. 260. Plenum Publishing Company, New York.

71. Scharrer, E., and Scharrer, B. (1954): Hormones produced by neurosecretory cells. *Recent Prog. Horm. Res.,* 10:183–240.

72. Schwabedal, P., and Bock, R. (1975): Influence of adrenalectomy, total body X-irradiation and dexamethasone on the amount of CRF-granules and "classical" neurosecretory material in the rat neurohypophysis. *Anat. Embryol.,* 148:267–278.

73. Scott, D. E., Kozlowski, G. P., and Sheridan, M. N. (1974): Scanning electromicroscopy in the ultrastructural analysis of the mammalian cerebral ventricular system. *Int. Rev. Cytol.,* 37:349–388.

74. Seif, S. M., Huellmantel, A. B., Platia, M. P., Haluszczak, C., and Robinson, A. G. (1977): Isolation, radioimmunoassay and physiologic secretion of rat neurophysins. *Endocrinology,* 100:1317–1326.

75. Seif, S. M., Robinson, A. G., Zimmerman, E. A., and Wilkins, J. (1977): Plasma neurophysin and vasopressin in the rat: Response to adrenalectomy and steroid replacement. *Endocrinology (in press).*

76. Sloper, J. C. (1966): The experimental and cytopathological investigation of neurosecretion in the hypothalamus and pituitary. In: *The Pituitary Gland, Vol. 3,* edited by G. W. Harris and B. T. Donovan, p. 131–239. Butterworths, London.

77. Sokol, H. W., Zimmerman, E. A., Sawyer, W. H., and Robinson, A. G. (1976): The hypothalamo-neurohypophysial system of the rat: Localization and quantification of neurophysin by light microscopic immunocytochemistry in normal rats and in Brattleboro rats deficient in vasopressin and a neurophysin. *Endocrinology,* 98:1176–1188.

78. Stillman, M. A., Recht, L. D., Rosario, S. L., Seif, S. M., Robinson, A. G., and Zimmerman, E. A. (1977): The effects of adrenalectomy and glucocorticoid replacement of vasopressin and vasopressin-neurophysin in the zona externa of the median eminence of the rat. *Endocrinology,* 101:42–49.

79. Sunde, D. A., and Sokol, H. W. (1975): Quantification of rat neurophysin by polyacrylamide gel electrophoresis (PAGE): Application to the rat with hereditary hypothalamic diabetes insipidus. *Ann. N.Y. Acad. Sci.,* 248:345–364.

80. Swann, R. W., and Pickering, B. T. (1976): Incorporation of radioactive precursors into the membrane and contents of the neurosecretory granules of the rat neurohypophysis as a method of studying their fate. *J. Endocrinol.,* 68:95–108.

81. Trygstad, O., Foss, I., and Sletten, K. (1975): Metabolic activities of human neurophysins. *Ann. N.Y. Acad. Sci.,* 248:304–316.

82. Turner, R. A., Pierce, J. G., and Du Vigneaud, V. (1951): The purification and amino acid content of vasopressin preparations. *J. Biol. Chem.,* 191:21–28.

83. Uttenthal, L. O., and Hope, D. B. (1970): The isolation of three neurophysins from porcine posterior pituitary lobes. *Biochem. J.,* 116:899–909.

84. Vandesande, F., De Mey, J., and Dierickx, K. (1974): Identification of neurophysin producing cells. I. The origin of the neurophysin-like substance-containing nerve fibres of the external region of the median eminence of the rat. *Cell Tissue Res.,* 151:187–200.

85. Vandesande, F., Dierickx, K., and De Mey, J. (1975): Identification of separate vasopressin-neurophysin II and oxytocin-neurophysin I containing nerve fibres in the external region of the bovine median eminence. *Cell Tissue Res.,* 158:509–516.

86. Van Dyke, H. B. (1970): Studies in neurohypophysial endocrinology. The Sir Henry Dale Lecture for 1970, Proceedings of the Society of Endocrinology, Meeting House, Zoological Society of London, pp. x–xix.

87. Van Wimersma, G. T. B., Bohus, B., and De Wied, D. (1975): The role of vasopressin in memory processes. *Prog. Brain Res.,* 42:135–141.

88. Van Wimersma, G. T. B., and De Wied, D. (1977): The physiology of the neuro-hypophysial system and its relation to memory processes. In: *Biochemical Correlates in Brain Function,* edited by A. N. Davison. Academic Press, New York (*in press*).
89. Van Wimersma, G. T. B., Dogterom, J., and De Wied, D. (1975): Intraventricular administration of anti-vasopressin serum inhibits memory consolidation in rats. *Life Sci.,* 16:637–644.
90. Vilhardt, H., and Robinson, I. C. A. F. (1975): Polyacrylamide gel electrophoresis of bovine neurophysins. *J. Neurochem.,* 24:1275–1276.
91. Walter, R., Audhya, T. K., Schlesinger, D. H., Shin, S., Saito, S., and Sachs, H. (1977): Biosynthesis of neurophysin proteins in the dog and their isolation. *Endocrinology,* 100:162–174.
92. Watkins, W. B. (1971): Neurophysins of the human pituitary gland. *J. Endocrinol.,* 51:595–596.
93. Watkins, W. B., Schwabedal, P., and Bock, R. (1977): Immunohistochemical demonstration of a CRF-associated neurophysin in the external zone of the rat median eminence. *Cell Tissue Res.* (*in press*).
94. Wuu, T., and Crumm, S. E. (1976): Characterization of porcine neurophysin III. Its resemblance and possible relationship to porcine neurophysin I. *J. Biol. Chem.,* 251:2735–1739.
95. Zimmerman, E. A. (1976): Localization of hypothalamic hormones by immunocytochemical techniques. In: *Frontiers in Neuroendocrinology, Vol. 4,* edited by L. Martini and W. F. Ganong, p. 25. Raven Press, New York.
96. Zimmerman, E. A., Carmel, P. W., Husain, M. K., Ferin, M., Tannenbaum, M., Frantz, A. G., and Robinson, A. G. (1973): Vasopressin and neurophysin: High concentrations in monkey hypophyseal portal blood. *Science,* 182:925–957.
97. Zimmerman, E. A., Defendini, R., Sokol, H. W., and Robinson, A. G. (1975): The distribution of neurophysin-secreting pathways in the mammalian brain: Light microscopic studies using the immunoperoxidase technique. *Ann. N.Y. Acad. Sci.,* 248:92–111.
98. Zimmerman, E. A., and Robinson, A. G. (1976): Hypothalamic neurons secreting vasopressin and neurophysin. *Kidney Int.,* 10:12–24.
99. Zimmerman, E. A., Robinson, A. G., Husain, M. K., Acosta, M., Frantz, A. G., and Sawyer, W. H. (1974): Neurohypophyseal peptides in the bovine hypothalamus: The relationship of neurophysin I to oxytocin, and neurophysin II to vasopressin in supraoptic and paraventricular regions. *Endocrinology,* 95:931–936.

Frontiers in Neuroendocrinology, Vol. 5,
edited by W. F. Ganong and L. Martini.
Raven Press, New York © 1978.

Chapter 3

The Brain Isorenin-Angiotensin System: Biochemistry, Localization, and Possible Role in Drinking and Blood Pressure Regulation

Detlev Ganten, Kjell Fuxe, M. Ian Phillips,
Johannes F. E. Mann, and Ursula Ganten

*Department of Pharmacology,
University of Heidelberg,
Heidelberg, Germany*

Extrarenal tissue of most mammals contains enzymes that are similar to kidney renin; they hydrolyze the substrate angiotensinogen to form the decapeptide angiotensin I (AI), and they do not lead to further degradation of AI (Fig. 3–1). The trivial name isorenin seems best suited to designate the extrarenal enzymes as opposed to kidney renin (EC 3.4.99.19). A systematic nomenclature [angiotensinogen hydrolase (angiotensin I forming)] has been proposed (50,54), but this would leave open the question of whether the tissue enzymes are biochemically identical to or different from the kidney enzyme. The literature on the tissue isorenins has recently been reviewed (7,39,41,42,48,50,54,82,96), and discussion of the brain isorenin-angiotensin system (iso-RAS) must be viewed in the context of information available in other tissues. Pure crystalline isorenin has been obtained from mouse submaxillary gland and its specificity has been proved (13,74,89,123). Isorenin concentration can be higher in extrarenal tissue than in kidney (7,50,54). Extrarenal tumors can secrete large amounts of isorenin into the plasma and lead to high blood pressure and suppression of kidney renin ("ectopic primary reninism") (54,55,61,137). *In vitro* synthesis of isorenin in cell cultures has been demonstrated (31,129), and stimulation of isorenin synthesis and release has been shown in nephrectomized animals (39,54,56).

The brain is the first and only organ in which all components of the renin angiotensin system have been investigated simultaneously. Isorenin, the enzyme substrate angiotensinogen, AI, AI-converting enzyme, angiotensin II (AII), AII receptors, and the angiotensin destroying enzymes angiotensinases have been shown to be present in brain tissue. In this chapter we briefly summarize the biochemical and biophysical characteristics of these brain iso-RAS components, discuss the distribution of AII-like peptides in brain, and con-

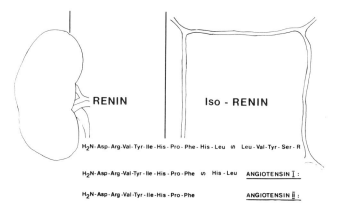

FIG. 3–1. Schematic outline of the renin-angiotensin system in kidney and the isorenin-angiotensin system in extrarenal tissue. The first of the 3 formulas at the bottom shows the renin substrate; R signifies the rest of the protein. The leucine-leucine bond is hydrolyzed by isorenin to form the decapeptide angiotension I. Converting enzyme hydrolyzes the phenylalanine-histidine bond of AI to form the effector peptide of the enzyme system, angiotensin II.

clude with discussion of the biological role of brain angiotensin in thirst and blood pressure regulating mechanisms.

ISORENIN IN BRAIN TISSUE

Isorenin was first described by Fischer-Ferraro et al. (30) and Ganten et al. (52,53) in the brains of intact and nephrectomized dogs and rats. Its presence was later confirmed in humans, sheep, and other species (28,39,41, 47,50,58,92,113). The biochemical characteristics of brain isorenin are similar to those of kidney renin: it is a protein, molecular weight between 40,000 and 60,000, nondialyzable, ammonium sulfate precipitable, stable in acid milieu, and unstable in heat. It probably has no metal prosthetic group and no serine residue in the active center. Chelating agents such as ethylenediaminetetraacetic acid (EDTA), dimercaprol, 8-OH-quinoline, and O-phenantroline as well as phenyl-methylsulfonylfluoride (PMSF) do not significantly affect isorenin activity (19,25,30,39,50,54). Antibodies raised against dog kidney renin also have an inhibitory effect on brain isorenin activity (39,52). Soybean trypsin inhibitor does not affect the activity of the brain and kidney enzyme, whereas pepstatin inhibits brain isorenin as well as kidney renin at low concentrations (25,39). Prostaglandins A and E inhibit brain isorenin and kidney renin of rats, and prostaglandin F2α has no effect on either enzyme from rat tissue (138). Brain isorenin of all species tested so far forms AI upon incubation with homologous, heterologous, and synthetic renin substrates and does not hydrolyze AI, i.e., has no angiotensinase activity. Brain isorenin has high affinity for the synthetic tetradecapeptide substrate, and in this respect it differs from kidney renin (39,52). Isorenin from rat brain has high affinity for dog substrate, whereas rat kidney renin hydrolyzes dog substrate more slowly. This fact has been exploited to obtain a sensitive rat tissue isorenin assay with minimal interference of kidney renin (43). Human brain isorenin has been measured using human, sheep (39,41), and hog plasma substrate (18). Dog brain isorenin reacts well with dog substrate extracted from dog plasma (19,39,52) and cerebrospinal fluid (105).

When isorenin from brain, purified according to the purification method of kidney renin, was injected intravenously into nephrectomized rats, a pressor response of 5 to 15 min duration was obtained (30). Tachyphylaxis, as typically seen with kidney renin, also occurred with repeated injections of isorenin, and the pressor activity was suppressed by heat denaturation as has been described for kidney renin; the same results were obtained if isorenin was purified from the brain of nephrectomized rats (30).

In the indirect assay, isorenin is incubated *in vitro* with excess exogenous substrate. The material formed during the incubation has been characterized as being mainly AI in the following ways: (a) The substance formed during the incubation of brain homogenate with angiotensinogen gives a blood pressure rise of short duration indistinguishable from that of angiotensin in the rat pressor assay. (b) Heating of the material for 2 hr at 90°C does not destroy its pressor activity. (c) The pressor effect in the rat bioassay is completely abolished after incubation with 2% trypsin. (d) The pressor material is dialyzable. (e) Dowex 50W-X2 NH_4^+ adsorbs the pressor material which can be eluted with diethylamine and ammonium hydroxide. (f) Immunological studies with specific AI and AII antibodies revealed that the pressor material formed during incubation consists of about 90% AI and 10% AII. Acidification of the antigen-antibody complex to pH 2 restored the full pressor activity of the incubation product. In radioimmunoassay the incubation product reacts with specific AI antibodies and not with AII antibodies (30,39,52). Like kidney renin, brain isorenin can be activated by acid or alcohol treatment. This suggests that a high molecular weight zymogen also occurs in brain tissue (25,138).

The pH optimum of enzyme activity has been described to be between 4.5 and 5.5 by most authors (19,39,52) and compares to a pH optimum of dog renal renin between 5.0 and 6 (52) and isorenin of the submaxillary of pH 8 (13,89). Fischer-Ferraro et al. (30) reported an optimum of the brain enzyme activity at pH 7.0 to 7.5. The pH optimum of 4.5 to 5.5 reported by Ganten et al. (39,52), Daul et al. (18), and Day and Reid (19) is not due to acid denaturation of the substrate since the same optimum has been found with tetradecapeptide synthetic substrate which is not denatured at acid pH (25,139). The low pH optimum of isorenin activity points to the possibility of other acid proteases interfering in the isorenin assay (39). Day and Reid (19) and Fahrer et al. (25) have found, indeed, that isorenin activity and cathepsin D activity copurify in various purification systems including salt precipitation, gel filtration, ion-exchange chromatography, and isoelectric focusing.

Pepstatin strongly inhibits isorenin, cathepsin D, as well as other acid proteases and has been used for purification of these enzymes by affinity chromatography (25) and for the calculation of enzyme purity (25,87). It thus appears that cathepsin D and tissue isorenin have many physicochemical properties in common, if they are not identical. This is also true for kidney renin. Many purified kidney renin preparations [hog renin, National Biochemical Corporation batch 256; human renin, National Institute for Biological Standards and Control (4); and pseudorenin from hog spleen (kindly supplied by Drs. L. Lentz and L. Skeggs)] copurify with cathepsin D activity (25). However, these enzyme preparations from kidney as well as purified fractions from brain do not contain angiotensinase activity. The substrate specificity especially of pseudorenin has been well studied with synthetic substrates and closely resembles that of kidney renin (120,121). Thus, enzymes which specifically hydrolyze angiotensinogens at the leucine-leucine bond to form AI and which do not further hydrolyze AI must be classified as renins or isorenins [angiotensinogen hydrolase (angiotensin I forming)] (54). Cathepsin D was named for a series of proteases found in beef spleen and in other tissues which did not hydrolyze the usual synthetic substrates acted on by other cathepsins (59,60,86). Cathepsin D is usually measured by the method of Anson (3) using denatured hemoglobin substrate; it is of interest to note that the β-chain of hemoglobin in positions 31 to 35 (Leu-Leu-Val-Val-Tyr) closely resembles the amino acid sequence of the synthetic tetradecapeptide renin substrate 10–13 (Leu-Leu-Val-Tyr), which is hydrolyzed by renin at the leucine-10-leucine-11 bond (120,121). It is therefore possible that specific leucine-leucinases such as renin and isorenin are being measured in both the isorenin assay using natural or synthetic angiotensinogen as substrate and in the cathepsin D assay (using denatured hemoglobin as substrate). The natural substrate for brain cathepsin D activity is not known, and it may well be that brain angiotensinogen is hydrolyzed and AI formed by this enzyme.

The question whether enzymes of low pH optimum can be physiologically active *in vivo* is discussed below, but a number of facts may be pointed out here. Enzyme characteristics depend on the testing conditions, among which substrate and environment are two important variables. *In vitro* testing conditions do not mirror *in vivo* conditions, and thus *in vitro* characteristics may be different from *in vivo* enzyme characteristics. For example, cathepsin D may have different characteristics with its unknown (natural) substrate than with the unphysiological denatured hemoglobin substrate in an even more unphysiological (acetic acid) buffer (3). If cathepsin D activity (hydrolysis of hemoglobin) and isorenin activity (AI formation from angiotensinogen) are indeed brought about by similar enzymes, then it would appear that the pH optimum is shifted from 3.5 (cathepsin D activity) to 4.5 to 5 (isorenin activity) by changing the substrates and buffer systems. It is conceivable that the tissue environment and physiologically available substrate would shift the pH optimum even more to neutral pH. It is of interest to note in this respect that enzymes rarely act at their pH optimum *in vivo*. Shifts in environmental pH or ionic strength can have regulatory functions, and if sufficiently large enzyme concentrations are available, product will be formed by isorenin *in vitro* at near neutral pH (39). On the other hand, a low pH optimum of enzyme activity *in vitro* need not be an argument against a possible physiological role *in vivo*, not only because enzyme characteristics may be different *in vivo* and *in vitro*, but also because true intracellular pH in various cell compartments has not been sufficiently studied. It is frequently lower than in blood, and acid proteases do find accommodating physiological environments intracellularly. The evidence for an active enzyme system will be discussed later. However, the most convincing evidence is that the effector peptide AII of the system apparently can be formed *in vivo* (Fig. 3–2), an observation that has been confirmed by several authors using different methods (12,30, 32,33,39,44,52,68).

Work on the purification and characterization of brain isorenin is presently

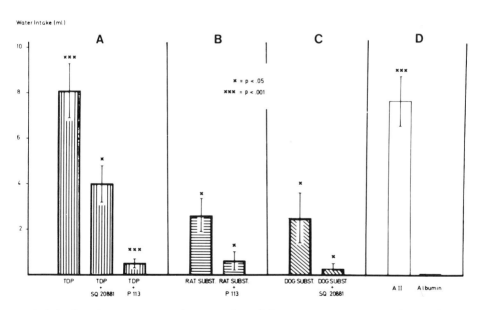

FIG. 3–2. Effect of angiotensinogen infusions into the medial preoptic region on water intake in nephrectomized rats. The purified substrates were free of AI and AII. Water intake of rats is given in ml per 10 min after start of testing. Values are means ± SE. A: synthetic tetradecapeptide substrate (TDP); B: rat plasma angiotensinogen; C: dog plasma angiotensinogen; D: intracranial albumin and angiotensin II control infusions. Statistical significance determined by Student's *t*-test for drinking after treatment vs albumin control, and for substrate plus the angiotensin I-converting enzyme inhibitor SQ 20881 or substrate plus the angiotensin II inhibitor saralasin (P 113) vs substrate infusions alone. Infusion rates were as follows: TDP, 14 ng/min; rat and dog substrate, 14 µg protein/min; SQ 20881, 10 µg/5 µl intracranial injection 2 min before start of substrate infusion; P 113, 5-min infusion before substrate at a rate of 1.4 µg/min; albumin, 14 µg protein/min; and AII, 14 ng/min(68).

being pursued (25), and it can be foreseen that better characterized enzyme fractions will be available in the near future. It is also important to consider the other components of the brain iso-RAS because the enzyme and its kinetics will not be definitely characterized as long as its natural substrate (brain angiotensinogen) is not available in pure form.

BRAIN ANGIOTENSINOGEN

The presence of angiotensinogen in brain tissue was first described by Ganten et al. (39,52). Using the same purification procedure as described for plasma angiotensinogen, they could generate 2.5 ng AI with 1 g brain tissue equivalent (52). Brain angiotensinogen reacted with both purified hog kidney renin and homologous dog kidney renin and brain isorenin (39,41). These results were confirmed by Printz (104) who found considerably higher angiotensinogen levels in brain tissue. Contamination with plasma angiotensinogen was avoided in both studies by thorough rinsing of the brains *in situ*. The physicochemical characteristics of brain tissue angiotensinogen appear to be similar to those of plasma angiotensinogen [glycoprotein, molecular weight 40,000 to 60,000, similar migration in an electrical field (52,104, 105)]. They seem to be regulated independently, however, since angiotensinogen concentrations in cerebrospinal fluid (CSF) remain unchanged

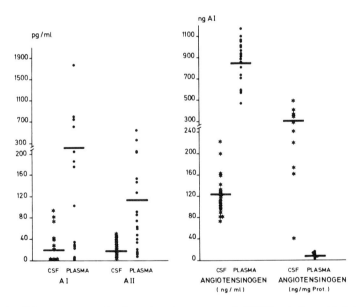

FIG. 3–3. Parallel measurements of renin-angiotensin components in CSF (*) and plasma (.) of dogs. Mean values are indicated by the horizontal bars. No correlation could be established between the plasma and CSF levels of angiotensin I, angiotensin II, or angiotensinogen. Note the high specific activity of angiotensinogen (ng AI equivalents per mg protein) in CSF as compared to plasma.

during maneuvers which increase plasma angiotensinogen and since there is no correlation between individual samples of plasma and CSF angiotensinogen (25,105,106). The specific activity of CSF angiotensinogen is higher than in plasma, although absolute concentrations in CSF are about one-fifth of plasma levels (Fig. 3–3). Chronic hepatectomy would have to be performed to fully exclude plasma angiotensinogen contamination. The independent regulation of brain angiotensinogen and its high molecular weight argue in favor of local synthesis of this protein in brain. Regardless of its origin, it is most important to remember that this large molecular weight precursor of AI is present in brain tissue and CSF and is biologically available since injection of exogenous renin into brain tissue or CSF results in AI formation (25,33,105). Angiotensinogen levels are sufficiently high to yield biologically active AII concentrations. Injection of 0.1 unit hog renin for example raised CSF levels of AI to more than 7,000 pg/ml. Plasma levels of AI for comparison were about 200 pg/ml in these experiments (25). On the other hand, brain angiotensinogen may be a rate-limiting and regulatory factor in AI production (103), since, as shown in Fig. 3–2, administration of exogenous angiotensinogen into brain tissue results in increased AI synthesis (68).

ANGIOTENSIN I CONVERTING ENZYME (EC 3.4.15.1)

Angiotensin I converting enzyme (CE) is a peptidyl-dipeptide hydrolase which cleaves histidyl-leucine from the carboxyl end of the decapeptide AI to yield the octapeptide AII (24). Enzyme concentrations in brain are lower than in lung but significantly higher than in plasma, liver, kidney, heart, and other tissues (43,102,107,135,136). CE was found to be unmeasurably low in CSF by the methods used (43). However, conversion of AI can possibly occur in CSF, since after injection of renin, the AI which is formed in CSF decreases with time while AII increases. Conversion may also occur on contact of AI with the ependymal lining of the brain ventricles (25). The enzyme requires chloride ion and is inhibited by EDTA and O-phenantroline, suggesting that it is a metalloprotein. The nonapeptide CE inhibitor (SQ 20881) inhibits the enzyme *in vitro* and *in vivo*. Brain CE activity has been measured with the following substrates: AI, Hip-His-Leu, Hip-Gly-Gly, Z-Gly-Gly-Val, and Z-Phe-His-Leu (135). The broad substrate specificity which has also been shown in other tissues suggests a role of CE with other naturally occurring peptides, such as those of the kininogenase-kinin system. CE activity was found to be high in striatum, cerebellum, and pituitary of rat brain (135), and reduced in a pituitary tumor (43). The posterior lobe of the pituitary contained higher activity than the anterior lobe (136). AI, on the other hand, was reported high in hypothalamic tissue (30). This gave rise to the speculation that AI (like antidiuretic hormone) is synthesized in hypothalamus, migrates along the hypothalamic-hypophyseal tract to the posterior lobe where it is converted to AII, and then releases antidiuretic hormone (136).

The microsomal subcellular fraction was rich in CE (135), whereas isorenin was concentrated in the mitochondrial fraction (18,39,90). The biological effects (thirst, blood pressure increase) produced by injection of renin, angiotensinogen, or AI into brain tissue cannot be obtained if CE is inhibited by SQ 20881 (33,68). The fact that AII injected directly into the brain still elicits these responses in the presence of SQ 20881 suggests that the responses produced by injection of AII precursors are mediated through formation of AII and that CE is biologically active in brain.

ANGIOTENSINASE ACTIVITY

All peptidases that hydrolyze AI or AII are angiotensinases. They may be amino-, carboxy-, and endopeptidases (80). They play an important role for terminating the action of AII. Brain tissue contains much higher angiotensinase activity than plasma and many other tissues (43,57). The enzymes are insufficiently investigated and need further characterization. If components of the iso-RAS are investigated *in vitro,* complete inhibition of angiotensinase activity is necessary. This can be achieved by a cocktail of the following substances, the optimum composition of which should be established for each *in vitro* system: 2.6 to 15 mM EDTA, 1.6 to 9.7 mM dimercaprol, 2.16 to 10 mM 8-OH-quinoline, 1 to 3.5 mM diisofluorophosphate (DFP), and 3.25 to 10% saturated alcoholic solution of PMSF.

BRAIN ANGIOTENSIN

The amino acid sequence of angiotensin-like peptides in the brain has not been established, and therefore brain angiotensin is not fully characterized. The similarity of brain angiotensin with synthetic AI and AII is discussed below. It may be that a peptide of slightly different amino acid sequence is cleaved from the natural brain angiotensinogen. The terms "brain angiotensin" and "brain AI or AII-like material" include this possibility.

The main problem in the extraction of angiotensin from brain is the short half-life of the peptide owing to high brain angiotensinase activity (43). The first reports on the presence of angiotensin in brain tissue by Fischer-Ferraro et al. (30) and Ganten et al. (52,53) indicated that mostly AI but also AII were present. The material corresponded by all classic criteria to angiotensin: it was water soluble and could be absorbed to Dowex 50W × 2 resin and Fullers earth. It produced a brief increase in blood pressure in rats, which was indistinguishable from that produced by AII or AI. The pressor effect could be inhibited by angiotensin antibodies. The activity remained after boiling but was destroyed after incubation with trypsin. The molecular weight as determined by gel filtration was below 2,000. Guinea pig ileum was contracted by the material, whereas rat uterus contracted only upon the addition of whole rat plasma that contained converting enzyme. Two peptides were separated by countercurrent distribution. One corresponded to synthetic AI and the other to AII. The AI material could be converted by incubation with plasma to AII, which was characterized by a second countercurrent distribution. Angiotensin concentrations in total brain were reported between 2.7 (39,52) and 11.2 (30) ng/g wet tissue. The highest concentration (85 ng/g) was found in the hypothalamus (30). Although these measurements cannot be considered strictly quantitative, brain angiotensin levels appear to be higher than in plasma (e.g., 100 pg/ml). Other authors (12,105) have confirmed the presence of immunoreactive AI-like material in brain tissue of dogs in concentrations of up to 85 ng/g tissue (30,105). The material described by Reid and Day (105) had a higher molecular weight, did not absorb to Fullers earth or Dowex, and was precipitated by boiling and acidification. This raises the possibility of protein binding of AI or interference of angiotensinogen in the angiotensin immunoassay. Protein binding, possibly to neurophysin-like proteins, is also indicated by some of the results reported by Baxter et al. (5). *In vivo* generation of angiotensin in brain is supported not only by the fact that angiotensin is generated by incubation *in vitro* without addition of angiotensinogen (47), but by the fact that the peptide can be extracted from the brains of nephrectomized animals (30,52). In addition, precursors of the enzyme system injected into brain tissue lead to AII formation as demonstrated by the occurrence of thirst and a rise in blood pressure, and the inhibition of these effects by specific AII blockade (33,68). The most important evidence for *in vivo* synthesis of AII in the brain is the fact that AII blockade reduces blood pressure and decreases thirst in models where interference with circulating AII is excluded by nephrectomy (49,50). The presence of angiotensin in brain demonstrates the existence of a biochemically active iso-RAS in brain, since the effector peptide can be synthesized enzymatically.

COMPONENTS OF THE RAS IN CEREBROSPINAL FLUID

Volicer and Loew (131) reported the presence of radioactivity in the CSF after ^{14}C-labeled AII had been injected intravenously. Johnson (75), using ^{3}H-labeled AII, similarly noted spread of radioactivity in the CSF and in the periventricular tissue after peripheral administration of AII. However, the radioactivity detected in these studies may have been attached to a fragment of the peptide chain. Many amino acids, especially tyrosine, which preferentially carries the radioactivity of labeled AII, are taken up freely by brain tissue (94,95). Volicer and Loew (131) concluded from their studies that intact AII had penetrated into the brain. However, they found only one radioactive fraction in plasma and in brain tissue homogenate 5 min after intravenous injection of AII. Since most of the AII is degraded into fragments after this time, it appears that no separation of intact AII from fragments was achieved in their characterization system. We have studied the permeability of the blood-cerebrospinal fluid barrier (BCB) in detail. Rats were infused intravenously with unlabeled (cold) AII, with ^{125}I-labeled AI and AII, and with ^{3}H-AII of high specific activity. The brain ventricular system was perfused with artificial CSF and the perfusate was collected from the cisterna magna and analyzed for AII by radioimmunological and biochemical methods. Experiments were performed in normotensive and hypertensive rats at various subpressor and pressor doses of AII (47,50,110,111). The results (110,111) provide no evidence for penetration of intact AII from blood into the CSF. Thus, the BCB appears to be impermeable to the intact AII molecule. In accord with previous studies, radioactivity was measured in the CSF perfusate. However, the activity was clearly characterized as small fragments of AII, rather than AII itself (50,111). The concentration of radioactivity in CSF increased after termination of the AII infusion when no intact AII was present in plasma. This indicated that fragments of AII (possibly tyrosine) are taken up by the brain. Furthermore, parallel measurements of AII as well as renin and angiotensinogen have been carried out in CSF and plasma of humans, dogs, and rats under normal conditions, after stimulation of the RAS, and in spontaneously hypertensive rats. No correlation was found between plasma and CSF RAS components (47,50,110,111). We conclude that neither AII nor the other components of the RAS freely cross the BCB. However, sudden, marked increases in systemic blood pressure with excessive doses of AII may force the peptide through cerebral capillaries (134). Evidence for this temporary breakdown of the BCB and blood brain barrier was obtained by Deshmukh and Phillips (20) who combined horseradish peroxidase and a 2-μg/kg intravenous injection of angiotensin. Five minutes later horseradish peroxidase could be detected in periventricular tissue and other brain sites. At normal blood pressures there was crossing of the horseradish peroxidase from periphery to brain only in the subfornical organ (SFO) and organum vasculosum lamina terminalis (OVLT). These organs have an incomplete blood brain barrier (see Chapter 4).

Another approach to this question has been the use of competitive antagonists of angiotensin such as 1-Sar-8-Ala-AII (saralasin, P 113) (14,15,33, 34,78,98,124). Intravenous infusions of saralasin effectively block the dipsogenic action of intravenous infusions of AII (14,15,78). Likewise, intracerebroventricular (IVT) infusions of the peptide and its antagonist effectively cancel one another. It has also been shown that intracranial saralasin blocks the dipsogenic effect of raised peripheral angiotensin levels (22,78). High intravenous doses of saralasin (72-μg bolus injections) antagonize the central effect of AII (67). The integrity of the blood brain barrier may be important before assuming that the peripheral and central routes lead to the same receptor sites. Intravenous saralasin in a bolus injection of 50 ng or more causes an agonistic effect which increases blood pressure by more than 30 mm Hg. Dose response curves (85,101) showed that lower doses of saralasin were ineffective in blocking central angiotensin effects even though these doses would have been antagonistic to the same dose of intravenous AII. Thus, the evidence for systemic angiotensin reaching the same sites as central angiotensin remains inconclusive when one considers levels of AII that do not cause excessive blood pressure increases.

In rats with high renin experimental hypertension, increased plasma renin coincided with decreased brain isorenin (47). A negative feedback of plasma AII with CSF AII has also been reported (108) but could not be confirmed (23). High concentrations of angiotensin-like peptide have been reported in CSF of patients with essential hypertension (29) and in spontaneously hypertensive rats of the New Zealand strain (49,50). We believe that components in CSF represent an overflow from the intracellular iso-RAS in brain tissue. On the other hand, several AII-sensitive receptor sites are located periventricularly (76,77), and angiotensinogen is present in CSF in high amounts (25,84,106). Despite many attempts, no pathophysiological regulatory role for RAS components in CSF has been discovered.

ANGIOTENSIN RECEPTORS

Angiotensin receptors in brain have been defined biochemically by binding characteristics *in vitro* (6,88) and by their biological effect *in vitro* (10,109) and *in vivo* (34,97,125,126).

Bennet and Snyder (6) and McLean et al. (88) identified high-affinity binding sites for ^{125}I-AII on bovine and rat brain membranes. AII binding was saturable and reversible. Analogues and fragments of AII competed for the binding sites, and their potency *in vitro* correlated with their potency *in vivo*. AI and the 3-8 hexapeptide and 4-8 pentapeptide showed less affinity, whereas des-asp-AII (AIII) and various position-8-substituted AII antagonists were slightly more potent than AII. In calf brain most AII receptors were localized in the cerebellar cortex and deep nuclei of the cerebellum. Less binding was found in the choroid plexus of the fourth ventricle and in the superior colliculus (6). In rats, AII binding was highest in the thalamus, hypothalamus and midbrain (6,88).

Electrophysiological recording from brain cells has revealed localized groups of neurons which are sensitive to AII specifically (26,97–100). Using microiontophoresis, investigators applied AII to cells in the subfornical organ of the cat. A dose response curve was established over an ejection current range of 5 to 150 nA. AII-sensitive units were not stimulated by bradykinin. The specificity of the response was demonstrated when saralasin was ejected during angiotensin application and the response of the cells was antagonized. Some units were responsive to both angiotensin and acetylcholine, but only the angiotensin sensitivity was antagonized by saralasin. Saralasin alone tended to slow the spontaneous activity of the neurons. This could be taken to mean that firing rate was maintained by endogenous brain angiotensin

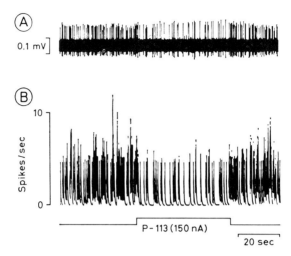

FIG. 3–4. Effect of angiotensin blockade by saralasin on unit firing in neurons of the subfornical organ of a cat. A: unit activity; B: integrated activity of the recording in A. Saralasin (P 113) was applied by an ejection current of 150 nA.

(Fig. 3–4). In other areas such as cortex and hippocampus, no angiotensin-sensitive cells were found (26,97). Earlier electrophysiological studies *in vivo* (93) and *in vitro* (109) had shown that the supraoptic nucleus contains angiotensin-sensitive neurons. These cells may be responsible for the release of vasopressin which is induced by centrally applied angiotensin II.

The most sensitive sites for the dipsogenic response to AII in cats were reported to be the septal region, anterior hypothalamus, and preoptic area. Less sensitive was the mesencephalic gray, and least sensitive was the intra-ventricular route (126). However, other authors working on rats (77) found the ventricles to be as sensitive to angiotensin as all other routes. The main effective area was in the anterior third ventricle and not in the lateral ventricles, cerebral aqueduct, fourth ventricle, or posterior third ventricle. Two circumventricular organs, the subfornical organ and the organum vasculosum lamina terminalis, and periventricular structures which are located in the anterior third ventricle are presently being investigated as potentially important receptor sites for angiotensin-mediated thirst (see Chapter 4; 2,33,76,118).

Thus, there appear to be multiple AII-sensitive sites. The sites can be approached by the peptide from the brain side or the blood side. The dual availability of receptors, which was demonstrated by the ventricular plugging studies (98), suggests that they can be stimulated by endogenous brain AII. Weindl and Joynt (133) showed that upon intraventricular injection, horse-radish peroxidase reached periventricular tissue but did not penetrate the OVLT. This would suggest that whereas systemic angiotensin might reach the OVLT, intraventricular would not. It was also shown that rats did not drink when intraventricular angiotensin reached the surface of the SFO (65,66). Injections of the octapeptide into the intact SFO produced dipsogenic responses. Thus, although blood-borne AII may be able to reach angiotensin-sensitive brain sites, there are other sites which may be preferentially stimulated by the brain iso-RAS.

The possibility that the brain iso-RAS has a role in thirst is supported by the presence of angiotensin receptors and sensitive sites for the dipsogenic response in the brain. In addition, the threshold for intracranial or intraventricular injections of AII is lower than the threshold for intravenous AII (33,98). The high peripheral levels of AII needed for stimulation have raised the question whether plasma AII can act as a physiological thirst stimulus (1). However, additional evidence for participation of the brain iso-RAS in thirst has been obtained in other experiments. Blockade of central AII receptors and cholinergic receptors was achieved by infusion of saralasin and atropine into the brain ventricular system. Neither saralasin nor atropine had any effect on water intake when they were infused alone into the brain ventricles of water-deprived rats. However, when both blockers were given together, there was a significant decrease in water intake during the infusion period. This effect apparently was specific for thirst, since milk intake in 24 hr food-deprived rats was not significantly inhibited. Ninety minutes after the end of the infusion of saralasin alone or saralasin plus atropine, there was a significant rebound in the drinking response. This effect may be due to the end of the inhibitory effect of the antagonists. In a related experiment, we have observed increased isorenin concentration in hypothalamic tissue following 2-hr intracranial saralasin infusions. This suggests that the brain iso-RAS could be involved in the rebound drinking response. Water intake was also reduced by combined angiotensin and cholinergic blockade in rats with hypothalamic diabetes insipidus. These rats have increased isorenin in hypothalamic tissue (64).

In another series of experiments, nephrectomized rats were infused intracranially with AII, synthetic tetradecapeptide substrate, and purified rat and dog plasma substrates. Significant drinking responses were observed with all four substances, whereas no effect on drinking was seen when albumin was infused at the same rate and protein concentration (Fig. 3–2). It has been argued that brain isorenin or other acid proteases act at a low pH and therefore could not be of physiological importance (105). Our results indicate that the isorenin-substrate reaction occurs in intracellular compartments with acid milieu, or that the enzyme-substrate reaction does not occur at its pH optimum, or that the pH optimum determined for isorenin *in vitro* does not reflect its optimum *in vivo*. Brain isorenin thus has the ability to hydrolyze naturally occurring and synthetic angiotensinogens and to generate angiotensin *in vivo* at the locally prevailing pH. The tetradecapeptide produced the largest water intake values, with dog substrate second and rat substrate third.

This corresponds with the ability of rat brain isorenin to produce AI from these substrates *in vitro* (39,43). The results also indicate that brain angiotensin receptors play a role in the physiological mediation of thirst, probably in conjunction with other transmitter systems. Since the experiments described above were carried out in rats that had been nephrectomized for 24 hr, isorenin endogenous to the brain must be considered the enzyme producing the effects.

DISTRIBUTION OF ANGIOTENSIN-LIKE IMMUNOREACTIVITY IN THE CENTRAL NERVOUS SYSTEM OF RATS

Immunohistochemical methods have proved to be a useful tool to study the localization of peptides in tissue. The distribution of AII in certain brain areas was studied to give a clue to its function.

Antibodies were obtained by coupling 5-Ile-angiotensin II to bovine serum albumin and injecting this complex into rabbits. Cross-reactivity of the antibody with somatostatin, bradykinin, substance P, TRH, and LRH was less than 0.01%, and with des-Asp-8-Ala AII, 0.01%. For control of specificity the antibodies were adsorbed with bovine serum albumin and with AII before the immunohistochemical procedure. AII generally eliminated the immunofluorescence, whereas the fluorescence did not disappear following adsorption with bovine serum alone. The histochemical procedure involved the indirect technique of Coons (16), using fluorescein isothiocyanate-conjugated sheep antirabbit immunoglobulin as a marker (for details see 37,38). Perfusion fixation was performed by means of 4% ice cold formalin. Cryostat sections were used. The antiserum was usually used in a dilution of 1:32.

The distribution of angiotensin-like immunoreactivity in the central nervous system of rats is summarized in Table 3–1. Much of the information has been published (36), but we have also included unpublished findings obtained in collaboration with Drs. Haebara, Hökfelt, and Bolme.

TABLE 3–1. *Distribution of angiotensin II-like immunoreactivity in the central nervous system of male Sprague-Dawley rats*

High density: Substantia gelatinosa of the spinal cord, nucleus tractus spinalis nervi trigemini, median eminence (medial external layer), nucleus amygdaloideus centralis, sympathetic lateral column.

Low-moderate density: Nucleus dorsomedialis hypothalami, locus ceruleus, ventral and caudal part of nucleus caudatus putamen.

Scattered terminals: Periventricular mesencephalic gray, hypothalamus, preoptic area, subcortical limbic structures (amygdaloid cortex, septal area), limbic cortex, thalamus (midline area), ventral midbrain, substantia nigra, reticular formation including the region of norepinephrine and epinephrine cell groups AI and CI, respectively, in the ventrolateral reticular formation of medulla oblongata, raphe region, nucleus tractus solitarius, nucleus dorsalis motorius nervi vagi, periventricular area of pons and medulla oblongata.

No immunofluorescence: Parts of the neocortex, cortex cerebelli.

Areas Containing a High Density of Angiotensin II-Positive
Nerve Terminals

Median Eminence

At all levels of the median eminence except the most anterior portion, a dense network of AII-positive nerve terminals was found concentrated in the medial external layer (Fig. 3–5).

Many positive terminals were found in the lateral external layer and the infundibular stalk. The nerve terminals of the median eminence appear to arise from axon budles which originate from the paraventricular hypothalamic nucleus. The axons, which are varicose, run laterally and ventrolaterally from the paraventricular nucleus to reach the lateral hypothalamic region and the medial part of the subthalamus, after which most of them sweep ventrally and ventromedially along the ventral surface of the hypothalamus at the level of the retrochiasmatic region (Fig. 3–6). In some rats there was a weak specific AII-like immunoreactivity within some of the nerve cells of the parvo-

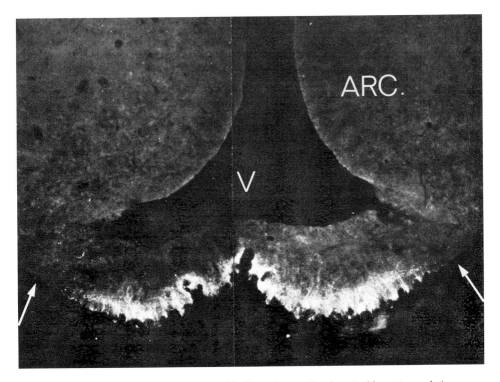

FIG. 3–5. Angiotensin II-like immunoreactivity. Median eminence of a 4-week-old spontaneously hypertensive rat of the Wistar Kyoto strain. The specific immunoreactivity is localized to a dense plexus of nerve terminals present in the medial palisade zone and the medial part of the lateral palisade zone (arrow). ARC., nucleus arcuatus; V, third ventricle. Magnification ×120.

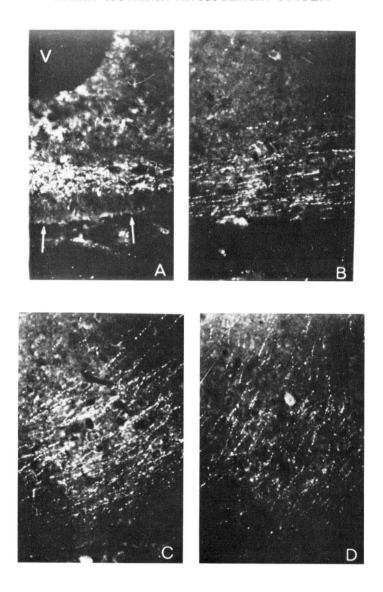

cellular portion of the nucleus paraventricularis hypothalami (Figure 3–7).

Thus, AII-like peptides may be secreted into the portal vessels to act at the pituitary level as releasing factors. It is not yet known if these nerve cells use neurophysins to store the AII-related peptides. This possibility is being explored by means of lesions of the paraventricular nucleus. Recently, axons have been observed which may originate from the supraoptic neurons, and some AII-positive cell bodies have been observed in nucleus dorsomedialis hypothalami and zona incerta. Therefore lesions should also be made in these nuclei. The axon bundles to the median eminence were particularly evident

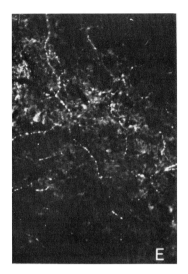

FIG. 3–6. Angiotensin II-like immunoreactivity. Retrochiasmatic area of a control rat of the Kyoto Wistar strain. A is the most medial part of the retrochiasmatic area, and E is the most lateral part of the retrochiasmatic area. The large bundles of varicose axons originating from the paraventricular hypothalamic region are seen to sweep from a dorsolateral position to a ventromedial location to innervate the rat median eminence. The arrows show that the most anterior part of the median eminence is not innervated by angiotensin II-positive nerve terminals. V, third ventricle. Magnification ×300.

in Wistar Kyoto normotensive rats of the strain that serves as a control in experiments involving spontaneously hypertensive rats of the Wistar Kyoto strain. The fluorescence was clearly stronger than in many of the Wistar Kyoto hypertensive rats, suggesting a possible change in the state of activity of these systems in relation to hypertension.

Substantia Gelatinosa

There was a high density of AII-positive nerve terminals within the substantia gelatinosa of the spinal cord and the spinal nucleus of the fifth nerve (Table 3–1). In the spinal cord, the nerve terminals were present at all levels. They appeared as dots when the spinal cord was transversely transected, and covered the substantia gelatinosa from its medial to its lateral part. This was also true for the substantia gelatinosa of the nucleus tractus spinalis nervi trigemini (Fig. 3–8). The terminals were present in lamina I and II. This suggests that AII-like peptides may exist in some types of primary sensory neurons.

Previous experiments have shown that two other types of peptides also exist in the substantia gelatinosa: substance P (70) and somatostatin (69). The distribution of AII-positive terminals in the substantia gelatinosa appears to be similar to that of substance P-positive terminals, whereas somatostatin-positive terminals have a more ventral location. Two subpopulations of dorsal ganglion cells have also been identified on a histochemical basis, one containing substance P and one containing somatostatin (69,70). These cell bodies appear to belong to the small cells in the spinal ganglia. There appear to be dorsal ganglion cells containing AII-like immunoreactivity in some ganglia. However, some of these cell bodies are definitely the large dorsal

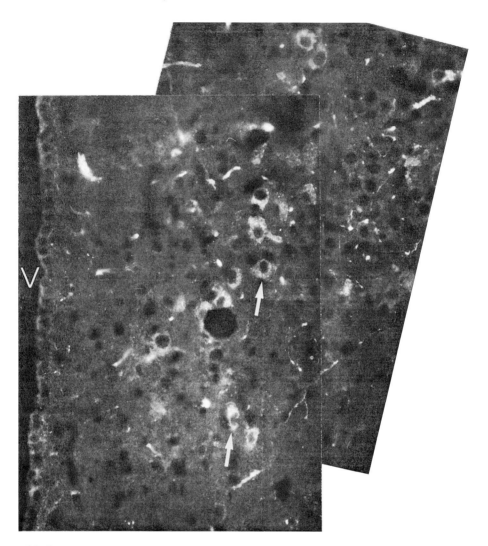

FIG. 3–7. Angiotensin II-like immunoreactivity. Nucleus paraventricularis hypothalami of male Wistar Kyoto rat. Nerve cell bodies *(arrows)* within the parvocellular part of the nucleus contain specific angiotensin II-like immunofluorescence. These nerve cell bodies probably give rise to the axons shown in Fig. 3–6. V, third ventricle. Magnification ×300.

root ganglion cells which are not supposed to innervate the substantia gelatinosa. Consequently, the specificity of this fluorescence is still being investigated. It is possible that a third type of dorsal root ganglion nerve cell body exists which contain AII-like peptides. In agreement with this view, it has been found that spinal cord transections do not cause any disappearance of AII-like immunoreactivity in the spinal cord, whereas transections of the dorsal roots lead to a disappearance of AII-like immunoreactivity in the

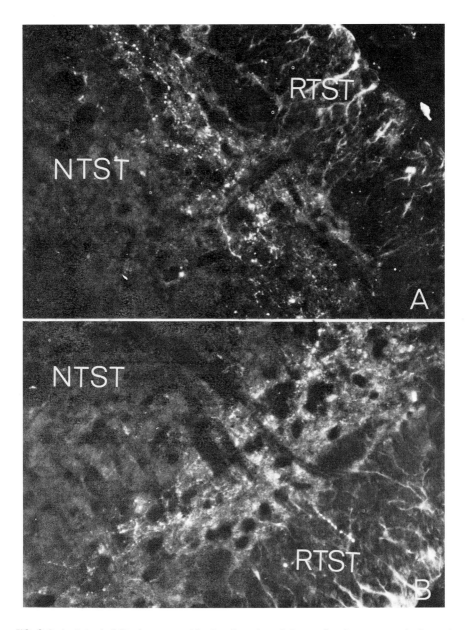

FIG. 3–8. Angiotensin II-like immunoreactivity in substantia gelatinosa of nucleus tractus spinalis nervi trigemini (NTST) of male Sprague-Dawley rat. A: dorsal part; B: ventral part. RTST, radix of the tractus spinalis nervi trigemini. Magnification ×300.

substantia gelatinosa. Taken together these findings suggest that AII-like peptides have a role as a transmitter or a modulator substance in certain types of primary sensory neurons.

Sympathetic Lateral Column

A high density of AII-positive nerve terminals exists within the sympathetic lateral column. These terminals appear to arise from axons descending in the lateral funiculus, since 1 week after transection of the spinal cord at the cervical level, the nerve terminals disappeared. At the same time, accumulation of immunoreactive material was observed within descending fibers in the lateral funiculus (Fig. 3–9).

Thus, supraspinal systems may exist which use AII peptides and which specifically control activity in the sympathetic lateral column. These AII-containing systems may be directly involved in central blood pressure control. AII-positive nerve terminal systems may also be involved in the control of the blood pressure via their innervation of regions within the reticular formation. They innervated the locus ceruleus, from which vasopressor responses can be elicited (132), and which is known to contain norepinephrine cell bodies (17,38). Norepinephrine pathways probably can be considered as vasopressor pathways (11,37). However, the angiotensin innervation of these regions was only weak to moderate. AII-like immunoreactivity was also found within terminals in the area of the norepinephrine cell group AI (17). The data support the view that centrally mediated hypertensive effects of angiotensin II may be mediated via activation of descending norepinephrine pathways to the spinal cord (56). In some spontaneously hypertensive rats of the Wistar Kyoto strain, a moderate innervation of AII-positive terminals was within the parasolitary nucleus, within the nucleus tractus solitarius, and within the dorsal motor nucleus of the vagus. The present immunohistochemical findings therefore support the view of Ganten et al. (49,50) that AII-related peptides may be of importance in central mechanisms of blood pressure regulation. In addition, they suggest that angiotensin may cause these effects via actions in the hypothalamus, medulla oblongata, and spinal cord.

Nucleus Amygdaloideus Centralis

This nucleus contained large numbers of AII-positive nerve terminals, many of which appear to establish axosomatic contacts in the posterior part of the nucleus (Fig. 3–10). Other parts of the amygdaloid complex contain scattered AII-positive nerve terminals, and single AII-positive nerve cells have been found in the medial nucleus. This is also true for other parts of the limbic system. For example, there were scattered nerve terminals within the limbic cortex and the septal area (Fig. 3–11). They were strongly fluorescent, of variable thickness, and had a clearly varicose appearance. It may be that

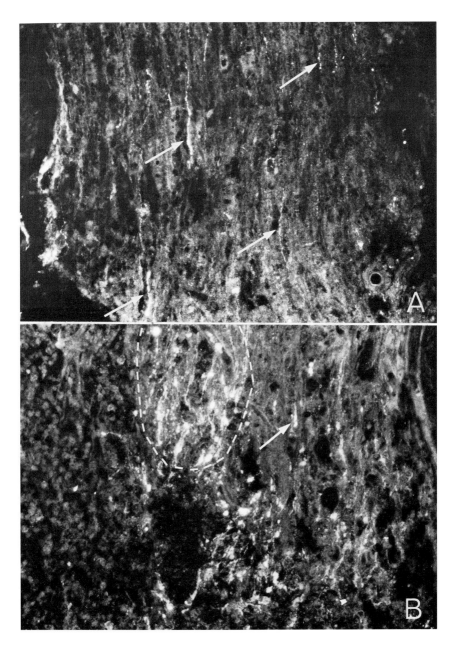

FIG. 3–9. Angiotensin II-like immunoreactivity. Lateral funiculus cranial to a spinal cord transection 7 days before killing. Male Sprague-Dawley rat. B: Lateral funiculus immediately above the spinal cord transection. A is taken 0.5 mm above the transection. The area of the highest accumulation of angiotensin II-positive material in axons is surrounded by a dashed line. Arrows point to individual angiotensin II-positive axons. Magnification ×120.

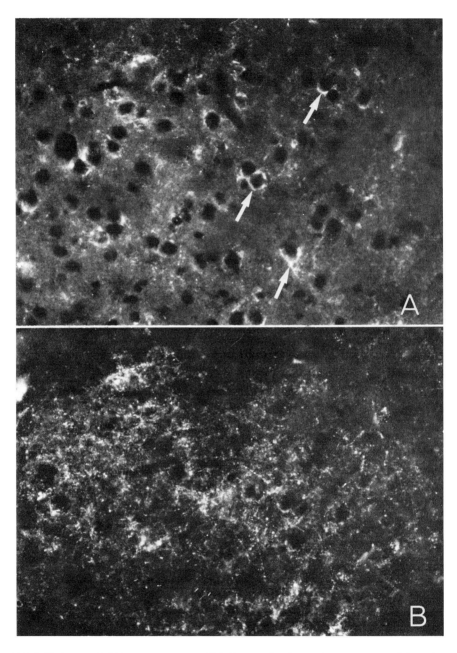

FIG. 3–10. Angiotensin II-like immunoreactivity. Male Sprague-Dawley rat. A: posterior part of the nucleus amygdaloideus centralis; B: anterior part. A large number of angiotensin II-positive nerve terminals are found in both regions. Arrows indicate apparent axosomatic contacts. Magnification ×300.

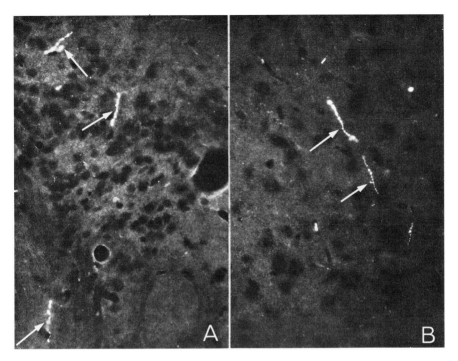

FIG. 3–11. Angiotensin II-like immunoreactivity. Normal male Sprague-Dawley rat. Single strongly fluorescent and varicose terminals containing angiotensin II-like immunoreactivity are observed within the nucleus septalis triangularis (A) and within the dorsal part of the nucleus interstitialis striae terminalis (B). Magnification ×300.

they represent preterminal axons and that the true nerve terminals in several regions may contain amounts of AII-like peptides too low to be discovered with the present method.

Brains of Wistar Kyoto rats appear to contain higher densities of AII-positive nerve terminals than brains of Sprague-Dawley rats. In Wistar Kyoto rats, a moderate to high innervation was found within the nucleus accumbens and within the septal area as well as within the nucleus interstitialis striae terminalis, ventral part and dorsal part. It is possible that the amounts of AII-like peptides present in the terminals vary from one strain of rats to another, allowing detection in some strains but not in others.

Areas Containing a Low to Moderate Density of Angiotensin II-Positive Nerve Terminals

Parts of the nucleus caudatus putamen (ventral and caudal) contain AII-positive nerve terminals suggesting that this peptide may participate in the functioning of the extrapyramidal motor system. A moderate density of innervation was found in the nucleus dorsomedialis hypothalami.

ANGIOTENSIN II-LIKE IMMUNOREACTIVITY WITHIN THE PERIPHERAL NERVOUS SYSTEM

Evidence presented above indicates that there is a subpopulation of dorsal root ganglion nerve cells which contain AII-like peptides. Other parts of the peripheral nervous system also seem capable of storing these peptides.

Gastrointestinal Tract

A large number of ganglion cells within Auerbach's plexus (plexus myentericus) contain a strong AII-like immunofluorescence. This was especially true in the duodenum, but some cells were observed in the colon and the stomach. Furthermore, AII-positive nerve terminals were found within Auerbach's plexus seemingly innervating AII-negative ganglion cells (Fig. 3–12). These terminals were found in the duodenum, the colon, and the stomach. In all three regions, AII-positive nerve terminals were located within the inner circular muscle layer and the outer longitudinal muscle layer. In the duodenum, some AII-positive terminals were found in Meissner's plexus and in the muscularis mucosa. Arteries of various sizes in the colon and in the duodenum appeared to be innervated by AII-positive nerve terminals approaching the outer surface of the media. These findings suggest that in the gastrointestinal tract, AII-related peptides serve as modulators or transmitters in local interneurons innervating blood vessels, muscles, and other nerve cells in the plexus myentericus. An important finding is the observation that local AII neurons may directly innervate arteries of the gastrointestinal tract, suggesting that the peptides participate in the control of blood flow in the gastroin-

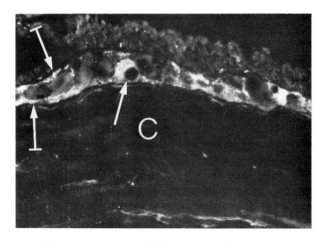

FIG. 3–12. Angiotensin II-like immunoreactivity. Colon of normal Sprague-Dawley rat. Arrow points to angiotensin II-positive nerve cell body in plexus myentericus. Arrows with one line point to angiotensin II-positive nerve terminals innervating nerve cells in the plexus myentericus containing no specific angiotensin II immunofluorescence. C, circular muscle layer. Magnification ×300.

testinal tract. It should be noted that isorenin has been found to be present in mesenteric arteries (46,62,63), and its concentration is increased by hypovolemia and mesenteric ischemia (46).

Superior Cervical Ganglion

In rats of the Wistar Kyoto strain, AII-positive immunofluorescence was found within some of the small intensely fluorescent (SIF) cells in the superior cervical ganglia. The specificity of this fluorescence needs further investigation, since it was difficult to completely remove it by adsorbtion of the antibodies with AII. In some adult spontaneously hypertensive rats of the Wistar Kyoto strain, there were plexuses of fiber-like structures within the superior cervical ganglion that contained AII-like immunoreactivity. Most of this activity could be removed by adsorbtion with AII (Fig. 3–13).

The frequency of the nerve terminals within the spontaneously hypertensive rats is being investigated. Significant increases in isorenin concentration have been observed in the superior cervical ganglia of spontaneously hypertensive rats (64). Angiotensin has also been found to stimulate the superior cervical ganglion (83).

Our preliminary analysis indicates that the distribution of AII-like immunoreactivity in the nervous systems of spontaneously hypertensive rats and Wistar Kyoto control rats is similar, but rats of the Wistar Kyoto strain appear to have more AII-positive terminals in the central nervous system than rats of the Sprague-Dawley strain.

Pituitary Gland

Practically all gland cells of the pars intermedia exhibit AII-like immunofluorescence (Fig. 3–14). The posterior pituitary does not contain any specific AII immunofluorescence (8). In the pars distalis, there are appreciable numbers of AII-positive gland cells, particularly in the normotensive and hypertensive Wistar Kyoto rats (Fig. 3–15).

The type of gland cell in the anterior pituitary which contains AII-like immunoreactivity has not been identified. The distribution and intensity of the AII-like immunoreactivity in the pars distalis are similar in spontaneously hypertensive rats and Wistar Kyoto control rats, but in the pars intermedia, the cells of the hypertensive rats appear to have a stronger reaction.

Reports from Other Laboratories

AII-positive staining of neural elements has also been reported by Nahmod et al. (91) in the spinal cord, cerebellum, midbrain, limbic system, and portions of the basal hypothalamic nuclei of rats. Using the peroxidase-antiperoxidase method, Changaris et al. (12) reported localization of AII in the

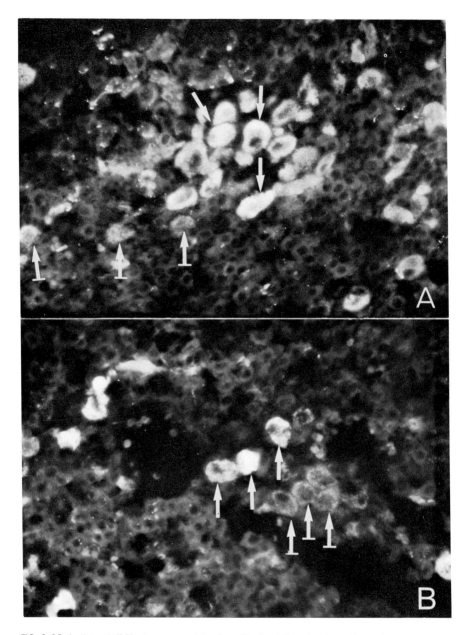

FIG. 3–15. Angiotensin II-like immunoreactivity. Pars distalis of the adenohypophysis of a spontaneously hypertensive rat (12 weeks old). The arrows show gland cells with a strong (*arrow*) and a weak (*arrow with a line*) specific immunofluorescence. A and B are taken from the same part of the pars distalis. Magnification ×300.

isorenin system might be involved in local or systemic electrolyte and volume regulation. However, there is no direct evidence for this hypothesis.

We have also measured isorenin levels in spontaneously hypertensive rats of the stroke-prone Wistar Kyoto strain. The isorenin concentration was high in posterior hypothalamic tissue, as well as in the superior cervical ganglia (64). This suggests that the isorenin system may be involved in neuroendocrine activity mediated by the hypothalamus in the control of sympathetic tone. The hypothalamus of rats with hereditary hypothalamic diabetes insipidus contained a high concentration of isorenin. It is not known whether these high levels are related to the lack of ability of the rats to secrete antidiuretic hormone or whether they are a primary factor in the increased water intake of these animals. Preliminary results with vasopressin substitution suggest that increased hypothalamic isorenin may be related to brain vasopressin content and a possible local feedback mechanism may be involved.

Changes in the isorenin concentration in choroid plexus have been noted with hemodynamic challenges. With an acute (3 hr) hemorrhage we have found a decrease in isorenin in this tissue. Since the rats were nephrectomized 24 hr previously, an interference of the peripheral system is unlikely. Decreased blood flow to the brain has similar effects. Unilateral or bilateral ligation of the internal carotid artery of rats for 24 hr produced a decrease in isorenin concentration in the choroid plexus without any significant changes in the hypothalamus or other brain regions tested. With chronic ligation, however, choroid plexus values increased again, and 1 week after unilateral ligation, isorenin concentration was above control levels(64).

Brain isorenin concentration was decreased in rats with experimental renal hypertension and high plasma renin concentration (coarctation of the aorta between both renal arteries), but unchanged in renal hypertension with normal plasma renin. In desert rats (Meriones shawi Duvernoy) which were subjected to 10 days of complete water deprivation, plasma renin increased, whereas brain isorenin decreased in the hypothalamus, hypophysis, and frontal cortex (47,64). These data suggest that there are feedback mechanisms between the local tissue isorenin systems and plasma renin. Contribution of the isorenin systems to plasma renin levels ("ectopic primary reninism") has also been shown in a case in which isorenin in the circulation came from a tumor (hemangiopericytoma) in the brain (137).

CENTRAL MECHANISMS OF BLOOD PRESSURE REGULATION

The participation of angiotensin in central mechanisms of blood pressure regulation is generally accepted (see 9,27,114). Among the proposed receptor sites for the mediation of central cardiovascular effects of angiotensin is the subnucleus medialis in the midbrain, which can be stimulated by AII in the cerebral aqueduct. Administration of AII into hypothalamic tissue also leads to an increase in blood pressure, and the anterior hypothalamus appears to be more sensitive than the posterior hypothalamus.

Recent evidence supports the hypothesis that the hypothalamus is involved in the blood pressure response to centrally administered angiotensin via release of antidiuretic hormone (50,72,73,79,115,116). In experiments in which AII was perfused through the brain ventricles, intraventricular AII produced a smaller pressor response in rats of the Brattleboro strain, which are homozygous for diabetes insipidus, than it did in Long-Evans controls. The dose response curve for intraventricular perfusion of AII in the rats heterozygous for diabetes insipidus was between the curves of the other two groups. Since rats homozygous for diabetes insipidus do not produce any antidiuretic hormone and heterozygous rats have a partial defect in antidiuretic hormone production, the data suggest that the central blood pressure response to angiotensin is due in part to vasopressin (49,50,72,73). The drinking response to AII was the same in diabetes insipidus rats and in controls, which indicates that the receptor sites or effector neurons for drinking and blood pressure regulation are different. It seems probable that increased sympathetic tone also contributes to the central blood pressure response to AII (9,27,115).

We have studied the possible participation of the brain isorenin system in central regulation of blood pressure in three different strains of spontaneously hypertensive rats. Male hypertensive rats derived from the New Zealand strain (SH-NZ) were perfused with artificial CSF through the brain ventricular system. The rats remained in the stereotaxic apparatus during the whole experiment after regaining consciousness from surgery under tribromoethanol anesthesia. Initial blood pressure in these rats was 179.4 ± 7.6 mm Hg. A significant decrease (31.6 ± 7.4 mm Hg; $p < 0.01$) occurred following perfusion of the brain ventricular system with saralasin at a rate of 200 ng/min. No change in arterial blood pressure was seen in control normotensive rats or after intravenous injection of $1 \mu g$ saralasin into the hypertensive rats (49, 50,71).

Spontaneously hypertensive rats originally derived from the Kyoto Wistar strain but bred by various commercial breeders (SH-BM) were implanted with a chronic cannula in the lateral brain ventricle. They received injections of the test substance in artificial CSF, and blood pressure was recorded, as in all experiments in these series, by a chronic femoral artery catheter. Injections of doses of saralasin up to 20 μg per rat did not lower arterial blood pressure in SH-BM rats; instead, this dose frequently produced an increase in blood pressure.

Hypertensive rats of the stroke-prone Wistar Kyoto strain (SH-SP) and age-matched Wistar Kyoto control rats (WKY) were implanted with a chronic cannula into the right lateral brain ventricle. A femoral vein catheter and a femoral artery catheter were inserted. Rats were awake, freely moving in a wooden box during testing and blood pressure recording. Three experimental groups were tested. In one group, 10 SH-SP and 6 WKY male and female rats, all 4 months old, were tested with intravenous and intracerebroventricular doses of saralasin. The second group consisted of 8-month-old female SH-SP rats. The third group consisted of 8-month-old females (7 SH-SP rats and 4 WKY rats) which had been nephrectomized 18 hr prior to the experiment. Saralasin was infused for 15 min intravenously in cumulative doses of 0.1, 1.0, 10.0, and 100 μg/kg/min. Sixty minutes after the infusion test, a bolus injection of 50 μg saralasin was given intravenously. After 2 to 3 hr recovery when blood pressure was stable, testing began with IVT injections of 5, 10, and 20 μg of saralasin. The order of testing was randomized and there was full recovery of the original blood pressure level between tests. The results are illustrated in Fig. 3–16. The mean starting arterial blood pressure of the SH-SP rats was 181.3 $\pm$ 9.2 mm Hg. Saralasin by the IVT route lowered blood pressure in a dose-response relationship in every rat tested. The fall in blood pressure in each case began within 1 min after the injection and reached a maximum at 5 to 7 min, with a return to the original blood pressure level in 15 to 30 min. Control Wistar Kyoto rats showed no response to IVT saralasin. Intravenous saralasin increased blood pressure in the SH and in the control rats. The bolus injection of 50 μg saralasin consistently produced an even more marked elevation in blood pressure in both SH rats (23.4 $\pm$ 2.5 mm Hg) and controls (35.3 $\pm$ 2.6 mm Hg). In nephrectomized SH-SP rats the mean lowering of blood pressure by 20 μg of IVT saralasin was 14.1 $\pm$ 3.8 mm Hg. No effect of intravenous saralasin was seen in the nephrectomized control rats (101).

There is little evidence for a role of plasma AII in the maintenance of hypertension (35,81,117,119,130). However, our data demonstrate a contribution of brain angiotensin to the elevated blood pressure in two strains of spontaneously hypertensive rats. Similar data have been reported by other authors (112,128), but negative results were reported by Elghozi et al. (21). Schoelkens et al. (112) reported an influence of age on the effect of central

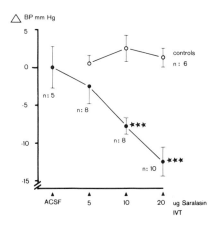

FIG. 3–16. Effect of intracerebroventricular (IVT) administration of saralasin on the arterial blood pressure of conscious spontaneously hypertensive rats of the stroke-prone Wistar Kyoto strain (SH-SP), 20 weeks old. The ordinate indicates the blood pressure decreases; doses of saralasin are indicated on the ordinate. *** p < 0.01; ACSF, control injection of artificial CSF.

AII blockade on arterial blood pressure. In other types of experimental hypertension with high circulating plasma renins, central AII blockade also lowers blood pressure (Fig. 3–17; 85,127). In experimental hypertension induced by salt loading such as deoxycorticosterone (DOCA) hypertension, central injections of saralasin lead to blood pressure increases.

On the basis of evidence available to date, it must be concluded that the AII receptors involved in central mechanisms of blood pressure regulation can be blocked and stimulated from outside and inside the blood brain barrier. The receptor area most probably stimulated by circulating plasma AII is the area postrema, which is not sensitive to AII from the CSF side. The subnucleus medialis and hypothalamus have already been discussed as receptor sites which can be stimulated from the brain ventricles. Both types of receptor sites appear to participate in the regulation of blood pressure. The degree of stimulation of the receptors inside or outside the blood brain barrier may depend on the levels of circulating plasma AII and local brain AII. This again varies in different models and stages of development of hypertension. In analogy to the high renin renal hypertension model, which shows blood pressure decreases on peripheral and central angiotensin blockade (85,127), and the low renin DOCA-salt hypertension model, which shows blood pressure increases in response to peripheral and central AII blockade (45), certain forms of spontaneous hypertension in rats have a more pronounced brain AII component (SH-NZ, SH-SP) and respond with blood pressure decreases to central but not to peripheral AII blockade. In other strains of spontaneously hypertensive rats (SH-BM) or at a later phase of development, other factors (e.g., salt, volume) may be important for the maintenance of high blood pressure. These hypertensive rats respond with blood pressure increases to central administration of saralasin. The importance of brain AII is documented by the following facts: (a) in some spontaneously hypertensive rats (NZ and SP strain) blood pressure decreases in response to intraventricular but not to intravenous saralasin; (b) blood pressure remains elevated after

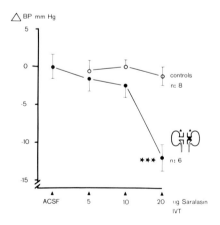

FIG. 3–17. Effect of intraventricular administration of saralasin on arterial blood pressure of conscious renal hypertensive rats. In this "high-renin" model one artery was stenosed by silver clip; the other kidney was intact. See legend for Fig. 3–16.

nephrectomy; (c) the blood pressure-decreasing effect of AII blockade persists after nephrectomy; (d) the AII-immunoreactive material is elevated in CSF of SH-NZ rats; and (e) the central and peripheral responses can be dissociated in spontaneously hypertensive rats and rats with some forms of renal hypertension(85).

CONCLUSION

In conclusion, the information available to date supports the view that AII-like peptides in brain as in other tissues may be involved in the control of a large number of biological functions. One important new aspect is the potential role of the peptide as a transmitter or a modulator substance within neurons of the central nervous system and the peripheral nervous system. This may be an additional way that angiotensin participates in blood pressure and thirst regulation.

ACKNOWLEDGMENTS

The work reported here was supported by grants from Deutsche Forschungsgemeinschaft "Cardiovaskuläres System, SFB 90" and the Swedish Medical Research Council. The authors wish to thank Dr. A. K. Johnson for his constructive criticisms in preparation of this manuscript. The competent secretarial help of Mrs. M. Funke is acknowledged.

REFERENCES

1. Abraham, S. F., Baker, R. M., Blaine, E. H., Denton, D. A., and McKinley, M. J. (1975): Water drinking induced in sheep by angiotensin—a physiological or pharmacological effect? *J. Comp. Physiol. Psychol.*, 88:503–518.
2. Andersson, B., Leksell, G., and Lishajko, F. (1975): Perturbations in fluid balance induced by medially placed forebrain lesions. *Brain Res.*, 19:261–275.
3. Anson, M. L. (1937): The estimation of cathepsin with hemoglobin and the partial purification of cathepsin. *J. Gen. Physiol.*, 20:565–574.
4. Bangham, R., Robertson, J., Robertson, J. I. S., Robinson, C. I., and Tree, M. (1975): An international collaborative study of renin assay: Establishment of the international reference preparation of human renin. *Clin. Sci. Mol. Med.*, 48:135–159.
5. Baxter, C. R., Horvath, J. S., Furby, F. H., and Tiller, D. J. (1976): Endogenous angiotensin in brain. Abstracts of V International Congress of Endocrinology, Hamburg, July 18–24.
6. Bennet, J. B., and Snyder, S. H. (1976): Angiotensin II binding to mammalian brain membranes. *J. Biol. Chem.*, 251:7423–7430.
7. Bing, J., and Poulsen, K. (1971): The renin system in mice. Effects of removal of kidneys or (and) submaxillary glands in different strains. *Acta Pathol. Microbiol. Scand. [A]*, 79:134–138.
8. Bloom, F., Battenberg, E., and Rossier, J., Ling, N., Leppaluoto, J., Vargo, T. M., and Guillemin, R. (1977): Endorphins are located in the intermediate and anterior lobes of the pituitary gland, not in the neurohypophysis. *Life Sci. (in press)*.
9. Buckley, J. P. (1972): Actions of angiotensin on the central nervous system. *Fed. Proc.*, 31:1332–1337.

10. Buranarugsa, P., and Hubbard, J. S. (1976): Angiotensin receptors in the rat sub-fornical organ in vitro. *Proc. Univ. Otago Med. School,* 54:3–4.
11. Chalmers, J. P. (1975): Neuropharmacology of central mechanisms regulating pressure. In: *Central Action of Drugs in Blood Pressure Regulation,* edited by D. Davies and J. L. Reid, pp. 36–60. Pitman Medical, London.
12. Changaris, D. G., Demers, L. M., Keil, L. C., and Severs, W. B. (1977): Immuno-pharmacology of angiotensin I in rat brain. In: *Symposium on the Central Actions of Angiotensin and Related Hormones,* edited by J. P. Buckley and C. M. Ferrario, pp. 233–243. Pergamon Press, New York.
13. Cohen, S., Taylor, J. M., Murakami, K., Michelakis, A. M., and Inagami, T. (1972): Isolation and characterization of renin-like enzymes from mouse submaxillary glands. *Biochemistry,* 23:4286–4292.
14. Cooling, M. J., and Day, M. D. (1973): Antagonism of central dipsogenic and peripheral vasoconstrictor responses to angiotensin II with sar^1-ala^8-angiotensin II in the conscious rat. *J. Pharm. Pharmacol.,* 25:1005–1010.
15. Cooling, M. J., and Day, M. D. (1974): Inhibition of renin-angiotensin induced drinking in the cat by enzyme inhibitors and by analogue antagonists of angiotensin II. *Clin. Exp. Pharmacol. Physiol.,* 1:389–396.
16. Coons, A. H. (1958): Flourescent antibody methods. In: *General Cytochemical Methods,* edited by J. F. Danielli, pp. 399–422. Academic Press, New York.
17. Dahlström, A., and Fuxe, K. (1964): Evidence for the existence of monoamine containing neurons in the central nervous system. I. Demonstration of monoamines in the cell bodies of brain system neurons. *Acta Physiol. Scand.* [*Suppl.* 232], 62: 1–55.
18. Daul, C. B., Heath, R. G., and Garey, R. E. (1975): Angiotensin-forming enzyme in human brain. *Neuropharmacology,* 14:75–80.
19. Day, R. P., and Reid, I. A. (1976): Renin activity in dog brain: Enzymological similarity to cathepsin D. *Endocrinology,* 99:93–100.
20. Deshmukh, P., and Phillips, M. I. (1977): Effect of horseradish peroxidase and angiotensin. *Anat. Rec.* (*in press*).
21. Elghozi, J. L., Altman, J., Devynck, M. A., Liard, J. F., Grunfeld, J. P., and Meyer, P. (1976): Lack of hypotensive effect of central injection of angiotensin inhibitors in spontaneously hypertensive and normotensive rats. *Clin. Sci. Mol. Med.,* 51:385s–389s.
22. Epstein, A. N., Fitzsimons, J. T., and Johnson, A. K. (1974): Peptide antagonists of the renin-angiotensin system and the elucidation of the receptors for angiotensin-in-duced drinking. *J. Physiol.* (*Lond.*), 238:34–35.
23. Epstein, A. N., and Ganten, D. (1977): *Unpublished observations.*
24. Erdös, E. G. (1975): Angiotensin I converting enzyme. *Circ. Res.,* 36:247–254.
25. Fahrer, A., Speck, G., Bayer, C., Sponer, G., Schelling, P., Ganten, U., and Ganten, D. (1977): *Unpublished observations.*
26. Felix, D., and Akert, K. (1974): The effect of angiotensin II on neurons of the cat subfornical organ. *Brain Res.,* 76:350–353.
27. Ferrario, C. M., Gildenberg, P. L., and McCubbin, J. W. (1972): Cardiovascular effects of angiotensin mediated by the central nervous system. *Circ. Res.,* 30:257–262.
28. Finkielman, S. (1973): The brain renin-angiotensin system. Its physiological role. *Acta Physiol. Lat. Am.,* 23:111.
29. Finkielman, S., Fischer-Ferraro, C., Diaz, A., Goldstein, D. J., and Nahmod, V. E. (1972): A pressor substance in the cerebrospinal fluid of normotensive and hyper-tensive patients. *Proc. Natl. Acad. Sci. USA,* 69:3341–3344.
30. Fischer-Ferraro, C., Nahmod, V. E., Goldstein, D. J., and Finkielman, S. (1971): Angiotensin and renin in rat and dog brain. *J. Exp. Med.,* 133:353–361.
31. Fischer, H., Flügel, R. M., Schelling, P., and Ganten, D. (1975): Differences in endogenous iso-renin in normal and SV 40 transformed 3T3 mouse cells: Correla-tion with cell growth. *Int. Res. Commun.,* 3:327.
32. Fitzsimons, J. T. (1972): Thirst. *Physiol. Rev.,* 52:468–561.
33. Fitzsimons, J. T. (1976): The physiological basis of thirst. *Kidney Int.,* 10:3–11.
34. Fitzsimons, J. T., Epstein, A. N., and Johnson, A. K. (1977): The peptide specificity of receptors for angiotensin-induced thirst. In: *Central Actions of Angiotensin and*

Related Hormones, edited by J. P. Buckley and C. Ferrario, pp. 405–415. Pergamon Press, New York.

35. Forman, B. H., and Mulrow, P. J. (1974): Effect of propranolol on blood pressure and plasma renin activity in the spontaneously hypertensive rat. *Circ. Res.,* 35:215–221.
36. Fuxe, K., Ganten, D., Hökfelt, T., and Bolme, P. (1976): Immunohistochemical evidence for the existence of angiotensin II containing nerve terminals in the brain and spinal cord of the rat. *Neurosci. Lett.,* 2:229–234.
37. Fuxe, K., Hökfelt, T., Bolme, P., Goldstein, M., Johansson, O., Johansson, G., Lidbrink, P., Ljungdahl, A., and Sachs, C. (1975): The topography of central catecholamine pathways in relation to their possible role in blood pressure control. In: *Central Action of Drugs in Blood Pressure Regulation,* edited by D. S. Davies and J. L. Reid, pp. 8–23. Pitman Medical, London.
38. Fuxe, K., Hökfelt, T., and Ungerstedt, U. (1970): Morphological and functional aspects of central monoamine neurons. *Int. Rev. Neurobiol.,* 13:93–126.
39. Ganten, D. (1972): Studies on the existence of an independent brain renin-angiotensin system: A model for extrarenal tissue renin. Ph.D. thesis, Department of Experimental Medicine, McGill University, Montreal, Canada.
40. Ganten, D., Boucher, R., and Genest, J. (1971): Renin activity in brain tissue of puppies and adult dogs. *Brain Res.,* 33:557–559.
41. Ganten, D., Boucher, R., Granger, P., and Genest, J. (1973): Quelques aspects nouveaux sur le système rénine-angiotensine. *Union Med. Can.,* 102:775–786.
42. Ganten, D., Ganten, U., Kubo, S., Granger, P., Nowaczynski, W., Boucher, R., and Genest, J. (1974): Iso-renin in rat adrenal glands: Influence of sodium, potassium and pituitary hormones. *Am. J. Physiol.,* 227:224–229.
43. Ganten, D., Ganten, U., Schelling, P., Boucher, R., and Genest, J. (1975): The renin and iso-renin angiotensin system in rats with experimental pituitary tumors. *Proc. Soc. Exp. Biol. Med.,* 148:568.
44. Ganten, D., Granger, P., Ganten, U., Boucher, R., and Genest, J. (1952): An intrinsic renin-angiotensin system in the brain. In: *Hypertension '72,* edited by J. Genest and E. Koiw, pp. 432–435. Springer-Verlag, Berlin.
45. Ganten, D., and Gross, F. (1976): Angiotensin-Antagonisten zur Diagnostik und Behandlung des reninabhängigen Hochdrucks. *Med. Klin.,* 71:2043–2050.
46. Ganten, D., Hayduk, K., Brecht, H. M., Boucher, R., and Genest, J. (1970): Evidence of renin release or production in splanchnic territory. *Nature,* 226:551–552.
47. Ganten, D., Hutchinson, J. S., Ganten, U., and Schelling, P. (1976): The intrinsic iso-renin angiotensin system in brain and its relationship to the classical kidney renin angiotensin system. In: *Central Nervous Control of Sodium Balance: Relation to the Renin Angiotensin System,* edited by W. Kaufmann and D. Krause, pp. 35–44. Thieme Verlag, Stuttgart.
48. Ganten, D., Hutchinson, J. S., Haebara, H., Schelling, P., Fischer, H., and Ganten, U. (1976): Tissue iso-renins. *Clin. Sci. Mol. Med.,* 51:117s–120s.
49. Ganten, D., Hutchinson, J. S., and Schelling, P. (1975): The intrinsic brain iso-renin angiotensin system: Its possible role in central mechanisms of blood pressure regulation. *Clin. Sci. Mol. Med.,* 48:265s–268s.
50. Ganten, D., Hutchinson, J. S., Sponer, G., Ganten, U., and Fischer, H. (1976): The iso-renin angiotensin systems in extrarenal tissue. *Clin. Exp. Pharmacol. Physiol.,* 2:103–126.
51. Ganten, D., Kusumoto, M., Constantopoulos, G., Ganten, U., Boucher, R., and Genest, J. (1973): Iso-renin, electrolytes and catecholamines in dog brain: Possible interrelationship. *Life Sci.,* 12:1–8.
52. Ganten, D., Marquez-Julio, A., Granger, P., Hayduk, K., Karsunky, K. P., Boucher, R., and Genest, J. (1971): Renin in dog brain. *Am. J. Physiol.,* 221:1733–1737.
53. Ganten, D., Minnich, J. L., Granger, P., Hayduk, K., Brecht, H. M., Barbeau, A., Boucher, R., and Genest, J. (1971): Angiotensin-forming enzyme in brain tissue. *Science,* 173:64–65.
54. Ganten, D., Schelling, P., Vecsei, P., and Ganten, U. (1976): Iso-renin of extrarenal origin. The tissue angiotensinogenase systems. *Am. J. Med.,* 60:760–772.
55. Genest, J., Rojo-Ortega, J. M., Kuchel, O., Boucher, R., Nowaczynski, W., Le-

febvre, R., Chrétien, M., Cantin, J., and Granger, P. (1975): Malignant hypertension with hypokalemia in a patient with renin-producing pulmonary carcinoma. *Trans. Assoc. Am. Physicians,* 88:192–201.

56. Goldstein, B. M., and Brody, M. J. (1976): Pressor response to intravertebral angiotensin II: Abolition by central catecholamine depletion. In: *Regulation of Blood Pressure by the Central Nervous System,* edited by G. Onesti, M. Fernandes, and K. E. Kim, pp. 183–189. Grune & Stratton, New York.
57. Goldstein, D. J., Diaz, A., Finkielman, S., Nahmod, V. E., and Fischer-Ferraro, C. (1972): Angiotensinase activity in rat and dog brain. *J. Neurochem.,* 19:2451–2452.
58. Goldstein, D. J., Fischer-Ferraro, C., Nahmod, V. E., and Finkielman, S. (1970): Angiotensin I in renal and extra-renal tissues. *Medicina,* 30:81–83.
59. Greenbaum, L. M. (1971): Cathepsins and kinin-forming and -destroying enzymes. In: *The Enzymes, Vol. III, Hydrolysis of Peptide Bonds, Ed. 3,* edited by P. D. Boyer, pp. 475–483. Academic Press, New York.
60. Grynbaum, A., and Marks, N. (1976): Characterization of a rat brain catheptic carboxypeptidase (cathepsin A) inactivating angiotensin II. *J. Neurochem.,* 26:313–318.
61. Hauger-Klevene, J. H. (1970): High plasma renin activity in an oat cell carcinoma: A renin secreting carcinoma? *Cancer,* 26:1112–1114.
62. Hayduk, K., Boucher, R., and Genest, J. (1970): Renin activity content in various tissues of dogs under different physiopathological states. *Proc. Soc. Exp. Biol. Med.,* 1:252–255.
63. Hayduk, K., Ganten, D., Boucher, R., and Genest, J. (1972): Arterial and urinary renin activity. In: *Hypertension '72,* edited by J. Genest and E. Koiw, pp. 435–443. Springer-Verlag, Berlin.
64. Hoffman, W. E., Ganten, D., Schelling, P., Haebara, H., Phillips, M. I., and Mann, J. F. E. (1977): In: Acquisitions récentes en radioimmunologie, compte-rendus du IIIᵉ colloque international de radioimmunologie de Lyon, 1976, edited by C. A. Bizollon, H. Bornet, B. Claustrat, J. Corniau, R. Mornex, J. Sassard, J. Tourniaire, and M. Vincent, pp. 47–82.
65. Hoffman, W. E., and Phillips, M. I. (1976): The effect of subfornical organ lesions and ventricular blockade on drinking induced by angiotensin II. *Brain Res.,* 108:59–73.
66. Hoffman, W. E., and Phillips, M. I. (1976): Regional study of cerebral ventricle sensitive sites to angiotensin II. *Brain Res.,* 109:1–18.
67. Hoffman, W. E., and Phillips, M. I. (1976): Evidence for sar¹-ala⁸-angiotensin crossing the blood cerebrospinal fluid barrier to antagonize central effects of angiotensin II. *Brain Res.,* 109:541–552.
68. Hoffman, W. E., Schelling, P., Phillips, M. I., and Ganten, D. (1976): Evidence for local angiotensin formation in brain of nephrectomized rats. *Neurosci. Lett.,* 3:299–303.
69. Hökfelt, T., Elde, R., Johansson, O., Luft, R., and Arimura, A. (1975): Immunohistochemical evidence for the presence of somatostatin, a powerful inhibitory peptide, in some sensory neurons. *Neurosci. Lett.,* 1:231–235.
70. Hökfelt, T., Kellerth, J.-O., Nilsson, G., and Pernow, B. (1975): Experimental immunohistochemical studies on the localization and distribution of substance P in cat primary sensory neurons. *Brain Res.,* 100:235–252.
71. Hutchinson, J. S., Schelling, P., and Ganten, D. (1975): Effect of centrally administered angiotensin II and P 113 on blood pressure in conscious rats. *Pflügers Arch.,* 355 (Suppl.):R28.
72. Hutchinson, J. S., Schelling, P., Möhring, J., and Ganten, D. (1976): Pressor action of centrally perfused angiotensin II in rats with hereditary hypothalamic diabetes insipidus. *Endocrinology,* 99:819–823.
73. Hutchinson, J. S., Schelling, P., Möhring, J., and Ganten, D. (1976): Effect of intraventricular perfusion of angiotensin II in conscious normal rats and in rats with hereditary hypothalamic diabetes insipidus. *Clin. Sci. Mol. Med.,* 51:391s–394s.
74. Inagami, T., Misono, K., and Michelakis, A. M. (1974): Definitive evidence for similarity in the active site of renin and acidic protease. *Biochem. Biophys. Res. Commun.,* 2:503–509.

75. Johnson, A. K. (1975): The role of the cerebral ventricular system in angiotensin-induced thirst. In: *Control Mechanisms of Drinking,* edited by G. Peters, J. T. Fitzsimons, and L. Peters-Haefeli, pp. 117–122. Springer-Verlag, Berlin.

76. Johnson, A. K., and Buggy, J. (1977): A critical analysis of the site of action for the dipsogenic effect of angiotensin II. In: *Central Actions of Angiotensin and Related Hormones,* edited by J. P. Buckley and C. Ferrario, pp. 357–386. Pergamon Press, New York.

77. Johnson, A. K., and Epstein, A. N. (1975): The cerebral ventricles as the avenue for the dipsogenic action of intracranial angiotensin. *Brain Res.,* 86:399–418.

78. Johnson, A. K., and Schwob, J. E. (1975): Cephalic angiotensin II receptors mediating drinking to systemic angiotensin II. *Pharmacol. Biochem. Behav.,* 3:1077–1084.

79. Keil, L. C., Summy-Long, J., and Severs, W. B. (1975): Release of vasopressin by angiotensin II. *Endocrinology,* 96:1063–1065.

80. Ledingham, J. G., and Leary, W. P. (1974): Catabolism of angiotensin II. In: *Angiotensin. Handbook of Experimental Pharmacology,* edited by I. H. Page and F. M. Bumpus, pp. 111–125. Springer-Verlag, Berlin.

81. Lee, D. R. (1973): Plasma renin activity in genetically hypertensive rats measured by a radioimmunoassay of angiotensin I. *Proc. Univ. Otago Med. School,* 51:34–35.

82. Lee, M. R. (1969): *Renin and Hypertension.* Lloyd-Luke, London.

83. Lewis, G. P., and Reit, E. (1966): Further studies on the actions of peptides on the superior cervical ganglion and suprarenal medulla. *Br. J. Pharmacol.,* 26:444–460.

84. Malayan, S. A., and Reid, I. A. (1976): Antidiuresis produced by injection of renin into the third cerebral ventricle of the dog. *Endocrinology,* 98:329–335.

85. Mann, J. F. E., Phillips, M. I., Haebara, H., Lüth, B., Dietz, R., and Ganten, D. (1976): Wirkung von intraventrikulär und intravenös injiziertem Saralasin auf den Blutdruck renal und spontan hypertoner Ratten. *Therapiewoche,* 26:7553.

86. Marks, N., and Lajtha, A. (1965): Separation of acid and neutral proteinases of brain. *Biochem. J.,* 97:74–83.

87. McKown, M. M., Workman, R. J., and Gregerman, R. I. (1974): Pepstatin inhibition of human renin kinetic studies and estimation of enzyme purity. *J. Biol. Chem.,* 748:7770–7774.

88. McLean, A. S., Sirett, N. E., Bray, J. J., and Hubbard, J. I. (1975): Regional distribution of angiotensin II receptors in the rat brain. *Proc. Univ. Otago Med. School,* 53:19–20.

89. Michelakis, A. M., Cohen, S., Taylor, J., Murakami, K., and Inagami, T. (1974): Studies on the characterization of pure submaxillary gland renin. *Proc. Soc. Exp. Biol. Med.,* 147:118–121.

90. Minnich, J. L., Ganten, D., Barbeau, A., and Genest, J. (1972): Subcellular localization of cerebral renin-like activity. In: *Hypertension '72,* edited by J. Genest and E. Koiw, pp. 432–435. Springer-Verlag, Berlin.

91. Nahmod, V. E., Finkielman, S., de Gorodner, O. S., Goldstein, D. J. (1977): On the neural localization and the physiological variations of brain angiotensin. In: *Central Actions of Angiotensin and Related Hormones,* edited by J. P. Buckley and C. Ferrario, pp. 573–578. Pergamon Press, New York.

92. Nahmod, V. E., Fischer-Ferraro, C., Finkielman, S., Diaz, A., and Goldstein, D. J. (1972): Renin and angiotensin in extrarenal tissues. *Medicina,* 32 (Suppl. 1):43–47.

93. Nicoll, R. A., and Barker, J. L. (1971): Excitation of supraoptic neurosecretory cells by angiotensin II. *Nature [New Biol.],* 233:172–173.

94. Oldendorf, W. H. (1971): Brain uptake of radiolabelled amino acids, amines, and hexoses after arterial injection. *Am. J. Physiol.,* 6:1629–1639.

95. Oldendorf, W. H. (1974): Blood-brain barrier permeability to drugs. *Annu. Rev. Pharmacol.,* 14:239–248.

96. Page, I. H., and McCubbin, J. W. (Eds.) (1974): *Renal Hypertension.* Year Book Medical Publishers, Chicago.

97. Phillips, M. I., and Felix, D. (1976): Specific angiotensin II receptive neurons in the cat subfornical organ. *Brain Res.,* 109:531–540.

98. Phillips, M. I., Felix, D., Hoffman, W. E., and Ganten, D. (1977): Angiotensin receptor sites in the brain ventricular system. In: *Neuroscience Symposium,* edited by

W. M. Cowan and J. A. Ferrendelli, pp. 308–339. Society for Neuroscience, Bethesda, Maryland.

99. Phillips, M. I. and Hoffman, W. E. (1977): Sensitive sites in the brain for the blood pressure and drinking responses to angiotensin II. In: *Central Actions of Angiotensin and Related Hormones,* edited by J. P. Buckley and C. Ferrario, pp. 325–356. Pergamon Press, New York.

100. Phillips, M. I., Hoffman, W. E., Felix, D., and Ganten, D. (1976): Nachweis von Angiotensinrezeptoren im Gehirn. *Therapiewoche,* 26:7548.

101. Phillips, M. I., Mann, H., Dietz, R., and Ganten, D. (1977): Lowering of hypertension by central saralasin in the absence of plasma renin: A role for brain isorenin-angiotensin. *Science (in press).*

102. Poth, M. M., Heath, R. G., and Ward, M. (1975): Angiotensin-converting enzyme in human brain. *J. Neurochem.,* 25:83–85.

103. Poulsen, K. (1973): Kinetics of the renin system. The basis for determination of the different components of the system. *Scand. J. Clin. Lab. Invest.,* 31 (Suppl. 132).

104. Printz, M. P., and Lewicki, J. A. (1977): Renin Substrate in the CNS: Potential Significance to Central Regulatory Mechanisms. In: *Central Actions of Angiotensin and Related Hormones,* edited by J. P. Buckley and C. Ferrario, pp. 57–64. Pergamon Press, New York.

105. Reid, I. A., and Day, R. P. (1977): Interactions and properties of some components of the renin-angiotensin system in brain. In: *Central Actions of Angiotensin and Related Hormones,* edited by J. P. Buckley and C. Ferrario, pp. 267–282. Pergamon Press, New York.

106. Reid, I. A., and Ramsay, D. J. (1975): The effects of intracerebroventricular administration of renin on drinking and blood pressure. *Endocrinology,* 97:536–542.

107. Roth, M., Weitzman, A. F., and Piquilloud, Y. (1969): Converting enzyme content of different tissues of the rat. *Experientia,* 25:1247, 1969.

108. Saad, W., Epstein, A. N., Simpson, J. B., and Camargo, L. A. (1975): Brain and blood-borne angiotensin II in the control of thirst. *Neurosci. Abstr.,* 1:470.

109. Sakai, K. K., Marks, B. H., George, J., and Koestner, A. (1974): Specific angiotensin II receptors in organ-cultured canine supra-optic nucleus cells. *Life Sci.,* 14:1337–1344.

110. Schelling, P., Ganten, D., Heckl, R., Hayduk, K., Hutchinson, J. S., Sponer, G., and Ganten, U. (1977): On the origin of angiotensin-like peptides in cerebrospinal fluid. In: *Central Actions of Angiotensin and Related Hormones,* edited by J. P. Buckley and C. Ferrario, pp. 519–526. Pergamon Press, New York.

111. Schelling, P., Hutchinson, J. S., Ganten, U., Sponer, G., and Ganten, D. (1976): Impermeability of the blood-cerebrospinal fluid barrier for angiotensin II in rats. *Clin. Sci. Mol. Med.,* 51:399s–402s.

112. Schoelkens, B. A., Jung, W., and Steinbach, R. (1976): Blood pressure response to central and peripheral injection of angiotensin II and 8-C-phenylglycine analogue of angiotensin II in rats with experimental hypertension. *Clin. Sci. Mol. Med.,* 51:403s–406s.

113. Sen, S., Ferrario, C. M., and Bumpus, F. M. (1974): Alteration in the feedback control of renin release by an angiotensin antagonist. *Acta Physiol. Lat. Am.,* 24:149–532.

114. Severs, W. B., and Daniels-Severs, A. E. (1973): Effects of angiotensin on the central nervous system. *Pharmacol. Rev.,* 25:415–449.

115. Severs, W. B., Summy-Long, J., Taylor, J. S., and Connor, J. D. (1970): A central effect of angiotensin: Release of pituitary pressor material. *J. Pharmacol. Exp. Ther.,* 27:174–186.

116. Shade, R. E., and Share, L. (1975): Vasopressin release during nonhypotensive hemorrhage and angiotensin II infusion. *Am. J. Physiol.,* 228:149–154.

117. Shiono, K., and Sokabe, H. (1973): Plasma renin activity in the spontaneously hypertensive rat of early hypertensive stage. *Jpn. Heart J.,* 14:168–169.

118. Simpson, J. B., Epstein, A. N., and Camardo, J. S. (1975): Ablation or competitive blockade of subfornical organ (SFO) prevents thirst of intravenous angiotensin. *Fed. Proc.,* 24:374.

119. Sinaiko, A., and Mirkin, B. L. (1974): Ontogenesis of the renin-angiotensin system in spontaneously hypertensive and normal Wistar rats. *Circ. Res.*, 34:693–696.
120. Skeggs, L. T., Dorer, F. E., Kahn, J. R., Lentz, K. E., and Levine, M. (1976): The biochemistry of the renin-angiotensin system and its role in hypertension. *Am. J. Med.*, 60:737–748.
121. Skeggs, L. T., Dorer, F. E., Kahn, J. R., Lentz, K. E., and Levine M. (1974): The biological production of angiotensin. In: *Handbook of Experimental Pharmacology*, edited by I. H. Page and F. M. Bumpus, pp. 1–16. Springer-Verlag, Berlin.
122. Slaven, B. (1975): Influence of salt and volume on changes in rat brain angiotensin. *J. Pharm. Pharmacol.*, 27:782–783.
123. Suketa, Y., and Inagami, T. (1975): Active site directed inactivators of mouse submaxillary renin. *Biochemistry*, 14:3188–3194.
124. Summy-Long, J., and Severs, W. B. (1974): Angiotensin and thirst: Studies with a converting enzyme inhibitor and a receptor antagonist. *Life Sci.*, 15:569–582.
125. Swanson, L. W., Marshall, G. R., Needleman, P., and Sharpe, L. G. (1973): Characterization of central angiotensin II receptors involved in the elicitation of drinking in the rat. *Brain Res.*, 49:441–446.
126. Swanson, L. W., and Sharpe, L. G. (1973): Centrally induced drinking: Comparison of angiotensin II- and carbachol-sensitive sites in rats. *Am. J. Physiol.*, 225:566–572.
127. Sweet, C. S., Columbo, J. M., and Gaul, S. L. (1976): Central antihypertensive effects of inhibitors of the renin angiotensin system in rats. *Am. J. Physiol.*, 231:1794–1799.
128. Sweet, C. S., Columbo, J. M., Gaul, S. L., Weitz, D., and Wenger, H. C. (1977): Inhibitors of the renin-angiotensin system in rats with malignant and spontaneous hypertension: Comparative antihypertensive effects of central vs. peripheral administration. In: *Central Actions of Angiotensin and Related Hormones*, edited by J. P. Buckley and C. Ferrario, pp. 283–292. Pergamon Press, New York.
129. Symonds, E. M., Stanley, M. A., and Skinner, S. L. (1968): Production of renin by in vitro cultures of human chorion and uterine muscle. *Nature*, 217:1152–1153.
130. Vincent, M., Sassard, J., and Cier, J. F. (1972): Méthode rapide de détermination radio-immunochimique de l'activité rénine du plasma. *Rev. Eur. Etud. Clin. Biol.*, 17:1001–1006.
131. Volicer, L., and Loew, C. G. (1971): Penetration of angiotensin II into the brain. *Neuropharmacology*, 10:631–636.
132. Ward, D. G., and Gunn, C. G. (1976): Locus coeruleus complex: Elicitation of a pressor response and a brain stem region necessary for its occurrence. *Brain Res.*, 107:401–406.
133. Weindl, A., and Joynt, R. J. (1971): The median eminence as a circumventricular organ. In: *Brain Endocrine Interaction*, edited by K. M. Knigge, D. E. Scott, and A. Weindl, pp. 280–297. S. Karger, Basel.
134. Wislocki, G. B., and King, L. S. (1936). The permeability of the hypophysis and hypothalamus to vital dyes. *Am. J. Anat.*, 58:421–472.
135. Yang, H.-Y., and Neff, N. H. (1972): Distribution and properties of angiotensin converting enzyme of rat brain. *J. Neurochem.*, 19:2443–2450.
136. Yang, H.-Y., and Neff, N. H. (1973): Differential distribution of angiotensin converting enzyme in the anterior and posterior lobe of the rat pituitary. *J. Neurochem.*, 21:1035–1036.
137. Yokoyama, H. (1976): Studies on the simultaneous measurement of plasma renin activity and plasma aldosterone concentration in patients with various endocrine, hypertensive, edematous diseases; Its clinical evaluation and significance. *Folia Endocrinol. Jpn.*, 52:729–750.
138. Zahn, P., and Ganten, D. (1976): Influence of $^{+}$H-ion concentrations and of prostaglandins on the activity of extrarenal angiotensinogenases. *Naunyn Schmiedebergs Arch. Pharmacol.*, 293 (Suppl.):R 36.

Frontiers in Neuroendocrinology, Vol. 5,
edited by W. F. Ganong and L. Martini.
Raven Press, New York © 1978.

Chapter 4

The Neuroendocrinology of Thirst and Salt Appetite

Alan N. Epstein

Institute of Neurological Sciences,
University of Pennsylvania,
Philadelphia, Pennsylvania 19174

Thirst is a phenomenon of motivated behavior and therefore cannot have a simple neurologic mechanism. It is aroused by at least two separate afferent systems, each linked to one of the water compartments of the body (53). It is obedient, in most mammals, to the daily light-dark cycle (155). It occurs in close contiguity with eating behavior (95). It is ruled by cognitive processes such as learning (112) and anticipation (69), and must also be controlled by the hedonic consequences of the fluid being drunk even when only water is ingested and especially when the chemical composition of the fluid alters its taste (55,154).

This chapter reviews the neuroendocrine aspects of thirst and focuses on the neural mechanism by which angiotensin arouses drinking. But the novelty and success of this research enterprise must not tempt us into repeating the error that discouraged research on the neuropsychology of thirst during the first half of this century when it was mistakenly asserted that because thirst was a sensation and drinking behavior was a reflex, an understanding of dryness of the oropharynx would provide the explanation for both (32,33). Angiotensin must not become the new oversimplification of the mechanism of thirst. It is not the hormone of thirst. It is, rather, the endocrine participant in a complex neurological process for which simple explanations no longer suffice.

The complex context of current research on the neurology of thirst began with Andersson's report (7) of the elicitation of drinking by hyperosmotic stimulation of the brain of the goat. Conscious animals showing no interest in water drank avidly, sometimes massively, when stimulated briefly in the anterior hypothalamus with small volumes of hypertonic saline or, in later experiments, with weak electric currents. In addition, simple tasks that the animals had previously learned in order to gain access to water after deprivation were performed in the absence of deprivation while stimulation was applied to the same sites in the goats' brains from which drinking had been obtained (11). The sites of effective injection or stimulation occupied a zone of hypothalamic tissue lying in the anterior and lateral hypothalamic region along the trajectory of the mammalothalamic tract. These reports, vividly demonstrating the arousal of thirst by stimulation of the brain, had two important conceptual consequences. First, they ended preoccupation with thirst as a mere sensation, and with drinking behavior as a simple association of reduced salivary flow with dehydration (32). And, second, they made a reality of predictions of a central neural basis for thirst as a form of instinctive (98) and motivated (153) behavior.

Lesion studies confirmed the existence of a "thirst center" (or more properly a major focus of the neurological systems for thirst) in the hypothalamus when dogs (10) and rats (107) were rendered adipsic by ablations of tissues within the medial forebrain bundle of the lateral hypothalamus. The failure to drink was prolonged and quite specific. The animals refused water for the rest of their postoperative lives but ate palatable diets and drank nutritive fluids such as beef broth and thereby maintained themselves alive and well.

In this work of the mid 1950s and early 1960s, emphasis was given almost exclusively to the thirst of cellular dehydration, first proposed by Wettendorff (173) and then established as a mechanism of thirst by Gilman's well-known experiments (79). Andersson's use within the brain of hyperosmotic solutions which dehydrated the cells that they superfused led quite naturally to widespread interpretation of his experiments as showing the behavioral effects of stimulation of detectors within the brain of water loss from cells analogous to the osmoreceptors that Verney (169) invoked for vasopressin release. With this work a neural basis for the thirst of cellular dehydration was clearly foreseen.

An endocrine basis for thirst was not accepted until Fitzsimons (59,60) established hypovolemia or reduced blood volume as an independent stimulus for thirst. He did so by eliciting water intake in rats with a variety of experimental manipulations (hemorrhage, ligation of the inferior vena cava, hyperoncotic colloid dialysis), all of which reduced the circulating blood volume without an increase in the osmolarity of the remaining plasma and therefore without withdrawal of water from cells. This essential point has since been confirmed by Tang (163) whose recent work shows, first, that hyperoncotic colloid dialysis reduces the plasma volume of rats without altering serum electrolytes or osmolarity, and, second, that if the reduction in intravascular volume is prevented by intravenous infusion of a plasma substitute, drinking is suppressed. Earlier work had shown that thirst was generated by deficits in serum sodium (34), which must have led to contraction of plasma volume accompanied by overhydration of cells, but interpretation of the drinking that followed sodium deficiency was limited to dry-mouth theorizing. Adolph et al. (4), on the other hand, had predicted with unusual prescience that thirst must be controlled by multiple factors. He pointed out that the stimulus for drinking could not be osmotic pressure alone and included changes in extracellular volume among the other stimuli that must be considered. But this did not express the idea of hypovolemia as a second and coequal stimulus of thirst capable of operating under normal conditions of dehydration and having an independent sensory system using detectors of reduced blood volume. This concept we owe to Fitzsimons (see 66 for a full summary). The hypovolemic stimulus has since been shown to have a low threshold for the initiation of drinking (156), to generate water intake as a function of the magnitude of the reduction in blood volume (156), to add its stimulation of thirst quantitatively to a concurrent stimulus to cellular dehydration (40,70), and to yield thirst with the expected properties of motivation (81,136). And, as this chapter emphasizes, the hormone system renin-angiotensin has been shown to be an important participant in its arousal (63,65).

The demonstration that both cellular dehydration and the loss of extracellular volume are each separately competent for the arousal of thirst has suggested the *double depletion hypothesis of thirst* (53), which assumes that water loss arouses thirst by two physiological mechanisms with afferent systems that are separately tuned either to the cellular or to the extracellular compartment for body water. The nature of the receptors for the two depletions, the portions of the brain devoted to their appreciation, and the manner of their joint function in the control of spontaneous drinking behavior are the major concerns of current research on the neurology of thirst (see 17, 48, and 66 for more general reviews).

DIPSOGENIC ROLE OF ANGIOTENSIN

The role of angiotensin in thirst and the several perspectives from which it is viewed must be introduced by a brief review of the work leading to the discovery of the dipsogenic role of angiotensin. As already noted, the discovery grew out of Fitzsimons' revival of the study of the thirst of hypovolemia. Having shown that an isotonic decrease in plasma volume aroused thirst in rats, Fitzsimons (60) found that several of the treatments he employed to produce hypovolemia depended on the maintenance of the circulation through the kidneys for their full dipsogenic effect (61). This is shown most clearly in the data reproduced in Fig. 4–1 and Table 4–1 from Fitzsimons' studies of the

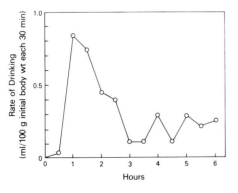

FIG. 4–1. Drinking induced in 6 hr immediately after caval ligation. See text. From Fitzsimons (61).

TABLE 4–1. *Drinking in the 6 hr following caval ligation in nephrectomized or ureteric ligated rats*

Treatment	Water drunk (ml/100 g initial body wt.)	Change in body wt. (g/100 g initial body wt.)
Caval ligation and bilateral nephrectomy (N = 15)	1.60 ± 0.25	+0.54 ± 0.21
Sham caval ligation and bilateral nephrectomy (N = 15)	1.20 ± 0.45	−0.25 ± 0.20
Caval ligation and bilateral ureteric ligation (N = 12)	3.04 ± 0.47	+1.76 ± 0.47
Sham caval ligation and bilateral ureteric ligation (N = 15)	1.12 ± 0.30	+0.13 ± 0.55

From Fitzsimons (61).

thirst that follows caval ligation. Figure 4–1 records the half-hourly water intake of rats after ligation of the inferior vena cava. The surgery was performed under ether, permitting the study of behavior within a short time after reduction of the circulating blood volume. Drinking began in the first hour, continued throughout most of the 6-hr observation period, and was considerable (data are given as milliliters drunk per 100 g body weight; the animals weighed 300 to 400 g). Table 4–1 shows that this impressive phenomenon occurs only if the kidneys remain in the circulation. In nephrectomized animals, caval ligation produced only a slight increase in the water intake generated by the removal of the kidneys *per se*. Caval ligation remained dipsogenic when the kidneys' excretory function was abolished by ureteric ligation (compare 3.04 ml/100 g intake in the caval and ureteric ligation group with 1.12 ml/100 g in the group subjected to ureteric ligation alone). These differences in intake are confirmed by the changes in body weight. Fitzsimons saw from these and similar data that the kidneys played a major role in the thirst of hypovolemia, but as an endocrine rather than as an excretory organ.

There were allusions to this idea in earlier work. A Spanish group (102), having found that extracts of kidney provoked excess water intake in rats, had, in fact, suggested that renin may be dipsogenic. Others (12,114) had reported the dipsogenic effect of renal extracts as an incidental finding. But the Spanish group (88) rejected their own suggestion when renal extracts that were presumed to contain renin did not yield increased drinking. Fitzsimons' meticulous and comprehensive work (62) avoided this error. Kidney extracts prepared in his laboratory and shown to contain renin by their pressor action were dipsogenic when given to rats by intraperitoneal injection. The dipsogenic action was destroyed by boiling and enhanced by prior nephrectomy as would be expected of renin. Renin was then shown to be dipsogenic in a dose-dependent manner, and angiotensin II infused intravenously stimulated thirst in the satiated rat (72). Equally as important as the experimental demonstrations themselves was Fitzsimons' clear recognition of the appropriateness of the renal hormone for the regulation of body water. He pointed out that renin is released from the kidney by hypovolemia, among other stimuli, and that in addition to sustaining blood pressure and releasing aldosterone the renin-angiotensin system provides the kidney with a means for participation in the control of thirst which is the behavioral defense against reduced blood volume. This occurs while the brain is appreciating the hypovolemic state by receipt of afferents from volume receptors and is orchestrating the kidney's primary response to hypovolemia by releasing vasopressin to promote the conservation of water from tubular urine. By fitting the renal hormone into the nexus of physiological and behavioral events that are mobilized by the brain and kidney to defend body water volume, Fitzsimons made the idea of a stimulus of thirst of renal origin both clear and attractive.

DIPSOGENIC EFFECT OF PHYSIOLOGICAL DOSES OF ANGIOTENSIN

A series of experiments has now shown that angiotensin stimulates thirst at reasonable physiologic doses when testing is done under conditions that mimic those that must prevail when the hormone participates in spontaneous drinking (87). When the hormone is given intravenously after full recovery from the artifacts of surgery, with the animal in its home cage and without the disturbance of restraint and manipulation, rats drink reliably to doses of the hormone (Fig. 4–2) that are the same as those that provoke a mild to moderate pressor response (83). These hormone doses are similar to or less than those employed to produce the other effects of the hormone in animals that have not been nephrectomized (120). Moreover, the dose-response relationship is linear until strong pressor doses are reached. As shown by the

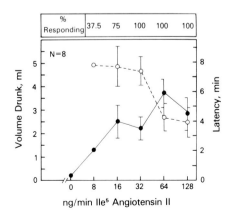

FIG. 4–2. Dose-response curve of drinking (*left ordinate*) and latency to the onset of drinking (*right ordinate*) as a function of intravenous dose of angiotensin II. Percent of animals responding at each dose is given in box above. From (87).

interrupted line in Fig. 4–2, latencies to the onset of drinking are short (6 to 8 min at the lowest 100% effective dose). The thirst induced by intravenous angiotensin is blocked by concurrent infusion of specific competitive inhibitors of angiotensin (52,164). Other pharmacological agents such as isoproterenol that are potent dipsogenic stimuli have been found to release renin (122) and to rely for their dipsogenic action on the receipt of angiotensin by the brain (127). Water deprivation provokes renin release (103) as does the ingestion of a meal (16), and both are reliable predictors of drinking behavior.

In addition, Hsiao, Epstein, and Camardo (87) showed that the dipsogenic dose of angiotensin is reduced to 4 ng/rat/min (10 ng/kg/min) when the hormone infusion is preceded by a pulse injection of sodium chloride that by itself is too small to be reliably dipsogenic. These results are shown in Table 4–2, which gives the individual data for each animal in the experiment. In four separate tests each animal received either the low dose of angiotensin or saline intravenously and each infusion was preceded either by the low dose of extracellular solute (1 ml of 0.3 M NaCl, s.c.) or by a subcutaneous injection of saline. The double saline condition (fourth column) produced very little drinking. Neither 4 ng/min/rat of angiotensin II (second column) nor 1 ml of 0.3 M NaCl (third column) induced drinking in more than half of the rats studied. The combined treatment resulted in drinking in all six. Latencies were short and the amounts drunk were quite representative of the size of the average draft taken by rats drinking spontaneously (95). When it is remembered that the infused hormone is diluted in approximately 20 ml of plasma in an adult rat, and that it is rapidly degraded, the 4 to 10 ng/rat/min dose is physiologically quite reasonable. The intact, uninfused animal has 30 pg/ml or 600 pg/rat of angiotensin II in its circulation at rest (80). This figure can

TABLE 4–2. Effect of a prior injection of 0.3 M NaCl on the dipsogenic response to intravenous angiotensin II

	Intravenous A II, 4 ng/min				Intravenous isotonic saline			
	0.3 M NaCl, s.c.		Iso. saline, s.c.		0.3 M NaCl, s.c.		Iso. saline, s.c.	
Animal	vol. (ml)	lat.	vol. (ml)	lat.	vol. (ml)	lat.	vol. (ml)	lat.
1	1.6	6'45"	0.0	17'30"	1.1	11'45"	0.9	9'40"
2	1.8	30"	0.5	4'30"	1.9	4'15"	0.0	17'30"
3	0.8	3'20"	0.0	17'30"	0.0	17'30"	0.0	17'30"
4	1.9	9'35"	2.0	1'25"	1.2	5'25"	0.2	45"
5	2.4	3'10"	0.0	17'30"	0.0	17'30"	0.0	17'30"
6	0.7	3'10"	0.3	9'50"	0.0	17'30"	0.0	17'30"
Mean	1.53	4'25"	0.47	11'23"	0.70	12'19"	0.18	13'24"
SE	0.27	1'19"	0.31	2'57"	0.33	2'32"	0.15	2'50"
Percent responding	100		50		50		33.3	

vol., volume drunk; lat., latency; iso., isotonic.

rise by an order of magnitude when renin is released (97) to reach levels of 6 ng/rat.

Drinking to physiological doses of angiotensin has also been shown in dogs (166). Animals were infused continuously for either 10 days at 13 ng/kg/min or 8 days at 26 ng/kg/min. Daily water intakes were clearly increased under both conditions, the average intake more than doubling at the lower dose. The increase was greater with the higher dose ($N = 2$, 302 and 903 ml/day during vehicle infusion, 657 and 1,705 ml/day during angiotensin infusion). The lower dose also produced a moderate and sustained elevation of blood pressure but did not increase plasma aldosterone levels. Levels of blood angiotensin that are attained by injection of 13 ng/kg/min for several hours (200 to 300 pg/ml plasma) are well within those that are produced by stimuli of renin release in the dog. Confirmation has recently been obtained by J. T. Fitzsimons, J. Kucharczyk, and G. Richards (*personal communication*), who have produced drinking in all dogs tested with as little as 3 ng/kg/min of angiotensin II infused into the carotid artery. The failure of sheep to drink to intravenous angiotensin (2) is the result of differences either of species or of experimental design.

Angiotensin appears to be dipsogenic in humans as well. Elevations of plasma renin produced by several pathological conditions (38) are associated with intense thirst and excessive water intake (26). Rogers and Kurtzman (134) reported that excess water intake disappeared in a patient with chronic kidney disease after both kidneys were removed and the renin level fell.

ELICITATION OF THIRST BY INTRACRANIAL ANGIOTENSIN

Direct action of angiotensin on the brain was shown first as an incidental finding by Booth (22), demonstrated definitively by Epstein et al. (51) and Severs et al. (142), and confirmed by Swanson and Sharpe (161). In these experiments rats drank copiously and repeatedly within tens of seconds or minutes after injection of angiotensin II into their brains. The response was quite specific, both behaviorally, because only drinking behavior was elicited, and chemically, because among the many agents tested (vasopressin, oxytocin, aldosterone, kallikrein, bradykinin, epinephrine, and cyclic AMP) only angiotensin was dipsogenic (51,64,65). Subsequent experiments showed that the precursors of angiotensin II (renin, renin substrate, and angiotensin I) were highly dipsogenic in the brain and that the first degradation product (des-asp angiotensin II) had 50% the dipsogenic potency of the intact octapeptide (64). Secondly, it was shown that the drinking was blocked or attenuated by prior treatment of the brain with antibodies against angiotensin II (49) and with competitive inhibitors of angiotensin or its precursors (39,50). Thirdly, it was found that the phenomenon was biologically ubiquitous. All species that have been tested drink to intracranial angiotensin. This includes a variety of rodents, several ungulates (sheep and goat), carnivores (dog and cat), the monkey, birds (ring-dove and chicken), and the iguana. Fourthly, it became clear that the brain is a uniquely sensitive site when drinking was obtained with doses of 1.2 ng (162). And, lastly, the thirst elicited by angiotensin was shown to have normal motivational characteristics (94,135,136). Intracranial administration of angiotensin suppresses feeding, produces drinking despite quinine adulteration of the water, and generates lever pressing for water in animals that have been trained to do so after water deprivation (81).

DISCOVERY OF THE ROLE OF THE SUBFORNICAL ORGAN

Fitzsimons' experiments, especially those employing intravenous infusion (72) made the dipsogenic action of angiotensin clear. But progress in understanding how it interacts with the brain was obstructed by the impenetrability of the blood-brain barrier to circulating peptides. If angiotensin could not reach cerebral tissue, how did it produce thirst? Where were the receptors for its dipsogenic action? The solution to this vexing problem was provided by the important work of Simpson and his colleagues who showed, beginning in 1973 (149), that the subfornical organ (SFO), which is in the brain but outside the barrier, contains the required receptors.

This problem of the means by which the hormone gains access to the brain was posed by the demonstration that angiotensin is excluded from the intrinsic tissues of the brain (119,144). Tritium-labeled angiotensin II with high biological activity, even when used in intravenous doses as high as 2 μg, did not concentrate in any portion of the parenchyma of the brain, including the anterior hypothalamic-septal region that Epstein et al. (51) had identified as the sensitive zone for the dipsogenic action of the hormone. Severs and colleagues (142) had previously used the lateral ventricle as a convenient site of injection in studies concerned with vasopressin release and the central pressor effect of the hormone, and autoradiographs suggested that the blood-borne hormone reached periventricular sites such as the area postrema (170). But the significance of the periventricular structures was not appreciated until Johnson and Epstein (90) showed that injection was effective only if it was made through cannulas that passed through a ventricular space, permitting the hormone to follow the outer wall of the cannula and enter the ventricular fluid. This process is shown in Fig. 4–3, which is an autoradiograph of adjacent sections through the tract left in a rat's forebrain by a cannula through which 4 ng of tritiated angiotensin II was injected several minutes before the animal was sacrificed. Note that the hormone has reached all parts of the cannula tract and has passed through the foramen of Monroe to perfuse the entire anterior ventricular system including the contralateral lateral ventricle. The conclusion drawn from earlier studies that angiotensin-sensitive sites were widely distributed in the anterior forebrain (51) could now be rejected as an artifact of ventricular leakage. When these same sites (preoptic area

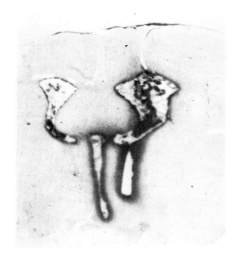

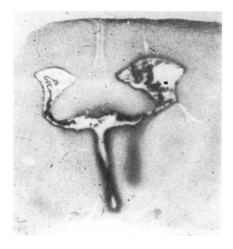

FIG. 4–3. Autoradiographs of adjacent sections from a rat's forebrain showing the spread of angiotensin throughout the ventricular system following injection of 1 μl of radioactive angiotensin solution through a cannula that transversed a lateral ventricle. All darkened areas (except the dorsal edge of the sections) are reduced grains. The cannula opened into the anterior hypothalamus-preoptic region as shown in the upper section. The lower section shows the confluence of the foramina of Monroe and the third ventricle with the subfornical organ in its roof at the midline. Note the absence of grains between the cannula tract and the wall of the third ventricle. Unstained sections autoradiographed while frozen. From (90).

and anterior hypothalamus) were reached in the Johnson and Epstein experiments (90) by cannulas that did not traverse a ventricle, they were inert for doses of angiotensin as high as 128 ng, and, unlike effective sites elsewhere in the brain, injection of radiolabeled angiotensin through them did not result in the appearance of radioactivity in the cisternal CSF. Moreover, periventricular sites were further implicated when Johnson and Schwob (91) found that ventricular injection of competitive inhibitors of angiotensin II were uniquely effective in suppressing thirst induced by angiotensin that had been injected peripherally.

Simpson and Routtenberg were led to their precedent-making work by an interest in the thirst induced by intracranial carbachol (84). Believing that it exerts its dipsogenic effect by acting on tissue lining the ventricles, they focused their attention on the subfornical organ of the third ventricle because of the richness of its choline acetyltransferase and acetylcholinesterase content. Ablation of the organ reduced or abolished the rat's drinking response to carbachol (148), and injection of cholinergic agents directly into the organ elicited drinking at low doses, with short latencies (150).

The subfornical organ is one of the family of circumventricular structures (6,172) which are midline specializations of the ependyma, richly vascularized, in contact over one surface with the cerebrospinal fluid, and outside the blood-brain barrier (175). This final characteristic made the subfornical organ an attractive candidate for the brain's sensor of angiotensin in its dipsogenic role. The area postrema, a circumventricular organ in the wall of the fourth ventricle, had already been shown to be a receptor organ for the central pressor response of angiotensin II (see 46 for review). The location of the subfornical organ at the dorsal-anterior extremity of the third ventricle between the foramina of Monroe placed it in an ideal position for exposure to angiotensin that was injected into the lateral ventricle. At the time of Simpson and Routtenberg's work (148), this was either deliberately or inadvertently the most frequent route of administration of the hormone. When the organ was ablated in rats that were drinking an average of 14 ml in response to 100 or 500 ng of angiotensin II injected into the anterior forebrain, six of seven animals did not drink postoperatively (149). Lesions in adjacent tissue had no effect. Moreover, drinking behavior (spontaneous drinking, drinking induced by water deprivation) was not disturbed by the subfornical organ ablations, except for a brief postoperative hypodipsia.

CONFIRMATION OF THE ROLE OF THE SUBFORNICAL ORGAN

Lesion studies by themselves, even when they produce specific deficits, cannot demonstrate hormone receptor structures in the brain. They must be complemented by a demonstration that the presumed receptor organ has uniquely high sensitivity to direct application of the active agent. The effect produced should be a faithful mimic of that which occurs when the hormone reaches the brain from the blood. In addition, direct application of specific inhibitors of the hormone to the presumed receptor organ should suppress its action. The suppression should be limited to the effects of the blood-borne hormone, and it should be reversible. The subfornical organ has now met all these criteria (146).

Figure 4–4 shows the dose-response curve for drinking elicited by angiotensin II injected directly into the subfornical organ of the rat. The hormone was injected (in a volume of 1.0 μl) from a remote syringe while the animal rested quietly in its home cage. Experiments were conducted during the daylight hours when spontaneous drinking is rare and were completed in 15 to 20

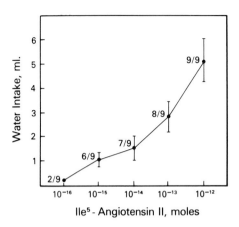

FIG. 4–4. Dose-response curve of drinking produced by injection of angiotensin II directly into the subfornical organ. See text. From (146).

min. Spontaneous drinking is very infrequent under these circumstances, and saline injection elicited only rare drinking of small volumes. In all nine animals studied, the tip of the injector opened into the body of the subfornical organ without rupture of the limiting ependyma of the third ventricle. The fractions adjacent to the curve in Fig. 4–4 are response fractions that give the number of animals tested at each dose (denominator) and the number drinking to that dose (numerator). The dose range explored extended from 10^{-16} to 10^{-12} moles. Figure 4–4 shows that the threshold dose (50% of animals responding) was between 0.1 and 1.0 pg of angiotensin II (10^{-16} to 10^{-15} moles). At 1 ng (10^{-12} moles), all animals drank and the average intake was considerably greater than the average draft size for the rat when it is drinking spontaneously (95). The behavior elicited at all doses was normal in all respects and indistinguishable from that which is elicited by low intravenous doses of the hormone (87). The animals roused themselves and moved, usually quite directly, to the water spout. They drank in one or two drafts, then groomed and retired to the rear of the cage, sometimes after a brief bout of restless motion. There were no behavioral artifacts and eating was not elicited. In other animals in which the cannulas had penetrated the ependyma and opened into the ventricular space, or had missed the body of the subfornical organ and lay in adjacent tissue such as the ventral commissure of the fornix, the threshold for drinking was two or three orders of magnitude higher. This threshold was similar to that reported by others (161) for ventricular injection or for injection into tissue adjacent to ventricular compartments. Thus, the sensitivity of the subfornical organ for the dipsogenic action of angiotensin is high, and it is unique among all other sites that have been tested within the brain. Responsiveness to 0.1 to 1.0 pg is reasonable for a hormone that circulates in the rat at a concentration of 30 to 100 pg/ml of plasma (1,80). Moreover, the angiotensin II antagonist saralasin (sarcosine-1, alanine-8 angiotensin II, or P113) in large doses (20 to 200 ng/min for 30 min) elicited very little drinking, showing that the requirements of the subfornical organ receptors are chemically quite specific.

The criterion of specific and reversible blockade was met in the Simpson, Epstein, and Camardo (146) experiments with the use of saralasin. This angiotensin analogue has been shown to block the pressor response of intravenous angiotensin II and the dipsogenic actions of both intravenous (164) and intraventricular angiotensin (50). The inhibitor was infused into the subfornical organ for a 30-min period, during the last 20 min of which the animal received an intravenous infusion of angiotensin II at a high dose (50 or 64 ng/min/rat). The data from 2 of the 27 rats studied in this way are shown in Fig. 4–5. When isotonic saline was infused into the subfornical organ, there was no inhibition of angiotensin-induced drinking. When the competitive inhibitor of angiotensin II perfused the organ, drinking induced by intravenous angiotensin was suppressed. The suppression was reversible, and at the highest dose shown (20 pg/min), it was complete. Infusion of the antagonist into the overlying ventral commissure of the fornix also blocked the drinking, but only at doses that were two orders of magnitude higher. Infusions into the third ventricle did not block the drinking until very high and debilitating doses were used. The effect of the inhibitor was specific for angiotensin-induced thirst; thirst induced by systemic cellular dehydration was not suppressed.

The Simpson, Epstein, and Camardo experiments (146) also show that ablation of the organ abolishes the drinking produced by intravenous infusion of angiotensin. This confirms the results of Simpson and Routtenberg (149), and avoids the artifact of injection of high doses of angiotensin. Instead, physiologically reasonable doses of angiotensin were given (87) by a technique that closely imitates the route by which the hormone normally reaches the brain. Animals that suffered a loss of 95% or more of the organ did not drink to intravenous angiotensin even when it was given in doses that were frankly hypertensive (128 ng/min/rat). The complete unresponsiveness of the animals whose subfornical organs had been ablated (lowest curve, labeled SFO in Fig. 4–6) contrasts with the normal responsiveness to intra-

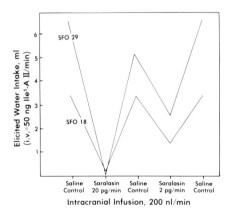

FIG. 4–5. Reversible blockade of drinking induced by intravenous angiotensin II produced by infusion of saralasin into the subfornical organ (SFO). Note complete blockade at higher dose and complete reversibility when saline is infused. From (146).

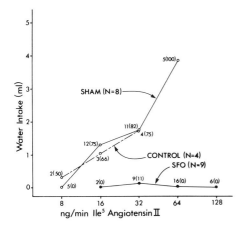

FIG. 4–6. The abolition of drinking induced by intravenous angiotensin II that follows ablation of the subfornical organ (SFO). See text. From (146).

venous angiotensin of animals without brain damage (sham) and those with damage to adjacent structures (control). Drinking to cellular dehydration and deprivation were not reduced, nor were there abnormalities of spontaneous drinking once the animals had recovered from the brief hypodipsia that follows damage to the subfornical organ. The failure to drink is therefore specific to angiotensin-induced thirst. Complete unresponsiveness to intravenous angiotensin II was found 80 to 84 days after subfornical ablation. The organ is therefore essential for the dipsogenic action of the hormone.

This impressive body of evidence is strengthened by the following additional demonstrations: (a) as shown by radioimmunoassay, blood levels of renin (105) and of angiotensin II (1,137) are elevated after hypovolemic thirst stimuli; (b) as shown by autoradiography using doses of hormone as low as 400 ng, tritiated angiotensin II can reach the circumventricular organs from the blood while being excluded from the intrinsic tissues of the brain (144); and (c) as shown by electrophysiology, there are cells within the subfornical organ that respond selectively to angiotensin II (see below).

ELECTROPHYSIOLOGICAL IDENTIFICATION OF ANGIOTENSIN-SENSITIVE UNITS IN THE SUBFORNICAL ORGAN

In important studies reported by Felix and Akert (58) and by Phillips and Felix (123), the subfornical organ of the cat was exposed *in situ* and studied by microiontophoretic application of angiotensin II, saralasin, and acetylcholine (Fig. 4–7). In one study (123), 50 spontaneously active units were studied. Twenty-two responded to angiotensin II. Of these, 19 increased their rate of discharge as the injection current increased, in confirmation of Felix and Akert's earlier demonstration of a dose-response relationship between ejected angiotensin II and unit discharge rate (Fig. 4–7, *left*). Eighteen of these units ceased their response to angiotensin II during concurrent ejec-

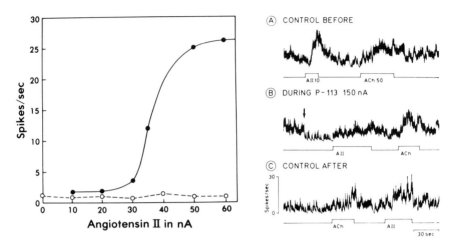

FIG. 4–7. *Left:* Dose-response curve to microiontophoretically applied angiotensin II of a single sensitive unit in the subfornical organ. Dotted line is absence of response to isotonic saline. From (58). *Right:* Specific blockade of angiotensin II-sensitive unit by concurrent application of saralasin (P-113). A II, angiotensin II; ACh, acetylcholine. From (123).

tion of the specific peptide antagonist. The unit shown in Fig. 4–7 (*right*) is responsive to both angiotensin II and acetylcholine (record A). Seven of the twenty-two units showed such dual responsiveness. The blocker produced an immediate slowing of the rate of spontaneous firing followed by a blockade of the excitation produced by exogenous angiotensin II (record B). The acetylcholine response was unaffected, and there was rapid recovery (record C). Ten units that responded exclusively to angiotensin II were completely suppressed by saralasin, whereas the same dose of saralasin did not completely inhibit the seven units with dual responsiveness. The selective response of units within the subfornical organ to angiotensin II and their great sensitivity to blockade by a specific angiotensin antagonist are what would be expected of cells bearing specific receptors for the hormone.

CONTROVERSIAL ISSUES IN RESEARCH ON ANGIOTENSIN-INDUCED THIRST

Role of Angiotensin in Spontaneous Drinking

Although there is general agreement that angiotensin is a potent dipsogen, and that it is more potent than agents such as carbachol and norepinephrine (100), objections have been raised to the proposal that it contributes to spontaneous drinking and to the thirst of water deprivation. Water deprivation depletes both the cellular and extracellular water compartments, and the action of the hormone can provide only part of the mechanism by which it produces thirst. Although intravenous infusion of a competitive inhibitor of angiotensin II has little or no effect on the water intake of water-deprived dogs (126) and sheep (3), infusion of the inhibitor into the cerebral ventricles of rats partially reduces deprivation-induced thirst (104). Similarly, intraventricular infusion of saralasin (138) or infusion of it directly into the subfornical organ reduces (146) and in some species may abolish (127) thirst generated by beta-adrenergic activation. Intravenous infusion of the inhibitor is said to be ineffective (164). The thirst of hyperoncotic colloid dialysis which survives nephrectomy and almost certainly employs afferents from the low-pressure baroreceptors is reduced 52% by infusion of saralasin into the subfornical organ prior to and during access to water (146). As expected, cellular dehydration thirst is not diminished by nephrectomy (59) and is unaffected by saralasin no matter how administered (146). Thus, it is clear that the thirst challenge presented to the animal, the species studied, and the technique employed to reduce or block circulating angiotensin are crucial to the outcome of experiments on this subject. It appears that pharmacological blockade of endogenously released angiotensin with techniques that deliver the blocker into extracellular fluid immediately adjacent to the dipsogenic receptors are to be preferred. In addition, studies of the dynamics of the renin-angiotensin system that are addressed to its role in thirst should employ infusion of the active hormone itself and its direct measurement rather than measurement of its precursors such as plasma renin activity (158), which tends to overestimate the contemporary angiotensin concentration.

Alternatives to Subfornical Organ Receptors

Objections have been raised to the claim of exclusivity of the subfornical organ as the site of the receptors for the dipsogenic action of angiotensin. Mogenson and his colleagues (106) have proposed additional receptors sites in the preoptic area. They recorded excitation of single units in the lateral hypothalamic area and the ventral tegmentum of the midbrain after injection of angiotensin into the ipsilateral preoptic area, and have reported (15) that lesions of the lateral hypothalamus ipsilateral to the preoptic cannula through which angiotensin is injected into the rat brain produce more severe impairment of drinking than symmetrical contralateral lesions. These findings are most easily interpreted as the result of damage to hypothalamic and midbrain pathways that are aroused by receptor tissue in the preoptic area. However, this idea is contradicted by the failure of angiotensin to elicit thirst when injected into the preoptic area, even in high doses, unless the cannula traverses the anterior ventricles (90).

Recovery of the dipsogenic action of angiotensin has been reported (30) within 10 to 14 days after what have been described as complete lesions of the subfornical organ. The hormone was injected into the lateral ventricle, and the temporary reduction of its dipsogenic action was attributed to blockade of the foramen of Monroe by lesion debris and edema. The proximity of the subfornical organ to the foramina makes the risk of such blockade a reality, but the issue of recovery once the blockade has been relieved rests on the completeness of subfornical organ destruction. Given the extreme sensitivity of the organ, even small portions of it could mediate thirst when doses of 100 ng or more of angiotensin II are used, as was the case in these experiments. Simpson et al. (146) produced complete and permanent abolition of the dispogenic effect of blood-borne angiotensin, and there can be no artifact of ventricular obstruction underlying these results.

Obstruction of the ventricular lumen with injected cold cream (29,86) has produced two results that can be explained only with recourse to hypothetical receptors for the dipsogenic action of angiotensin at some site in the brain other than the subfornical organ. In these experiments the high doses of the hormone that were used support the argument of the work. On the one hand, drinking occurred when the cold cream occluded access to the subfornical organ, and on the other hand, drinking did not occur when the cold cream covered the anterior-ventral third ventricle, in the region of the lamina terminalis and organum vasculosum lamina terminalis (OVLT), leaving the dorsal third ventricle and the subfornical organ uncovered and exposed to hormone reaching it through the foramen of Monroe. However, these findings rely on a technique that is not yet fully validated. It is not clear that postmortem examination reveals where the cold cream was at the time of the intraventricular injections, nor is it clear from published reports that the cream had selectively occluded the portions of the ventricular surface being studied. Both the subfornical organ and the OVLT lie in the anterior surface of the third ventricle and they are close together. Cold cream injections into the area may have occluded both structures [see, in particular, Fig. 5, rat 720 from (86)].

Angiotensin II acts on receptors in the area postrema (46,167) and in the central gray of the midbrain (45) for its central pressor action, and it is a potent releaser of vasopressin (109,121,140). It may act in the latter role and others at receptors that have been identified pharmacologically (14) and microiontophoretically (82,171) in many parts of the forebrain including the vicinity of the supraoptic nucleus (116). Research in hand does not exclude the possibility that alternative receptors for the dipsogenic action of the hormone exist within the parenchyma of the brain. But they cannot mediate thirst induced by blood-borne angiotensin because subfornical organ ablation completely abolishes that effect even when high intravenous doses are employed (146). In addition, they cannot be sensitive to blood-borne angiotensin that may reach the spinal fluid from the blood because this has now been excluded by careful radioimmunoassay of spinal fluid during intravenous infusion of high doses of angiotensin II (143). The alternative receptors, if they exist, may appreciate changes in the levels within the brain of angiotensin that has been generated by the cerebral isorenin system (77), but it must be noted that the proposals of such receptors (124) rest heavily on lesion studies and in no case do such lesions produce a specific loss of the thirst induced by angiotensin (9,89). Therefore, these studies have not distinguished between a receptor zone for angiotensin, a region containing transmission or integrative systems for thirst stimuli of several kinds, or brain damage that alters the readiness with which angiotensin that has been injected into the brain can reach subfornical organ receptors.

Andersson denies the necessity for specialized receptors for the dipsogenic action of angiotensin (8). He assumes that the hormone acts by rendering hypothetical sodium receptors more permeable to CSF sodium. He draws the suggestion from a multiplicative (rather than simply additive) relationship between the dipsogenic effects of intraventricular sodium chloride and angiotensin in his experiments with the goat (8). Although additive effects of combined sodium chloride and angiotensin stimulation have been reported (67), and cells have been found in the lateral hypothalamus and zona incerta that are excited by electrophoresis of both sodium ions and angiotensin II (118, 171), the multiplicative phenomenon on which Andersson's idea depends has not been confirmed in other species (28,67,162).

SATIETY SYSTEMS FOR ANGIOTENSIN-INDUCED THIRST

Septal Inhibitory System

Massive septal lesions in the rat enhance the drinking induced by dipsogenic treatments that are mediated in whole or in part by angiotensin. Such animals are spontaneously hyperdipsic postoperatively (85), but their excessive drinking is selective. They do not drink more to cellular dehydration and in most cases do not drink prandially as a consequence of a salivary deficit (19). They drink more than normal rats to ligation of the vena cava, release of endogenous renin by beta-adrenergic agonists, injection of exogenous renin, and intravenous infusion of angiotensin. Electrical stimulation of the septum has been reported to specifically suppress thirst in which the renin-angiotensin system participates (20). This has led to the suggestion that the septum contains a neural system that is specifically inhibitory for the thirst mediated by angiotenisn (19,21). Although this idea remains attractive, recent studies of this problem have left the full meaning and the neurologic basis of the phenomenon unclear. Cells have been found in the septum (25) that respond to thirst challenges, but they respond to both cellular dehydration and hypovolemia, implying a more general role in thirst. This is consistent with the finding that electrical stimulation of ventral portions of the septum suppresses thirst aroused by water deprivation (174) and drinking elicited by electrical stimulation of the lateral hypothalamus (145) without reducing food intake (108). Moreover, hyperdipsia without exaggeration of hypovolemic thirst has been produced in 55% of rats with ventral knife cuts of the septum (165). Curiously, the knife cuts that completely isolated the septum by interrupting its blood supply and resulting in its disappearance from the brain did not increase daily water intake. In addition, we have no explanation for the fact that the electrolytic lesions that produce the hyperdipsia by massive ablation of virtually the entire septum produce decreases in whole brain acetylcholine content that correlate with the degree of hyperdipsia (151). Such lesions may also alter the blood supply of the subfornical organ, which is adjacent to the triangular nucleus of the septum posterior to the septal complex, or make this organ more susceptible to angiotensin in the blood or spinal fluid. Therefore, the full meaning of this interesting phenomenon and its relationship to angiotensin-induced drinking are still unclear.

Prostaglandins of Cerebral Origin

The prostaglandin Es (PGE) synthesized within the brain provide another interesting possibility for inhibitory control of thirst, and particularly of those thirsts in which angiotensin plays a role. Kenney and Epstein (92,93) reported that when injected into the lateral cerebral ventricle prostaglandins E_1 and E_2 (but not the prostaglandins A or F_{2a}) suppress drinking induced by angiotensin. The suppression is effective at doses as low as 10 ng/rat (Fig. 4–8) and is not an artifact of anorexia or of the pyrexic effects of the intracranial injection of the PGEs. The data shown in Fig. 4–8 were generated from experiments in which all animals received 5 ng of angiotensin II into the lateral cerebral ventricle accompanied by the vehicle solution for the prostaglandins (bar labeled VEH). On a subsequent day they received both the angiotensin and prostaglandin E_1 at the dose indicated. They were then tested again without prostaglandin, and if their original drinking response

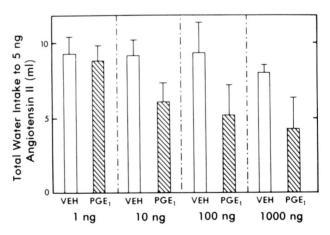

FIG. 4–8. Dose-response relationship between the suppression of angiotensin-induced drinking and prostaglandin E_1 (PGE$_1$). In all experiments rats received 5 ng angiotensin II into the lateral cerebral ventricle accompanied by the vehicle for PGE$_1$ (VEH), or PGE$_1$ at the doses shown. From (93).

was unimpaired their data were used. The finding has been confirmed. Phillips and Hoffman (124) have prolonged the drinking induced by intracranial angiotensin with prior injection of a prostaglandin synthetase inhibitor, and Nicolaïdis and Fitzsimons (115) have shown that the suppressive effect can be produced by vasoplegic drugs such as nitroprusside and papavarine as well as PGE_1. N. J. Kenney, S. Fluharty, and A. N. Epstein (*unpublished observations*) tested the suppressive effects of the PGEs against those of other thirst challenges and found that as the dose of prostaglandin increased, the range of the antidipsogenic effect of the hormone expanded. All thirsts tested (intracranial angiotensin, intracranial carbachol, systemic hypovolemia, and water deprivation) were affected except the thirst of cellular dehydration. The effectiveness of the suppression appeared to increase with increasing dependence of the thirst stimulus on angiotensin. These investigators proposed that as angiotensin activates the subfornical organ it concurrently stimulates the synthesis of the prostaglandin Es, perhaps in the organ itself. The prostaglandins then participate in the suppression of thirst by their vasodilator action. This has the interesting conceptual corollary that the activation of thirst by angiotensin itself may be vasoactive; as suggested by Epstein and Hsiao (52) and Nicolaïdis and Fitzsimons (115), the hormone may act on specialized vascular beds in the brain just as it does in the peripheral blood vessels. It may produce vasoconstriction which is then transduced into a neural signal contributing to the arousal of thirst. A recent report of increased drinking during prostaglandin infusion of the cerebral ventricle (101 cannot be reconciled with Kenney's work. It occurred only during exposure of the brain to large doses of prostaglandin (approximately 1 μg/min for 30 min).

G. DeCaro, L. G. Micossi, and M. Massi (*personal communication*) have reported similar results with eledoisin, a peptide of amphibian origin that resembles substance P. They found that intraventricular eledoisin (250 to 1,000 ng) had a marked antidipsogenic effect without depressing food intake or producing other behavioral modifications. The thirsts induced by angiotensin II and carbachol as well as by water deprivation were depressed. Substance P was also antidipsogenic in these experiments, and the authors suggest that since substance P is found in the brain in mammals, it may be a natural satiator of thirst. The possibility of a physiological role for antidipsogens that are endogenous to the brain is a most promising one for future research, and there may be several having different modes of action.

The most well-established satiator of the thirst induced by angiotensin and, in fact, of all thirst is rehydration either by drinking or by passive administration of water. Stricker (157) has shown that both cellular and extracellular thirst are best satiated by water ingestion, and Blass and Hall (18) have added the important insight that maximum satiety is achieved when the rehydration occurs in contiguity with the act of water ingestion. The neurology and possible endocrinology of the satiety produced by water itself is unknown.

Nature of Cerebral Receptors for Angiotensin

Neuropharmacological work has made a very clear contribution to the question of the nature of the receptors within the brain for the dipsogenic action of angiotensin. When Fitzsimons (64,65) showed that all of the precursors of angiotensin (renin, artificial renin substrate, and angiotensin I) were dipsogenic in the brain, the possibility was opened of multiple receptors for the dipsogenic effect, in particular receptors for both angiotensin I and angiotensin II. He also demonstrated that des-aspartyl angiotensin II (angiotensin III) had half the dipsogenic potency of angiotensin II. Lehr et al. (99) demonstrated enhancement of the dipsogenic effect of several thirst stimuli (beta-adrenergic stimulation, caval ligation, hypovolemia of hyperoncotic colloid, and water deprivation) when conversion of angiotensin I to II was prevented by peripheral administration of a blocker of the converting enzyme. Furthermore, the enhancement did not occur for thirsts heavily dependent on renin when the converting enzyme blocker was given into the cerebral ventricles. These findings suggested that when unconverted angiotensin I is in excess in the circulation it reaches receptors in the brain and contributes to the thirst of some but not all dipsogens.

A series of experiments, recently concluded, has clarified this issue by defining the dipsogenic receptor as one that best accommodates angiotensin II (68). The strategy of the work is shown in Fig. 4–9, which recapitulates the synthetic cascade leading from renin substrate to angiotensin II and depicts a model receptor for the octapeptide harbored within the brain, but outside the

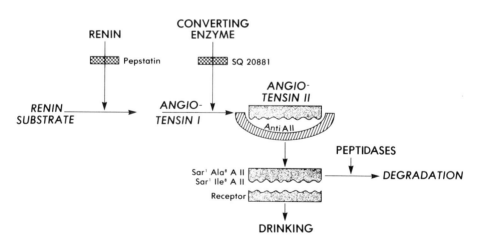

FIG. 4–9. Schematic summary of experiments demonstrating the octapeptide specificity of the receptor for the dipsogenic action of angiotensin. Synthetic sequence begins with renin substrate *(left)* and ends with degradation products *(right)* of angiotensin II. Competitive inhibitors of renin (pepstatin) and converting enzyme (SQ 20881) suppress drinking induced by renin and angiotensin I, respectively. Anti-angiotensin II antibodies (Anti-A II) block drinking induced by angiotensin II, as do competitive analogues (Sar[1] Ala[8] and Sar[1] Ile[8] A II) of angiotensin II. From (68).

blood-brain barrier (see discussion of subfornical organ). In all the work summarized in Fig. 4–9, a component of the renin-angiotensin system was delivered into the anterior ventricles of the rat brain just after an anti-angiotensin II antibody, or a pharmacological blocker or a competitive inhibitor of angiotensin II, in the pairings shown in Fig. 4–9. Carbachol was used throughout and its dipsogenic effect was not reduced, demonstrating that the suppressions obtained were quite specific for the interactions between the pharmacological agents and the components of the renin-angiotensin system. Treatments that prevented the generation of angiotensin II (competitive inhibition of substrate or converting enzyme) or that interfered with angiotensin II access to receptors (anti-angiotensin II antibodies or competitive analogues of angiotensin II) reduced or abolished the drinking. These studies confirmed an early suggestion of Severs et al. (141) who combined angiotensin I or II and a blocker of conversion in the ventricles of rats and found that only the dipsogenic effect of angiotensin I was impaired. Conflicting reports (27,31, 160) have been based on molal ratios of blocker to agonist that were too low to be effective.

A complete renin-angiotensin system has been identified within the brain, including an isoenzyme of renin, a renin substrate, and a converting enzyme, and it appears that angiotensin can be produced endogenously within the brain (Chapter 3; *this volume*). Moreover, high-affinity binding sites for angiotensin II have been identified in cell fractions of rat and calf brain (14). Although limited almost exclusively to the cerebellum in the calf, they are widely distributed in the rat, being found in membrane fractions from the diencephalon, midbrain, and brainstem. Moreover, angiotensin II has been identified by immunofluorescence within axons with wide distribution in the rat brain (75). An early report (147) that renin substrate was highly dipsogenic in the brain of nephrectomized rats has now been contradicted by the failure of natural angiotensinogen to induce thirst by intracranial injection in both rats and dogs (128, J. T. Fitzsimons, *personal communication*). The early report used artificial tetradecapeptide substrate and was the only direct evidence for a role of the cerebral renin-angiotensin system in thirst. We are therefore left with an important unanswered question concerning the part played by the cerebral system in the neural mechanisms of thirst.

NEUROCHEMICAL MEDIATION OF ANGIOTENSIN-INDUCED THIRST

Although cholinergic agents and angiotensin share the same anatomical structure, the thirsts they induce do not have a direct relationship. We have known since 1960 that carbachol is dipsogenic when injected into the brain of the rat (84), and we know now, as the result of the work of Simpson and Routtenberg (148), that this results from cholinergic activation of the subfornical organ. Despite this close anatomical association, angiotensin-induced thirst is not cholinergic. It is not blocked by atropine (43,62,78) or by nicotinic antagonists (71) when both the anticholinergic agents and the angiotensin are given into the cerebral ventricles. Nevertheless, there may be a cholinergic component in the neuropharmacology of angiotensin-induced thirst, perhaps in the neural system for its satiety. The septal lesions that result in hyperdipsia linked to thirst in which angiotensin is a participant are correlated with decreased brain acetylcholine (151), and Myers and his colleagues have reported an intriguing overlap of nicotinic and angiotensin-sensitive sites for thirst in the monkey brain (110). These are the only fragments of current evidence for a cholinergic system for thirst. They invite further investigation.

A strong case has been made for mediation by dopamine of the thirst induced by angiotensin (71,139). The dipsogenic action of angiotensin is blocked by prior application to the brain of haloperidol, but not by either an alpha- or beta-adrenergic blocker; and selective depletion of dopamine, but not norepinephrine, reduces the dipsogenic effectiveness of intracranial angiotensin without affecting the thirst induced by carbachol. Furthermore, deprivation-induced drinking (but not feeding) is reduced by intracranial haloperidol, unaffected by alpha- or beta-adrenergic blockers, and is increased, relative to food-intake after overnight starvation, by a combination of drugs within the brain that increases the amount of available dopamine (a beta-hydroxylase inhibitor plus L-DOPA). Dopamine itself is dipsogenic when given into the lateral ventricle, but very high doses must be used (circa 200 μg) that produce weakness and ataxia. It is most remarkable that animals drink during such treatments despite the disabling artifacts of the amine. Norepinephrine in similarly high doses in the ventricle is not dipsogenic.

These experiments relate directly to Ungerstedt's (168) important observations of severe deficits in thirst and hunger that follow destruction of the biogenic amine pathways of the midbrain. With local injections of 6-hydroxy-dopamine and subsequent histochemical verification, he showed that rats with combined loss of both dopamine and norepinephrine ascending pathways suffered a syndrome of aphagia and adipsia that mimicked the early stages of the lateral hypothalamic syndrome (47). Depletion of norepinephrine alone did not impair ingestive behavior. Similar animals prepared by others (117, 152) have many of the residual deficits that characterize the lateral hypothalamic syndrome. These include failure to drink to all thirst challenges and failure to eat to glucoprivation. The thirst deficits, in particular, have been associated with damage to the nigrostriatal bundle and subsequent depletion of forebrain dopamine (117). It has been proposed (159) that the failure of animals with lateral hypothalamic damage to drink and eat to acutely imposed metabolic imbalances is caused by depletion of forebrain monamines (dopamine, in particular), rather than by disruption of specific systems for response to deficit signals. By this interesting argument, the loss of the monamines deprives the brain of a background of neurochemical activation that is essential for rapid mobilization of homeostatic behaviors.

POSSIBLE ROLE FOR ANGIOTENSIN
IN SODIUM APPETITE

By controlling the secretion of aldosterone (44,76), angiotensin plays a major role in the homeostasis of sodium. A role has therefore been sought for the renin-angiotensin system in the homeostasis that is achieved behaviorally by sodium ingestion, particularly that which accompanies sodium deficits.

There are two phenomena of sodium ingestion and they must be distinguished from each other. Most mammals have an innate preference for weak solutions of sodium salts and will drink more of them than water across a wide range of concentrations (0.2% to 2.0%) in the absence of a need for sodium (154). Stronger solutions are avoided. These preferences and aversions are purely hedonic and depend on peripheral gustatory input (23). The kidney plays an unidentified role here because nephrectomy produces an aversion for all sodium chloride solutions including those in the range of concentrations preferred by normal rats (73). However, this effect is not mediated via the renin-angiotensin system because the aversion for salt is produced by ureteric ligation or experimental uremia without nephrectomy.

When a sodium deficit is imposed on the animal (or when it is subjected to an excess of mineralocorticoid), an appetite for sodium grows out of its natural preference. It now drinks more salt at all concentrations, and the range of acceptable concentrations expands to include both those that were too low to be preferred and those that were so high that they were previously avoided. This enhancement of sodium intake has been studied in detail by Richter (132). It requires no experience (54,111). It appears to be due to the arousal of an internal state that enhances the palatability of salt solutions at all detectable concentrations (54). The state requires the taste of salt solutions for its satiation (113).

A sodium appetite occurs under the special circumstances of pregnancy and lactation (133). Estradiol treatment or induction of pseudopregnancy can produce increases in the ingestion of hypertonic salt solutions (41), suggesting that the female steroids contribute to the arousal of a sodium appetite. Solutions containing potassium, magnesium, and calcium salts are also ingested, but the increases in sodium intake are more reliable and long lasting.

Sodium appetite, like water intake, has complex causes that are both hydrational and endocrinological (131). It is not produced simply by a deficiency of plasma sodium because it occurs during treatment with sodium-retaining hormones (129). And it is not produced simply by an excess of such hormones because it is produced by adrenalectomy (130). It is not reversed by chronic intragastric infusion of salt over several days (96) or by direct infusion of salt into the central circulation (13). It appears to be aroused by internal events that are related to changes in body water and specifically to those produced by hypovolemia. This was shown by Falk (56) and confirmed by Fitzsimons (62), who emphasized the onset of a sodium appetite after caval ligation and other hypovolemic treatments. In both instances the sodium intake is accompanied by excess water intake. In Fitzsimons' reports, the sodium appetite followed the hyperdipsia. A tentative neurological circuit has been proposed for the appetite that involves the hypothalamus and limbic structures (42). Lateral hypothalamic lesions diminish the preference for salt solutions and prevent the appearance of the appetite after imposed sodium deficits or pharmacological doses of DOCA. Medial lesions of the anterior hypothalamus increase sodium intake. Septal damage limited to the medial or lateral nuclear groups increases intake, and damage to the amygdala reduces it. Both of these effects appear to depend on intact hypothalamic tissue (42). An adrenergic system may be involved because intrahypothalamic implants of alpha-adrenergic agonists encourage the consumption of salt solutions (37).

Angiotensin may enhance sodium intake but this is controversial. Intracranial injection (28) or infusion (125) of angiotensin has been reported to increase the ingestion of sodium chloride solutions, but this has not been confirmed (74). The strongest evidence for a role for angiotensin in sodium appetite has been provided by Chiaraviglio (35,36), who confirmed the abolition of sodium appetite by nephrectomy and then showed that the excess intake of a preferred salt solution (1% NaCl w/v) that is produced acutely by peritoneal dialysis is restored to nephrectomized rats by systemic injection of renin or by intracranial injection of angiotensin. She also showed that the excess intake is absent in rats whose catecholamine synthesis has been interrupted by alpha-methyl-p-tyrosine and is restored to them by combined intraventricular injection of norepinephrine and angiotensin II. This effect is abolished by an alpha-adrenergic antagonist (dibenamine). Neither the nephrectomy nor the treatment with alpha-methyl-p-tyrosine interferes in these experiments with water intake. Chiaraviglio (35,36) suggests that angiotensin interacts with an alpha-adrenergic system in the forebrain to generate the sodium appetite. The interaction may resemble that which has been demonstrated in the periphery where angiotensin releases catecholamines from the adrenal medulla (57) and from sympathetic terminals (176). However, Fitzsimons and his colleagues find only a weak role for intracranial angiotensin (74) and none for the peripheral renin-angiotensin system (73) in the generation of the appetite. This confirms the failure of angiotensin to stimulate sodium appetite in the sodium-deficient sheep (24). However, unlike Chiaraviglio (35,36), Bott et al. (24) and Fitzsimons and his co-workers (59,74) used animals suffering from chronic sodium deficiencies, and their most frequently used sodium chloride solutions were from the range of concentrations that is normally avoided.

The complexity and fascination of this problem of sodium appetite are emphasized by recent work from Wolf's laboratory (5) showing that although lesions of the thalamic taste relay prevent the appearance of a sodium appetite (induced by combined treatment with furosemide and DOCA), they do so only in animals that have not tasted strong salt solutions preoperatively. Experience with salt solutions and their taste during sodium deficiency are clearly major factors in the phenomenon and will have to be taken into account in future research. Experiments that employ acute challenges in animals that have not tasted salt and those that employ animals that have had ample opportunity to drink salt both before and during sodium deficiency may not be comparable (23).

OTHER HORMONES

Several hormones other than angiotensin have been proposed as dipsogens. It has been suggested that insulin, prolactin and thyroid hormone are dipsogenic and that vasopressin is antidipsogenic, but none has been shown to affect thirst by direct action. The increased or decreased water intake associated with each is best understood as a consequence of their primary effects on water excretion (vasopressin, prolactin), metabolism (thyroid), and renin release (insulin). The relevant evidence has been exhaustively reviewed by Fitzsimons (66).

SUMMARY AND CONCLUSIONS

The discovery of the dipsogenic role of angiotensin grew from Fitzsimons' demonstration of the independence and potency of hypovolemia as a stimulus of thirst. Renin is released by hypovolemia and it is now clear that angiotensin is an effective dipsogen in all species tested as well as being implicated in the control of water intake in humans.

The arousal of thirst by intravenous doses that are physiologically reasonable in both rats and dogs establishes angiotensin as a possible participant in spontaneous drinking behavior. The effect is a direct and specific action of the hormone because it is completely abolished by concurrent administration of competitive analogues.

The hormone acts directly on the brain to contribute to the arousal of thirst. It acts via the subfornical organ which it reaches directly from the blood. The receptors in the subfornical organ accommodate best the octapeptide angiotensin II, but also respond to angiotensin III. Other receptors for the other central neural actions of the hormone (central pressor response, vasopressin release) exist elsewhere in the brain, but alternative receptors for the dipsogenic effect have not yet been demonstrated.

In the brain, the activation of the subfornical receptor system may arouse thirst through a catecholamine circuit in which dopamine appears to be the dominant amine.

The satiation of the thirst aroused by angiotensin may involve physiological inhibition by prostaglandin Es of cerebral origin of a privileged vascular bed that has been constricted by angiotensin. This competition of endogenous vasoactive agents may take place within the subfornical organ. In addition, inhibition of the thirst in which angiotensin participates may arise from the septum. The strong inhibition produced by rehydration awaits a neurologic explanation.

The hormone's well-established role in sodium metabolism invites speculation about its contribution to both sodium preference and sodium appetite. Evidence has been provided implicating it in sodium appetite, but other factors such as the nature of the treatment that provokes the sodium deficit and the animal's experience with strong salt solutions complicate the issue.

The establishment of the hormone as a physiological dipsogen and the identification of its receptor system in the brain prepare us for answers to the two major questions that must be addressed before the hormone can be assigned its role in natural drinking behavior. First, we must know when and with what magnitude the hormone contributes to the thirsts that arise spontaneously. We must know what part it plays in the several kinds of drinking behavior that are emitted by mammals and we must know how much it contributes to the arousal of each. For example, does it play the same role in the drinking that is closely associated with feeding, on the one hand, and in the drinking that occurs in the midst of an intermeal interval on the other? This topic is discussed further in other reviews (53,66). And what role does angiotensin play during drinking induced by water deprivation when deficit signals would dominate the control of the behavior? Secondly, we must know the nature of the neurologic system by which the hormonal input is integrated with the several other controls of drinking behavior such as cellular dehydration, palatability of the fluids drunk, and circadian factors. Where does this occur? What is its mechanism? And how do the cognitive and hedonic aspects of thirst arise from neurologic action? All that can be said at present is that lateral hypothalamic lesions abolish all thirsts of physiological origin including that induced by angiotensin (47). Tissue in that part of the brain, perhaps some component of the medial forebrain bundle, may serve the required integrative function.

Finally, it is necessary to repeat the caveat with which this chapter began. We are now free of the burden of oversimplified explanations of thirst (53). Not only are there many causes of drinking behavior which interact redundantly, but thirst itself may be several qualitatively different neural states which are all expressed as the same behavior. For example, the drinking evoked by the palatability of fluids in satiated animals in water balance is different from the drinking stimulated by dehydration and redistribution of body water in animals that have suffered water losses. It would be regressive if the attractiveness of the idea of angiotensin as a hormone of thirst misled us into returning to the false conclusion that thirst is a simple behavior with a single cause. Emphasis on the stimulation of drinking by angiotensin should not obscure the important fact that it is not the hormone of thirst but only a participant in the complex phenomenon of thirst.

ACKNOWLEDGMENTS

The author's research is supported by NINCDS 03469 and by aid from the Institute of Neurological Sciences. Saralasin was generously supplied by Dr. Alan Castellion, Norwich Pharmacal, Norwich, New York. Prostaglandins were generously supplied by Dr. John E. Pike, the Upjohn Company, Kalamazoo, Michigan. My colleagues James Fitzsimons, Bruce MacFarlane, and Steve Fluharty made valuable suggestions for improvement of this chapter. I am grateful to them.

REFERENCES

1. Abdellal, A. E., Mercer, P. F., and Mogenson, G. J. (1976): Plasma angiotensin II levels and water intake following β-adrenergic stimulation, hypovolemia, cellular dehydration and water deprivation. *Pharmacol. Biochem. Behav.*, 4:317–321.
2. Abraham, S. F., Baker, R. M., Blaine, E. H., Denton, D. A., and McKinley, M. J. (1975): Water drinking induced in sheep by angiotensin—a physiological or pharmacological effect? *J. Comp. Physiol. Psychol.*, 8:503–518.
3. Abraham, S. F., Denton, D. A., McKinley, M. J., and Weisinger, R. S. (1976): Effect of an angiotensin antagonist, Sar^1-Ala^8-angiotensin II on physiological thirst. *Pharmacol. Biochem. Behav.*, 4:243–247.
4. Adolph, E. F., Barker, J. P., and Hoy, P. A. (1954): Multiple factors in thirst. *Am. J. Physiol.*, 178:538–562.
5. Ahern, G. (1976): Escape from deficits in sodium appetite following gustatory thalamic lesions as a function of preoperative experience. Senior thesis, State University of New York, Purchase.
6. Akert, K. (1969): The mamalian sub-fornical organ. *J. Neuro-Visc. Relat. [Suppl.]*, IX:78–93.
7. Andersson, B. (1953): The effect of injections of hypertonic NaCl-solutions in different parts of the hypothalamus of goats. *Acta Physiol. Scand.*, 28:188–201.
8. Andersson, B. (1975): The central control of water and salt balance. In: *Neural Integration of Physiological Mechanisms and Behavior*, edited by G. J. Mogenson and F. R. Calaresu, pp. 213–225. University of Toronto Press, Toronto.
9. Andersson, B., Leksell, G., and Lishajko, F. (1975): Perturbations in fluid balance induced by medially placed forebrain lesions. *Brain Res.*, 99:261–275.
10. Andersson, B., and McCann, S. M. (1956): The effect of hypothalamic lesions in the water intake of the dog. *Acta Physiol. Scand.*, 35:312–320.
11. Andersson, B., and Wyrwicka, W. (1957): The elicitation of a drinking motor conditioned reaction by electrical stimulation of the hypothalamic "drinking area." *Acta Physiol. Scand.*, 41:194–198.
12. Asscher, A. W., and Anson, S. G. (1963): A vascular permeability factor of renal origin. *Nature*, 198:1097–1099.
13. Beilharz, S., Bott, E., Denton, D. A., and Sabine, J. R. (1965): The effect of intracarotid infusions of the 4 M NaCl on the sodium drinking of sheep with a parotid fistula. *J. Physiol.*, 178:80–91.
14. Bennett, J. P., Jr., and Snyder, S. H. (1976): Angiotensin II binding to brain membranes. *J. Biol. Chem.*, 251:7423–7430.
15. Black, S. J., Kucharczyk, J., and Mogenson, G. J. (1974): Disruption of drinking to intracranial angiotensin by a lateral hypothalamic lesion. *Pharmacol. Biochem. Behav.*, 2:515–522.
16. Blair-West, J. R., and Brook, A. H. (1969): Circulatory changes and renin secretion in sheep in response to feeding. *J. Physiol. (Lond.)*, 204:15–30.
17. Blass, E. M. (1974): The physiological, neurological and behavioral bases of thirst. In: *Nebraska Symposium of Motivation*, edited by M. R. Jones, pp. 1–47. University of Nebraska Press, Lincoln.

18. Blass, E. M., and Hall, W. G. (1974): Behavioral and physiological bases of drinking inhibition in water deprived rats. *Nature,* 249:485–486.
19. Blass, E. M., and Hanson, D. G. (1970): Primary hyperdipsia in the rat following septal lesions. *J. Comp. Physiol. Psychol.,* 70:87–93.
20. Blass, E. M., and Moran, J. S. (1975): Specific inhibition of angiotensin mediated drinking in rats by stimulation of the septum. *Neurosci. Abstr.,* 1:470.
21. Blass, E. M., Nussbaum, A. I., and Hanson, D. G. (1974): Septal hyperdipsia: Specific enhancement of drinking to angiotensin in rats. *J. Comp. Physiol. Psychol.,* 81:422–439.
22. Booth, D. A. (1968): Mechanism of action of norepinephrine in eliciting an eating response on injection into the rat hypothalamus. *J. Pharmacol. Exp. Ther.,* 160: 336–348.
23. Borer, K. T. (1968): The disappearance of preferences and aversions for sapid solutions in rats ingesting untasted fluids. *J. Comp. Physiol. Psychol.,* 65:213–221.
24. Bott, E., Denton, D. A., and Weller, S. (1967): The effect of angiotensin II infusion, renal hypertension, and nephrectomy on salt appetite of sodium-deficient sheep. *Aust. J. Exp. Biol. Med. Sci.,* 45:595–612.
25. Bridge, J. S., and Hatton, G. I. (1973): Septal unit activity in response to alterations in blood volume and osmotic pressure. *Physiol. Behav.,* 10:769–774.
26. Brown, J. J., Curtis, J. R., Lever, A. F., Robertson, J. I. S., DeWardener, H. E., and Wing, A. J. (1969): Plasma renin concentration and the control of blood pressure in patients on maintenance haemodialysis. *Nephron,* 6:329–349.
27. Bryant, R. W., and Falk, J. L. (1973): Angiotensin I as a dipsogen: Efficacy in brain independent of conversion to angiotensin II. *Pharmacol. Biochem. Behav.,* 1:469–475.
28. Buggy, J., and Fisher, A. E. (1974): Evidence for a dual central role for angiotensin in water and sodium intake. *Nature,* 250:733–735.
29. Buggy, J., and Fisher, A. E. (1976): Anteroventral third ventricle site of action for angiotensin induced thirst. *Pharmacol. Biochem. Behav.,* 4:651–660.
30. Buggy, J., Fisher, A. E., Hoffman, W. E., Johnson, A. K., and Phillips, M. I. (1975): Ventricular obstruction: Effect of drinking induced by intracranial angiotensin. *Science,* 190:72–74.
31. Burkhardt, R., Peters-Haefeli, L., and Peters, G. (1975): The mechanism of thirst-induction by intrahypothalamic renin. In: *Control Mechanisms of Drinking,* edited by B. Peters, J. T. Fitzsimons, and L. Peters-Haefeli, pp. 103–107. Springer-Verlag, New York.
32. Cannon, W. B. (1918): The physiological basis of thirst. *Proc. Roy. Soc. Lond.* [*Biol.*], 90:283–301.
33. Cizek, L. J. (1968): Total water balance: Thirst, fluid deficits, and excesses. In: *Medical Physiology,* edited by V. B. Mountcastle, pp. 350–369. C. V. Mosby, St. Louis.
34. Cizek, J. L., Semple, R. E., Huang, K. C., and Gregersen, M. I. (1951): Effect of extracellular electrolyte depletion on water intake in dogs. *Am. J. Physiol.,* 164: 415–422.
35. Chiaraviglio, E. (1976): Angiotensin-norepinephrine interaction on sodium intake. *Behav. Biol.,* 17:411–416.
36. Chiaraviglio, E. (1976): Effect of renin-angiotensin system on sodium intake. *J. Physiol. (Lond.),* 255:57–66.
37. Chiaraviglio, E., and Taleisnik, S. (1969): Water and salt intake induced by hypothalamic implants of cholinergic and adrenergic agents. *Am. J. Physiol.,* 216:1418–1422.
38. Conn, J. W., Cohen, E. L., Lucas, C. P., McDonald, W. J., Mayor, G. H. Blough, W. M., Jr., Eveland, W. C., Bookstein, J. J., and Lapides, J. (1972): Primary reninism. *Arch. Intern. Med.,* 130:682–686.
39. Cooling, M. J., and Day, M. D. (1973): Antagonism of central dipsogenic and peripheral vasoconstrictor responses to angiotensin II with Sar^1-Ala^8-angiotensin in the conscious cat. *J. Pharm. Pharmacol.,* 25:1005–1006.
40. Corbit, J. D. (1968): Cellular dehydration and hypovolaemia are additive in producing thirst. *Nature,* 218:886–887.

41. Covelli, M. D., Denton, D. A., Nelson, J. F., and Shulkes, A. A. (1973): Hormonal factors influencing salt appetite in pregnancy. *Endocrinology,* 93:423–429.
42. Covian, M. R., Antunes-Rodrigues, J., Gentil, C. G., Saad, W. A., Camargo, L. A., and Silva Neto, C. R. (1975): Central control of salt balance. In: *Neural Integration of Physiological Mechanisms and Behaviour,* edited by G. J. Mogenson and F. R. Calaresu, pp. 267–282. University of Toronto Press, Toronto.
43. Covian, M. J., Gentil, C. G., and Antunes-Rodrigues, J. (1972): Water and sodium chloride intake following microinjections of angiotensin II into the septal area of the rat. *Physiol. Behav.,* 9:373–377.
44. Davis, J. O. (1962): The control of aldosterone secretion. *Physiologist,* 5:65–86.
45. Deuben, R. R., and Buckley, J. P. (1970): Identification of a central site of action of angiotensin II. *J. Pharmacol. Exp. Ther.,* 175:139–146.
46. Dickinson, C. J., and Ferrario, C. M. (1974): Central neurogenic effects of angiotensin. In: *Angiotensin,* edited by I. H. Page and F. M. Bumpus, pp. 408–414. Springer-Verlag, Heidelberg.
47. Epstein, A. N. (1971): The lateral hypothalamic syndrome. In: *Progress in Physiological Psychology,* edited by E. Stellar and J. M. Sprague, pp. 263–317. Academic Press, New York.
48. Epstein, A. N. (1977): The neurology of thirst. In: *Handbook of Behavioral Neurobiology, Volume on Motivation,* edited by E. Satinoff and P. Teitelbaum. Plenum Press, New York (*in press*).
49. Epstein, A. N., Fitzsimons, J. T., and Johnson, A. K. (1972): Prevention by angiotensin II antiserum of drinking induced by intracranial angiotensin. *J. Physiol. (Lond.),* 230:42–43P.
50. Epstein, A. N., Fitzsimons, J. T., and Johnson, A. K. (1974): Peptide antagonists of the renin-angiotensin system and the elucidation of the receptors for angiotensin-induced thirst. *J. Physiol. (Lond.),* 238:34–35P.
51. Epstein, A. N., Fitzsimons, J. T., and Rolls, B. J. (1970): Drinking induced by injection of angiotensin into the brain of the rat. *J. Physiol. (Lond.),* 210:457–474.
52. Epstein, A. N., and Hsiao, S. (1975): Angiotensin as dipsogen. In: *Control Mechanisms of Drinking,* edited by G. Peters, J. T. Fitzsimons, and L. Peters-Haefeli, pp. 108–116. Springer-Verlag, Heidelberg.
53. Epstein, A. N., Kissileff, H. R., and Stellar, E. (1973): *The Neuropsychology of Thirst.* V. H. Winston, Washington, D.C.
54. Epstein, A. N., and Stellar, E. (1955): The control of salt preference in the adrenalectomized rat. *J. Comp. Physiol. Psychol.,* 48:167–172.
55. Ernits, T., and Corbit, J. D. (1973): Taste as a dipsogenic stimulus. *J. Comp. Physiol. Psychol.,* 83:27–31.
56. Falk, J. L. (1961): The behavioral regulation of water-electrolyte balance. In: *Nebraska Symposium on Motivation,* edited by M. R. Jones, pp. 1–33. University of Nebraska Press, Lincoln.
57. Feldberg, W., and Lewis, P. (1964): The action of peptides on the adrenal medulla. Release of adrenaline by bradykinin and angiotensin. *J. Physiol. (Lond.),* 171:98–108.
58. Felix, D., and Akert, K. (1974): The effect of angiotensin II on neurons of the cat subfornical organ. *Brain Res.,* 76:350–353.
59. Fitzsimons, J. T. (1961): Drinking by nephrectomized rats injected with various substances. *J. Physiol. (Lond.),* 155:563–579.
60. Fitzsimons, J. T. (1961): Drinking by rats depleted of body fluid without increase in osmotic pressure. *J. Physiol. (Lond.),* 159:297–309.
61. Fitzsimons, J. T. (1964): Drinking caused by constriction of the inferior vena cava in the rat. *Nature,* 204:479–480.
62. Fitzsimons, J. T. (1969): The role of a renal thirst factor in drinking induced by extracellular stimuli. *J. Physiol. (Lond.),* 201:349–369.
63. Fitzsimons, J. T. (1970): The renin-angiotensin system in the control of drinking. In: *The Hypothalamus,* edited by L. Martini, M. Motta, and F. Franschini, pp. 195–212. Academic Press, New York.
64. Fitzsimons, J. T. (1971): The effect on drinking of peptide precursors and of

shorter chain peptide fragments of angiotensin II injected into the rat's diencephalon. *J. Physiol. (Lond.),* 214:295–303.

65. Fitzsimons, J. T. (1971): The hormonal control of water and sodium intake. In: *Frontiers in Neuroendocrinology,* 1971, edited by L. Martini and W. F. Ganong, pp. 103–128. Oxford University Press, New York.

66. Fitzsimons, J. T. (1972): Thirst. *Physiol. Rev.,* 52:468–561.

67. Fitzsimons, J. T. (1973): Angiotensin as a thirst regulating hormone. In: *Endocrinology,* edited by R. D. Scow, F. J. G. Ebling, and I. W. Henderson, pp. 711–716. Excerpta Medica, Amsterdam.

68. Fitzsimons, J. T., Epstein, A. N., and Johnson, A. K. (1977): The peptide specificity of receptors for angiotensin-induced thirst. In: *Central Actions of Angiotensin and Related Hormones,* edited by J. P. Buckley and C. Ferrario, pp. 405–415. Pergamon Press, New York.

69. Fitzsimons, J. T., and Le Magnen, J. (1969): Eating as a regulatory control of drinking in the rat. *J. Comp. Physiol. Psychol.,* 67:273–283.

70. Fitzsimons, J. T., and Oatley, K. (1968): Additivity of stimuli for drinking in rats. *J. Comp. Physiol. Psychol.,* 66:450–455.

71. Fitzsimons, J. T., and Setler, P. E. (1975): The relative importance of central nervous catecholamine and cholinergic mechanisms in drinking in response to angiotensin and other thirst stimuli. *J. Physiol. (Lond.),* 250:613–631.

72. Fitzsimons, J. T., and Simons, B. J. (1969): The effect on drinking in the rat of intravenous infusion of angiotensin, given alone or in combination with other stimuli of thirst. *J. Physiol. (Lond.),* 203:45–57.

73. Fitzsimons, J. T., and Stricker, E. M. (1971): Sodium appetite and the renin-angiotensin system. *Nature [New Biol.],* 231:58–60.

74. Fitzsimons, J. T., and Wirth, J. B. (1976): The neuroendocrinology of thirst and sodium appetite. In: *Central Neuron Control of Na⁺ Balance—Relations to the Renin-Angiotensin System,* edited by D. K. Krause, pp. 80–93. G. Thieme Verlag, Stuttgart.

75. Fuxe, K., Ganten, D., Hökfelt, T., and Bolme, P. (1976): Immunohistochemical evidence for the existence of angiotensin II containing nerve terminals in the brain and spinal cord in the rat. *Neurosci. Lett.,* 2:229–234.

76. Ganong, W. F., Mulrow, P. J., Borycka, A., and Cera, G. (1962): Evidence for a direct effect of angiotensin II on adrenal cortex of the dog. *Proc. Soc. Exp. Biol. Med.,* 109:381–384.

77. Ganten, D., Hutchinson, J. S., Schelling, P., Ganten, U., and Fischer, H. (1975): The iso-renin angiotensin systems in extrarenal tissue. *Clin. Exp. Pharmacol. Physiol.,* 2:127–151.

78. Giardina, A. R., and Fischer, A. E. (1971): Effect of atropine on drinking induced by carbachol, angiotensin and isoproterenol. *Physiol. Behav.,* 1:653–655.

79. Gilman, A. (1937): The relations between blood osmotic pressure, fluid distribution and voluntary water intake. *Am. J. Physiol.,* 120:323–328.

80. Goodwin, F. J., Kirshman, J. D., Sealey, J. E., and Laragh, J. H. (1970): Influence of the pituitary gland on sodium conservation, plasma renin and renin substrate concentration in the rat. *Endocrinology,* 86:824–834.

81. Graeff, F. G., Gentil, C. G., Perez, V. L., and Covian, M. R. (1973): Lever-pressing behavior caused by intraseptal angiotensin II in water satiated rats. *Pharmacol. Biochem. Behav.,* 1:357–359.

82. Gronan, R. J., and York, D. H. (1976): Effects of angiotensin on cells in the preoptic area of rats. *Neurosci. Abstr.,* 2:300.

83. Gross, F., Bock, K. D., and Turrian, H. (1961): Untersuchen über die Blutdruckwirkung von Angiotensin. *Helv. Physiol. Acta,* 19:42–57.

84. Grossman, S. P. (1960): Eating or drinking elicited by direct adrenergic or cholinergic stimulation of hypothalamus. *Science,* 132:301–302.

85. Harvey, J. A., and Hunt, H. F. (1965): Effect of septal lesions on thirst in the rat as indicated by water consumption and operant responding for water reward. *J. Comp. Physiol. Psychol.,* 59:49–56.

86. Hoffman, W. E., and Phillips, M. I. (1976): Regional study of cerebral ventricle sensitive sites to angiotensin II. *Brain Res.,* 110:313–330.

87. Hsiao, S., Epstein, A. N., and Camardo, J. S. (1977): The dipsogenic potency of intravenous angiotensin. *Horm. Behav.,* 8:129–140.
88. Jiméniz-Diaz, C., Linazasoro, J. M., and Merchante, A. (1959): Further study of the part played by the kidneys in regulation of thirst. *Bull. Inst. Med. Res. Madrid,* 12:50–57.
89. Johnson, A. K., Buggy, J., and Housh, M. W. (1976): Effects of lesions surrounding the antero-ventral third ventricle (AV3V) on fluid homeostasis. *Neurosci. Abstr.,* 2:301.
90. Johnson, A. K., and Epstein, A. N. (1975): The cerebral ventricles as the avenue for the dipsogenic action of intracranial angiotensin. *Brain Res.,* 86:399–418.
91. Johnson, A. K., and Schwob, J. E. (1974): Cephalic angiotensin receptors mediating drinking to systemic angiotensin II. *Pharmacol. Biochem. Behav.,* 3:1077–1084.
92. Kenney, N. J., and Epstein, A. N. (1975): The antidipsogenic action of prostaglandin E₁ (PGE₁). *Neurosci. Abstr.,* 1:469.
93. Kenney, N. J., and Epstein, A. N. (1977): The antidipsogenic role of the E-prostaglandins. *J. Comp. Physiol. Psychol. (in press).*
94. Kirkstone, B. J., and Levitt, R. A. (1974): Comparison between drinking induced by water deprivation or chemical stimulation. *Behav. Biol.,* 11:547–559.
95. Kissileff, H. R. (1969): Food associated drinking in the rat. *J. Comp. Physiol. Psychol.,* 67:284–300.
96. Kissileff, H. R., and Hoefer, R. (1975): Reduction of saline intake in adrenalectomized rats during chronic intragastric infusions of saline. In: *Control Mechanisms of Drinking,* edited by G. Peters, J. T. Fitzsimons, and L. Peters-Haefeli, pp. 22–24. Springer-Verlag, New York.
97. Laragh, J. H., and Sealey, J. E. (1973): The renin-angiotensin-aldosterone hormonal system and regulation of sodium, potassium, and blood pressure homeostasis. In: *Renal Physiology: Section 8, Handbook of Physiology,* pp. 831–908. American Physiological Society, Washington, D.C.
98. Lashley, K. S. (1938): The experimental analysis of instinctive behavior. *Psychol. Rev.,* 45:445–471.
99. Lehr, D., Goldman, H. W., and Casner, P. (1973): Renin-angiotensin role in thirst: Paradoxical enhancement of drinking by angiotensin converting enzyme inhibitor. *Science,* 182:1031–1033.
100. Leibowitz, S. F. (1976): Brain catecholamine mechanisms for control of hunger. In: *Hunger: Basic Mechanisms and Clinical Implications,* edited by D. Novin, W. Wyrwicka, and G. Bray, pp. 1–18. Raven Press, New York.
101. Leksell, L. G. (1976): Influence of prostaglandin E₁ on cerebral mechanisms invoked in the control of fluid balance. *Acta Physiol. Scand.,* 98:85–93.
102. Linazasoro, J. M., Jiménez-Diaz, C., and Castro-Mendoza, H. (1954): The kidney and thirst regulation. *Bull. Inst. Med. Res. Madrid,* 7:53–61.
103. Maebashi, M., and Yoshinaga, K. (1967): Effect of dehydration on plasma renin activity. *Jpn. Circ. J.,* 31:609–613.
104. Malvin, R. L., Mouw, D., and Vander, A. J. (1977): Angiotensin: Physiological role in water deprivation induced thirst of rats. *Science,* 197:171–173.
105. Miselis, R., Nicolaïdis, S., Menard, M., and Siatitsas, Y. (1976): Concurrent measures of renin and drinking in response to hypovolemia. *Neurosci. Abstr.,* 2:305.
106. Mogenson, G. J., and Kucharczyk, J. (1975): Evidence that the lateral hypothalamus and midbrain participate in the drinking response elicited by intracranial angiotensin. In: *Control Mechanisms of Drinking,* edited by G. Peters, J. T. Fitzsimons, and L. Peters-Haefeli, pp. 127–131. Springer-Verlag, New York.
107. Montemurro, D. G., and Stevenson, J. A. F. (1957): Adipsia produced by hypothalamic lesions in the rat. *Can. J. Biochem. Physiol.,* 35:31–37.
108. Moran, J. S., and Blass, E. M. (1976): Inhibition of drinking by septal stimulation in rats. *Physiol. Behav.,* 17:23–27.
109. Mouw, D., Bonjour, P., Malvin, R. L., and Vander, A. (1971): Central action of angiotensin in stimulating ADH release. *Am. J. Physiol.,* 220:239–242.
110. Myers, R. D., Hall, G. H., and Rudy, T. A. (1973): Drinking in the monkey

evoked by nicotine or angiotensin II microinjected in hypothalamic and mesencephalic sites. *Pharmacol. Biochem. Behav.,* 1:15–22.

111. Nachman, M. (1962): Taste preferences for sodium salts by adrenalectomized rat. *J. Comp. Physiol. Psychol.,* 55:1124–1129.

112. Nachman, M. (1963): Learned aversion to the taste of lithium chloride and generalization to other salts. *J. Comp. Physiol. Psychol.,* 56:343–349.

113. Nachman, M., and Valentino, D. A. (1966): Roles of taste and postingestional factors in the satiation of sodium appetite in rats. *J. Comp. Physiol. Psychol.,* 62:280–283.

114. Nairn, R. C., Masson, C. M. C., and Corcoran, A. C. (1956): The production of serous effusions in nephrectomized animals by the administration of renal extracts and renin. *J. Pathol. Bacteriol.,* 71:155–163.

115. Nicolaïdis, S., and Fitzsimons, J. T. (1975): La dependence de la prise d'eau induite par l'angiotensine II envers la fonction vasomotrice cerebrale locale chez le Rat. *C. R. Acad. Sci. [D] (Paris),* 281:1417–1420.

116. Nicoll, R. A., and Barker, J. L. (1971): Excitation of supraoptic neurosecretory cells by angiotensin II. *Nature [New Biol.],* 233:172–174.

117. Oltmans, G. A., and Harvey, J. A. (1972): LH syndrome and brain catecholamine levels after lesions of the nigrostriatal bundle. *Physiol. Behav.,* 8:69–78.

118. Oomura, Y., Ono, T., Ooyama, H., and Wayner, M. J. (1969): Glucose and osmosensitive neurones of the rat hypothalamus. *Nature,* 222:282–284.

119. Osborne, M. J., Pooters, N., Angles d'Auriac, G., Epstein, A. N., and Worcel, M. (1971): Metabolism of tritiated angiotensin II in anaesthetized rats. *Pflügers Arch.,* 326:101–114.

120. Page, I. H., and Bumpus, F. M. (1974): *Angiotensin.* Springer-Verlag, New York.

121. Peck, J. W., and Epstein, A. N. (1971): Antidiuresis following intracranial injections of angiotensin II into rats. *Fed. Proc.,* 30:113.

122. Peskar, B., Meyer, D. K., Tauchmann, U., and Hertting, G. (1970): Influence of isoproterenol, hydralazine and phentolamine on the renin activity of plasma and renal cortex of rats. *Eur. J. Pharmacol.,* 9:394–396.

123. Phillips, M. I., and Felix, D. (1976): Specific angiotensin II receptive neurons in the cat subfornical organ. *Brain Res.,* 109:531–540.

124. Phillips, M. I., and Hoffman, W. E. (1977): Sensitive sites in the brain for the blood pressure and drinking responses to angiotensin II. In: *Central Actions of Angiotensin and Related Hormones,* edited by J. P. Buckley and C. Ferrario, pp. 325–356. Pergamon Press, New York.

125. Radio, G. J., Summy-Long, J., Daniels-Severs, A., and Severs, W. B. (1972): Hydration changes produced by central infusions of angiotensin II. *Am. J. Physiol.,* 223:1221–1226.

126. Ramsay, D. J., and Reid, I. A. (1975): Some central mechanisms of thirst in the dog. *J. Physiol. (Lond.),* 253:517–525.

127. Ramsay, D. J., Reid, I. A., and Ganong, W. F. (1976): Evidence that the effects of isoproterenol on water intake and urine production are mediated by angiotensin. *Fed. Proc.,* 35:620.

128. Reid, I. A., Simpson, J. B., Ramsay, D. J., and Kipen, H. M. (1977): Mechanism of dipsogenic action of tetradecapeptide renin substrate. *Fed. Proc.,* 36:482.

129. Rice, K. K., and Richter, C. P. (1943): Increased sodium chloride and water intake of normal rats treated with desoxycorticosterone acetate. *Endocrinology,* 33:106–115.

130. Richter, C. P. (1941): Sodium chloride and dextrose appetite of untreated and treated adrenalectomized rats. *Endocrinology,* 29:115–125.

131. Richter, C. P. (1942–3): Total self-regulatory functions in animals and human beings. *Harvey Lect.,* 38:63–103.

132. Richter, C. P. (1956): Salt appetite of mammals: Its dependence on instinct and metabolism. In: *L'instinct dans le Comportement des Animaux et de l'Homme,* edited by Masson et Cie, pp. 577–629. Libraires de l' Academie de Medecine, Paris.

133. Richter, C. P., and Barelare, B. (1938): Nutritional requirement of pregnant and lactating rats studied by the self-selection method. *Endocrinology,* 23:15–24.

134. Rogers, P. W., and Kurtzman, N. A. (1973): Renal failure, uncontrollable thirst and hyperreninemia. *J.A.M.A.*, 225:1236–1238.
135. Rolls, B. J., and Jones, B. P. (1972): Cessation of drinking following intracranial injections of angiotensin in the rat. *J. Comp. Physiol. Psychol.*, 80:26–29.
136. Rolls, B. J., Jones, B. P., and Fallows, D. J. (1972): A comparison of the motivational properties of thirst induced by intracranial angiotensin and by water deprivation. *Physiol. Behav.*, 9:777–782.
137. Russell, P. J. D., Abdellal, A. E., and Mogenson, G. J. (1975): Graded levels of hemorrhage, thirst, and angiotensin II in the rat. *Physiol. Behav.*, 15:117–119.
138. Schwob, J. E., and Johnson, A. K. (1975): Evidence for involvement of the renin-angiotensin system in isoproterenol dipsogenesis. *Neurosci. Abstr.*, 1:467.
139. Setler, P. E. (1973): The role of catecholamines in thirst. In: *The Neuropsychology of Thirst,* edited by A. N. Epstein, H. R. Kissileff, and E. Stellar, pp. 279–291. H. V. Winston, Washington, D.C.
140. Severs, W. B., and Daniels-Severs, A. E. (1973): Effects of angiotensin on the central nervous system. *Pharmacol. Rev.*, 25:415–449.
141. Severs, W. B., Summy-Long, J., and Daniels-Severs, A. E. (1973): Effect of a converting enzyme inhibitor (SQ 20881) on angiotensin-induced drinking. *Proc. Soc. Exp. Biol. Med.*, 142:203–204.
142. Severs, W. B., Summy-Long, J., Taylor, J. S., and Connor, J. D. (1970): A central effect of angiotensin: Release of pituitary pressor material. *J. Pharmacol. Exp. Ther.*, 174:27–34.
143. Shelling, P., Ganten, D., Heckl, R., Hayduk, K., Hutchinson, J. S., Sponer, G., and Ganten, U. (1976): On the origin of angiotensin-like peptides in cerebrospinal fluid. In: *Central Actions of Angiotensin and Related Hormones,* edited by J. P. Buckley and C. Ferrario, pp. 519–526. Pergamon Press, New York.
144. Shrager, E. E., Osborne, M. J., Johnson, A. K., and Epstein, A. N. (1975): Entry of angiotensin into cerebral ventricles and circumventricular structures. In: *Central Action of Drugs in Blood Pressure Regulation,* edited by D. S. Davies and J. L. Reid, pp. 65–67. University Park Press, Baltimore.
145. Sibole, W., Miller, J. J., and Mogenson, G. J. (1971): Effects of septal stimulation on drinking elicited by electrical stimulation of the lateral hypothalamus. *Exp. Neurol.*, 32:466–477.
146. Simpson, J. B., Epstein, A. N., and Camardo, J. S. (1977): The localization of receptors for the dipsogenic action of angiotensin II in the subfornical organ. *J. Comp. Physiol. Psychol. (in press).*
147. Simpson, J. B., Gordon, J., and Epstein, A. N. (1974): Dipsogenic potency of intracranial renin substrate after nephrectomy. *Fed. Proc.*, 33:417.
148. Simpson, J. B., and Routtenberg, A. (1972): The subfornical organ and carbachol-induced drinking. *Brain Res.*, 45:135–152.
149. Simpson, J. B., and Routtenberg, A. (1973): Subfornical organ: Site of drinking elicitation by angiotensin II. *Science,* 818:1172–1174.
150. Simpson, J. B., and Routtenberg, A. (1974): Subfornical organ: Acetylcholine application elicits drinking. *Brain Res.*, 79:157–164.
151. Sorenson, J. P., Jr., and Harvey, J. A. (1971): Decreased brain acetylcholine after septal lesions in rats: correlation with thirst. *Physiol. Behav.*, 6:723–725.
152. Smith, G. P., Strohmayer, A. J., and Reis, D. J. (1972): Effect of lateral hypothalamic injections of 6-hydroxydopamine on food and water intake in rats. *Nature,* 235:27–29.
153. Stellar, E. (1954): The physiology of motivation. *Psychol. Rev.*, 61:5–22.
154. Stellar, E., Hyman, R., and Samet, S. (1954): Gastric factors controlling water and salt solution drinking. *J. Comp. Physiol. Psychol.*, 47:220–226.
155. Stephan, F. K., and Zucker, I. (1972): Circadian rhythms in drinking behavior and locomotor activity of rats are eliminated by hypothalamic lesions. *Proc. Natl. Acad. Sci. USA,* 69:1583–1586.
156. Stricker, E. M. (1968): Some physiological and motivational properties of the hypovolemic stimulus for thirst. *Physiol. Behav.*, 3:379–385.
157. Stricker, E. M. (1969): Osmoregulation and volume regulation in rats: Inhibition of hypovolemic thirst by water. *Am. J. Physiol.*, 217:98–105.

158. Stricker, E. M., Bradshaw, W. G., and McDonald, R. H., Jr. (1976): The renin-angiotensin system and thirst: A reevaluation. *Science*, 194:1169–1171.
159. Stricker, E. M., and Zigmond, M. J. (1976): Recovery of function after damage to central calecholamine-containing neurons: A neurochemical model for the lateral hypothalamus syndrome. In: *Progress in Psychobiology and Physiological Psychology,* edited by J. M. Sprague and A. N. Epstein, pp. 121–188. Academic Press, New York.
160. Swanson, L. W., Marshall, G. R., Needleman, P., and Sharpe, L. G. (1973): Characterization of central angiotensin II receptors involved in the elicitation of drinking in the rat. *Brain Res.,* 49:441–446.
161. Swanson, L. W., and Sharpe, L. G. (1973): Centrally induced drinking: Comparison of angiotensin II and carbachol-sensitive sites in rats. *Am. J. Physiol.,* 225:566–572.
162. Swanson, L. W., Sharpe, L. G., and Griffin, D. (1973): Drinking to intracerebral angiotensin II and carbachol: Dose-response relationships and ionic involvement. *Physiol. Behav.,* 10:595–600.
163. Tang, M. (1976): Dependence of polyethylene glycol-induced dipsogenesis on intravascular fluid volume depletion. *Physiol. Behav.,* 17:811–816.
164. Tang, M., and Falk, J. L. (1974): Sar^1-Ala^8 angiotensin II blocks renin-angiotensin but not beta-adrenergic dipsogenesis. *Pharmacol. Biochem. Behav.,* 2:401–408.
165. Tondat, L. M., and Almli, C. R. (1975): Hyperdipsia produced by severing ventral septal fiber systems. *Physiol. Behav.,* 15:701–716.
166. Trippodo, N. C., McCaa, R. E., and Guyton, A. C. (1976): Effect of prolonged angiotensin II infusion on thirst. *Am. J. Physiol.,* 230:1063–1066.
167. Ueda, H., Katayama, S., and Kato, R. (1972): Area postrema-angiotensin-sensitive site in brain. *Adv. Exp. Biol. Med.,* 17:109–116.
168. Ungerstedt, U. (1971): Adipsia and aphagia after 6-hydroxydopamine induced degeneration of the nigro-striatal dopamine systems. *Acta Physiol. Scand. [Suppl.],* 367:95–122.
169. Verney, E. B. (1947): The antidiuretic hormone and the factors which determine its release. *Proc. R. Soc. Lond. [Biol.],* 135:25–106.
170. Volicer, L., and Loew, C. G. (1971): Penetration of angiotensin II into the brain. *Neuropharmacology,* 10:631–636.
171. Wayner, M. J., Ono, T., and Nolley, D. (1973): Effects of angiotensin II on central neurons. *Pharmacol. Biochem. Behav.,* 1:679–691.
172. Weindl, A. (1973): Neuroendocrine aspects of circumventricular organs. In: *Frontiers in Neuroendocrinology,* 1973, edited by W. F. Ganong and L. Martini, pp. 3–32. Oxford University Press, New York.
173. Wettendorff, H. (1901): Modifications du sang sous l'influence de la privation d'eau. Contribution a l'etude de la soif. *Trav. Lab. Physiol. Inst. Solvay,* 4:353–484.
174. Wishart, T. B., and Mogenson, G. J. (1970): Reduction in water intake by electrical stimulation of the septal region of the rat brain. *Physiol. Behav.,* 5:1399–1404.
175. Wislocki, G. B., and Leduc, E. H. (1952): Vital staining of the hematoencephalic barrier by silver nitrate and trypan blue and cytological comparisons of the neurohypophysis, pineal body, area postrema, intercolumnar tubercle and supraoptic crest. *J. Comp. Neurol.,* 96:371–413.
176. Zimmerman, B. G., Gomer, S. K., and Chia Liao, J. (1972): Action of angiotensin on vascular adrenergic nerve endings: Facilitation of norepinephrine release. *Fed. Proc.,* 31:1344–1350.

Frontiers in Neuroendocrinology, Vol. 5,
edited by W. F. Ganong and L. Martini.
Raven Press, New York © 1978.

Chapter 5

Neurophysiology and Neuropharmacology of the Hypothalamic Tuberoinfundibular System

Leo P. Renaud, Howard W. Blume, and Quentin J. Pittman

*Division of Neurology,
The Montreal General Hospital and McGill University,
Montreal, Quebec, Canada*

Hypothalamic regulation of adenohypophyseal secretion is mediated by specific peptides released into the pituitary portal circulation from median eminence nerve terminals of tuberoinfundibular neurons (14,64,65,69,71, 160,170,187). These tuberoinfundibular "neurosecretory" cells release the various peptides in response to appropriate neural stimuli. Therefore, the *tuberoinfundibular tract* forms the structural basis for the final neuro-hormonal link between hypothalamus and anterior pituitary. Neurosecretion in the tuberoinfundibular system is analogous to events associated with the release of vasopressin and oxytocin from the magnocellular neurohypophyseal system (4,31,38,43,44,103,173,174). From a neurophysiological viewpoint, we now have a modest understanding of the neural mechanisms associated with neurosecretion of oxytocin and vasopressin (31). Recent electrophysio-logical investigations of the tuberoinfundibular system have achieved some definition of the location and activity of neuronal elements considered to constitute the neurosecretory system for the regulation of adenohypophyseal secretion. The aim of this chapter is to review the available morphological and neurophysiological data on the tuberoinfundibular system, and perhaps to broaden the definition of this system. We wish to emphasize the electro-physiology of tuberoinfundibular neurons and incorporate available pharma-cological data relevant to an understanding of neural integration in this puta-tive peptidergic neural network.

DEFINITION OF TUBEROINFUNDIBULAR NEURON

The term "tuberoinfundibular neuron" was initially introduced into the anatomical literature in reference to a specific population of parvicellular hy-pothalamic neurons whose axons terminated on portal capillaries in the me-dian eminence (169,170). A substantial increase in our knowledge of both the location and function of the tuberoinfundibular neuronal system has occurred because of some rather striking advances recently achieved with immunocytochemical techniques. It is therefore appropriate to review briefly the relevant anatomical and immunohistochemical data on this system, since this will provide a conceptual framework against which one can compare the electrophysiological observations to be described in a later section.

Anatomical Considerations

The tuberoinfundibular tract is a fine unmyelinated fiber system that divides into short branches prior to termination on capillary loops in the zona externa of the median eminence (71,130,168,170). In Golgi preparations, axons of this system are seen to arise from small fusiform neurons in the arcuate nucleus, the ventral part of the anterior periventricular area, and the medial part of the retrochiasmatic area (66,169,170). Anatomical studies of the rat hypothalamus suggest that few neurons located outside the areas described above contribute significantly to nerve terminal populations found in the external palisade zone of the median eminence (66,154). However, in the cat and in man, sources of the tuberoinfundibular tract have been described in the ventromedial, paraventricular, and posterior hypothalamic nuclei (30,111).

Functional Considerations

Both dopamine and norepinephrine are present in nerve terminals within the median eminence (11–13,56,57,77). The adrenergic endings do not appear to come from local neurons, but rather to arise from neurons in the brainstem. However, some dopaminergic terminals are considered to arise from short axon neurons in the arcuate nucleus and periventricular area. These cells display intense fluorescence for dopamine and are therefore part of a dopaminergic tuberoinfundibular system, most probably responsible for the dopamine found in the portal circulation (10). This dopaminergic system may be but a part of a more extensive catecholaminergic tuberoinfundibular system originating from areas outside of the mediobasal hypothalamus (12).

The peptidergic nature of the tuberoinfundibular system has received clarification as a result of recent progress in immunocytochemical and immunohistochemical technology, made possible by the structural characterization and synthesis of three hypothalamic peptides, i.e., thyrotropin releasing hormone (TRH) (25,124), luteinizing hormone releasing hormone (LRH) (2,159), and somatostatin (17). These peptides are localized not only in the hypothalamus but also in certain extrahypothalamic regions of brain as well as in the spinal cord and the peripheral nervous system, and some nonneural tissues (21,73,74,76). In the brain, these peptides are localized to neurons rather than neuroglia. Subcellular fractionation studies indicate their presence in synaptosomes (7,52,137,140,171,172,181), similar to the subcellular localization of other putative neurotransmitter agents (177). In the median eminence, these peptides appear to be associated with a population of dense granules (61,122,135,136) located in nerve terminals.

TRH-containing nerve fibers are located in the more medial part of the external palisade zone of the median eminence, the dorsomedial hypothalamic nucleus, periformical areas, and in certain extrahypothalamic regions (73,79, 80). At the moment, the source of this extrahypothalamic and hypothalamic TRH is uncertain since few neuronal perikarya containing TRH have yet been visualized. Neurons located outside of the mediobasal hypothalamus are considered responsible for the synthesis and transport of median eminence TRH since hypothalamic deafferentation drastically reduces hypothalamic TRH content without having a significant effect on extrahypothalamic TRH levels (23). TRH-producing neurons are presumably located in the rostral hypothalamus or preoptic area since lesions of the periventricular region result in a decrease in median eminence TRH (49) and electrical stimulation of the anterior hypothalamic area evokes a rise in plasma TSH (110).

LRH-containing nerve fibers are present in the lateral part of the external palisade zone of the median eminence, anterior periventricular region, medial preoptic area, and organum vasculosum of the lamina terminalis (9,73,78,81, 92,95,100,163–166,188–190,193). Several observations indicate that these LRH nerve fibers originate from neuronal perikarya located both in the mediobasal hypothalamus and at rostral levels. Studies in different species have demonstrated neuronal perikarya containing immunoreactive LRH in the medial preoptic and suprachiasmatic region (8,9,164) as well as in the arcuate and ventromedial nuclei (100,123,165,192,193). Anterior hypothalamic deafferentation produces a decrease in mediobasal hypothalamic LRH [whether measured by radioimmunoassay (20, but see ref. 165) or immunohistochemistry (164)] and a slight rise in preoptic LRH levels (83).

Somatostatin has a widespread distribution in both peripheral and central neuronal tissues, and in extraneural tissues such as the gut and pancreas (19,74). In the nervous system, somatostatin is in highest concentration in the hypothalamus, particularly in the median eminence (19), where it is observed in nerve fibers scattered throughout the external palisade zone (73, 81,91). Elsewhere in the hypothalamus, somatostatin immunoreactive nerve fibers have been reported in the arcuate and ventromedial nuclei, the periventricular region, and preoptic area (41,42,49,73–75,162). Neuronal perikarya immunoreactive for somatostatin have now been described in the anterior periventricular and anterior hypothalamic area (1,42,134), the rostral part of the suprachiasmatic nucleus, and the posterior arcuate nucleus (134). Lesions in the anterior periventricular region (49) and anterior hypothalamic deafferentation (18) both reduce the levels of somatostatin within the median eminence indicating that cells located at these rostral hypothalamic levels are probably responsible for synthesis and transport of most of the median eminence somatostatin.

In summary, TRH, LRH, and somatostatin have been identified in nerve fibers in both hypothalamic and extrahypothalamic regions, and in neuronal perikarya in the mediobasal and rostral hypothalamus in the approximate location for the origin of the tuberoinfundibular tract.

ELECTROPHYSIOLOGICAL IDENTIFICATION AND LOCALIZATION OF TUBEROINFUNDIBULAR NEURONS

Cross and Green (32) pioneered the electrophysiological analysis of recordings from single hypothalamic magnocellular neurosecretory neurons, and demonstrated that these neurons generated electrical impulses identical to those recorded from other central neurons. Subsequent electrophysiological studies in preoptic neurosecretory neurons of goldfish (84) and the magnocellular neurohypophyseal system of rat (182) and cat (82) have confirmed the neuron-like electrical characteristics of neurosecretory neurons. In these and subsequent investigations (6,31,38,39,43,44,93,103,117,121,125–129,173, 174,185), the technique of antidromic invasion, i.e., retrograde activation of cell somata by electrical excitation of axon terminals, has been used as a precise means for identifying neurosecretory cells that project to the neural hypophysis.

Similar methods have been used with some success to define components of the tuberoinfundibular system. Thus the terminals of tuberoinfundibular neurons can be activated by stimulation of the surface of the median eminence near the junction with the pituitary stalk (70,104,115,116,119,141,142,144– 147,151,156–158,184,185). In pentobarbital- or urethane-anesthetized rats, neurons displaying features of antidromic invasion have been located in the region of the mediobasal hypothalamus (arcuate, ventromedial, and dorsal premammillary nuclei), the periventricular region, the anterior hypothalamic area, and at more rostral levels (suprachiasmatic nucleus and medial preoptic area) (Fig. 5–1; see also refs. 70,104,119,144,148,157).

It is of interest that some neurons in the paraventricular nucleus (see Fig. 5–1) also demonstrate antidromic invasion from median eminence stimulation (104,144). Current spread and subsequent activation of magnocellular neurosecretory neurons projecting to the neural hypophysis could explain this observation. However, there are two other possibilities: first, that neurons containing releasing factors (e.g., TRH) are present in the paraventricular nucleus (55); second, that neurons containing oxytocin, vasopressin, or neurophysins project to the median eminence. In support of the latter possibility are the following observations: (a) the neurohypophyseal peptides (vasopressin, oxytocin, and neurophysins) have been found in fibers in the zona externa of the median eminence in several species (188–190); (b) vasopressin and neurophysin have been demonstrated by immunoelectron microscopy in nerve terminals on or near portal capillaries in the guinea pig (167) and rat (62); (c) vasopressin is present in high concentration in the

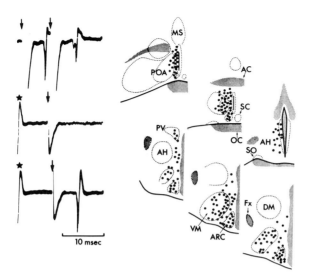

FIG. 5–1. Identification and localization of tuberoinfundibular neurons.

Left: Three oscilloscope sweeps illustrate the criteria for antidromic invasion used during this study. The upper trace illustrates action potentials of a tuberoinfundibular neuron that occur with constant latency after a pair of stimuli *(arrows)* are delivered to the median eminence at a frequency of 150 Hz. In the middle and lower traces, a spontaneous action potential *(star)* from this tuberoinfundibular neuron is used to trigger the median eminence stimulus *(arrow).* In the middle trace, the stimulus is set to occur within the critical time interval for cancellation of the antidromic action potential, whereas in the lower trace, the interval between the spontaneous action potential and the median eminence stimulus is 1 msec longer and results in the reappearance of the antidromic action potential. Negativity is indicated by an upward deflection in these and all subsequent traces.

Right: The dots refer to approximate sites within the medial hypothalamus and preoptic area where tuberoinfundibular neurons, identified by antidromic invasion, were localized. Abbreviations: AC, anterior commissure; AH, anterior hypothalamic area; ARC, arcuate nucleus; DM, hypothalamic dorsomedial nucleus; Fx, fornix; MS, medial septum; OC, optic chiasm; POA, preoptic area; PV, paraventricular nucleus; SC, suprachiasmatic nucleus; SO, supraoptic nucleus; VM, hypothalamic ventromedial nucleus. Reproduced from (148).

portal blood (191). The paraventricular nucleus is the most likely source for this portal blood vasopressin, since unilateral lesions in the paraventricular nucleus result in a marked reduction of vasopressin and neurophysin in the ipsilateral median eminence zona externa (3). Others have already suggested that vasopressin may be involved in the regulation of adenohypophyseal secretion (97,188).

ELECTRICAL PROPERTIES OF TUBEROINFUNDIBULAR NEURONS: ACTIVITY PATTERNS

In anesthetized preparations, 60 to 80% of the tuberoinfundibular neurons display little or no spontaneous activity. Action potentials from active tuberoinfundibular neurons seldom exceed frequencies of 3/sec (104,144).

Their activity patterns have not been examined in detail. Some cells appear to discharge randomly, others display activity in the form of bursts of 5 to 8 action potentials at frequencies of 300 Hz, and few cells are sporadically active with phasic periods of activity lasting 30 to 40 sec, separated by relatively silent intervals of 20 to 40 sec (144).

Axon Conduction Velocity

Tuberoinfundibular neurons display a wide range of antidromic invasion latencies: 0.5 to 14.0 msec for those in the mediobasal hypothalamus, and 4.0 to 25.0 msec for those in the anterior hypothalamic and medial preoptic area. When the latencies are converted to conduction velocities, it is apparent that the axons of tuberoinfundibular neurons conduct impulses slowly, i.e., at velocities under 2.0 msec (104). Tuberoinfundibular neurons located less than 0.5 mm from the portal capillary plexus within the arcuate nucleus and ventral portion of the ventromedial nucleus display conduction velocities under 0.2 msec (144,146). Since this area also contains dopaminergic tuberoinfundibular neurons (11–13,56,57,77,102), there could be a correlation between the slowest conducting tuberoinfundibular neurons and the dopaminergic tuberoinfundibular system.

Action Potentials of Tuberoinfundibular Neurons

The spontaneous orthodromic or antidromic action potentials of tuberoinfundibular neurons are generally biphasic with an initial positivity and a later negative component, similar to the action potentials recorded from neighboring hypothalamic or other central neurons. All cells display an inflexion on the rising phase of the action potential, presumably a reflection of sequential depolarization beginning with the initial axon segment, followed by the soma-dendrite complex (48).

Varying the interval between two successive suprathreshold stimuli delivered to the median eminence provides useful information about the refractory period of tuberoinfundibular neurons. As the interstimulus interval is shortened below 10 to 30 msec, the inflexion on the rising phase of the second antidromic spike is usually more obvious because it occurs in the relative refractory period of the first antidromic spike. At intervals under 5 msec, both the latency and the threshold of the second antidromic potential are increased (Fig. 5–2 A through C). At intervals under 2 msec, the second antidromic action potential can no longer be generated due to its occurrence within the absolute refractory period of the first action potential (144,157). Thus, for tuberoinfundibular cells the absolute refractory period is between 1.5 and 2.0 msec, whereas the relative refractory period may extend up to 10 to 30 msec.

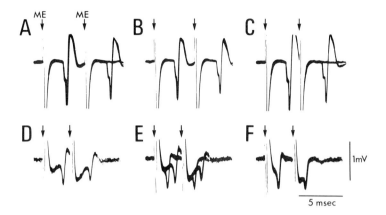

FIG. 5–2. Oscilloscope traces from two different tuberoinfundibular neurons.

A–C: Superimposed oscilloscope sweeps illustrate changes in threshold for antidromic invasion after paired median eminence stimuli. (A): At stimulus intensities barely suprathreshold for antidromic invasion (0.06 mA), there are occasional failures in antidromic invasion from the second stimulus when interstimulus intervals are less than 5 msec. This is resolved in (B) by a slight increase in stimulation intensity to 0.07 mA. However, a further shortening of interstimulus intervals (C) results in an increase in threshold for antidromic invasion from the second stimulus, and once again some failures of the second antidromic spike occur.

D–F: The superimposed traces illustrate one example of two latencies for antidromic invasion, depending on stimulation intensity, for a periventricular tuberoinfundibular neuron. At low intensities (0.18 mA) of median eminence stimulation (D), the cell displays antidromic invasion at a latency of 2.1 msec. (E): An increase in stimulus intensity to 0.195 mA reaches threshold for the appearance of antidromic invasion at either a shorter latency of 1.2 msec or the longer latency of 2.1 msec. A further increase in stimulation intensity (F) produces consistent antidromic invasion at the shorter of the two latencies observed. Reproduced from (144).

EVIDENCE FOR AXON COLLATERALS IN THE TUBEROINFUNDIBULAR SYSTEM

Intrahypothalamic

The majority of tuberoinfundibular neurons display but one antidromic invasion latency following median eminence stimulation. However, on occasional instances in both neurohypophyseal (supraoptic and paraventricular) neurons and tuberoinfundibular neurons (Fig. 5–2 D through F) stimulation to the pituitary stalk or median eminence, respectively, at suprathreshold intensities evokes antidromic invasion at two distinctly different latencies (6,31, 125,144). These observations suggest either that the axon pursues a tortuous course through the focus of stimulation (31) or that there are axon branches or axon collaterals spaced at different distances from the stimulating electrode with different threshold intensities for activation (6,31,144). Anatomical descriptions confirm that fibers in the tuberoinfundibular system do indeed divide into short branches prior to termination (130,168,169). Similar evidence for axon collaterals is seen in records from rostral hypothalamic neurons after stimulation of the arcuate-ventromedial nuclear complex (45) and from mediobasal hypothalamic neurons after stimulation in the medial pre-optic area (147).

A small number of tuberoinfundibular cells evidently have projections to other sites in the hypothalamus in addition to their projections to the median eminence. Studies in independent laboratories have reported that some tu-beroinfundibular neurons display antidromic invasion from stimulation sites in the anterior hypothalamic area (70,142,144,151) and the paraventricular nucleus (70).

Recordings from spontaneously active tuberoinfundibular neurons indi-cate that most cells have a period of decreased excitability following median eminence stimulation (Fig. 5–3C). Evidently, this silent period is not a sim-ple postactivation depression, but rather it displays all the characteristics of a postsynaptic inhibitory process: the decrease in excitability is observed at both sub- and suprathreshold stimulation intensities for antidromic invasion; and the duration of the silent period increases from 40 to 150 msec as the stimulus intensity is increased. If one assumes that only the axons of tuberoin-fundibular neurons are activated by median eminence stimulation, this post-synaptic inhibition must be mediated through axon collaterals in the tuberoinfundibular tract.

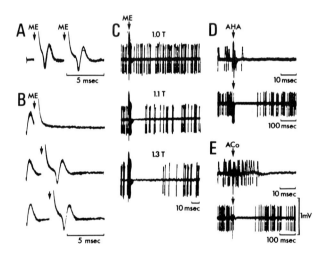

FIG. 5–3. Responses of a ventromedial nucleus tuberoinfundibular neuron to various stimuli.

In (A) and (B) superimposed oscilloscope traces illustrate that two criteria for antidromic invasion have been satisfied for this tuberoinfundibular neuron. (A) illustrates the ability for this neuron to follow high-frequency median eminence stimuli at constant latency. (B) illustrates cancellation of the antidromic action potential where the stimulus is delivered within a critical interval after a spontaneous action potential that occurs at the onset of the sweep. Note that the latency for antidromic invasion is prolonged slightly as the stimulus is delivered closer to the critical interval (A, second stimulus, and B, middle and lower traces). In (C), superimposed sweeps illustrate a progressively longer silent interval following median eminence (ME) stimulation as intensities are increased above threshold for antidromic invasion. In (D) and (E), stimulation in the anterior hypothalamic area (AHA) and cortical nucleus of the amygdala (ACo) also evoked short-latency silent intervals with a duration of 100 msec. Reproduced from (147).

Some nontuberoinfundibular neurons located within the mediobasal hypothalamus (144) and medial preoptic area (184) demonstrate short latency orthodromic responses following median eminence stimulation. Certain cells display a decrease in excitability, characteristic of postsynaptic inhibition, at latencies of 2 to 12 msec with durations up to 120 msec. Other neurons display activation at variable latencies, depending on stimulus intensity. Both response patterns are presumed to be mediated transsynaptically through axon collaterals of the tuberoinfundibular system, and are seen with stimulus intensities similar to those used to evoke antidromic invasion of neighboring tuberoinfundibular neurons.

Extrahypothalamic

In a series of studies designed to characterize the connections of neurons in the hypothalamic ventromedial nucleus, we have determined that many of these cells display antidromic invasion from several extrahypothalamic sites, notably the amygdala, preoptic area, midline thalamic nuclei, and midbrain periaqueductal gray (147,149,151). Some of these same hypothalamic neurons project not only to one of these extrahypothalamic regions, but also to

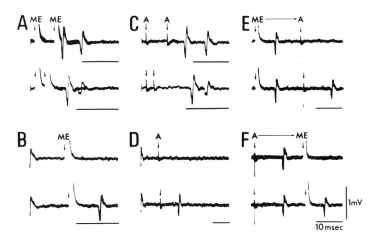

FIG. 5–4. Electrophysiological evidence for axon branching in a tuberoinfundibular neuron.
This cell displays antidromic invasion from both the median eminence (ME) and the cortical nucleus of amygdala (A). In (A) and (C), superimposed oscilloscope traces illustrate constant latency responses to paired stimuli at frequencies over 200 Hz from both sites. In (B) and (D) a spontaneous action potential, seen at the onset of each trace, is used to trigger the stimulator and deliver current pulses to the median eminence and amygdala, respectively. In the upper traces, the stimulus is set to occur within the critical interval for cancellation of the antidromic action potential. In the lower traces, the time interval is longer and the antidromic action potential reappears. Traces in (E) and (F) illustrate that stimulation of one axon branch followed by suprathreshold stimulation of a second axon branch results in cancellation of the second antidromic potential if the time interval between the two stimuli is sufficiently short. In the lower traces, the longer interstimulus intervals permit reappearance of the second antidromic potential. Reproduced from (146).

the median eminence, i.e., in each instance cells display all the criteria for antidromic invasion from both sites (Fig. 5–4; 142,144–146). A detailed study of the critical stimulation intervals required to produce cancellation of the antidromic spike evoked from one area by a suprathreshold stimulus to the other area (Fig. 5–4 E and F) indicates that these axons bifurcate close to the cell soma (147; see Table 5–1).

Recent studies have raised the possibility that these neurons may be "bipolar" neurons, with two separate axons (16,46,51). Although the available morphological literature provides many examples of fusiform neurons and axonal arborization in the hypothalamus (28,66,113,114,170), substantial evidence for two separate axons is lacking. Therefore, the use of the term "bipolar" to describe hypothalamic neurons with a dual projection seems inappropriate.

TABLE 5-1. Summary of data obtained from hypothalamic neurons that demonstrate antidromic invasion from either the medial preoptic area or anterior hypothalamic area and one other stimulation site

Location	Antidromic latencies (msec)						Cancellation interval
	MPOA	AHA	ME	AMG	MDT	PAG	
ARC	20.0	—	6.0	—	—	—	—
ARC	28.0	—	1.5	—	—	—	30
ARC	12.0	—	—	—	—	14.5	26
HVM	8.2	—	4.2	—	—	—	13
HVM	12.3	—	—	31.5	—	—	41
HVM	0.5	—	—	3.8	—	—	5
HVM	13.0	—	—	14.5	—	—	—
HVM	6.2	—	—	18.5	—	—	25
HVM	8.2	—	—	8.0	—	—	16
HVM	—	0.5	—	3.5	—	—	5
HVM	—	1.9	—	—	10.0	—	—
HVM	—	2.5	—	—	13.0	—	—
HVM	—	3.0	—	—	15.6	—	19
HVM	—	4.3	1.5	—	—	—	6
HVM	—	5.0	1.3	—	—	—	7
HVM	12.8	—	—	—	—	21.8	32
HVM	6.0	—	—	—	—	8.5	—
HVM	6.0	—	—	—	—	22.0	—
HVM	4.7	—	—	—	—	3.0	7
HVM	5.5	—	—	—	—	2.5	8

The column on the left denotes the location of neurons within the arcuate (ARC) or ventromedial (HVM) nucleus. The center columns list the antidromic invasion latencies from medial preoptic area (MPOA), anterior hypothalamic area (AHA), median eminence (ME), basolateral-basomedial amygdala (AMG), medialis dorsalis nucleus of the thalamus (MDT), and midbrain periaqueductal gray (PAG). The column on the right refers to data (where available) from interaction experiments (see Fig. 5–4) and lists the critical interval (in msec) between suprathreshold stimulation at each site that resulted in cancellation of the antidromic response to the second stimulus. Note that the cancellation interval approximates the sum of the individual antidromic latencies, suggesting axon bifurcation close to the cell soma. Reproduced from (147).

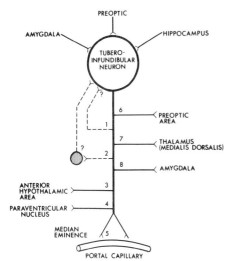

FIG. 5–5. Summary sketch of known connections of the tuberoinfundibular system.

Efferent connections are shown in the lower half of this diagram. The heavy vertical line refers to the main peptidergic or dopaminergic axon connecting the cell soma to the portal capillary plexus, thus identifying the cell as a tuberoinfundibular neuron. Intrahypothalamic axon collaterals are referred to by Nos. 1–5; 1 and 2 depict either direct or indirect recurrent pathways whose transmitter agent is unknown (?); 3 and 4 refer to axon collaterals to the anterior hypothalamic area and paraventricular nucleus; 5 refers to terminal branching in the vicinity of the portal plexus. Extrahypothalamic axon collaterals are depicted as Nos. 6–8 on the right side of the diagram. Afferent connections from at least three areas are illustrated at the top of the figure. Reproduced from (148).

In summary (see Fig. 5–5), electrophysiology has yielded evidence that axons of tuberoinfundibular neurons not only project to the median eminence but also have central axon collaterals. Within the hypothalamus, these axon collaterals participate in prominent recurrent inhibitory (and excitatory) circuits that can dramatically modify the behavior of the parent neuron or adjacent neurons. Tuberoinfundibular neurons with extrahypothalamic projections to the medial preoptic area, amygdala, and midline thalamus are no doubt involved in far more complex neural processes yet to be characterized.

AFFERENT CONNECTIONS OF TUBEROINFUNDIBULAR NEURONS

The mediobasal hypothalamus evidently functions with a certain degree of autonomy in its control of adenohypophyseal secretion, since surgical deafferentation fails to interfere with either basal or certain pulsatile adenohypophyseal secretory patterns (15,65,67,179). However, surgical deafferentation does result in the loss of an adaptive flexibility normally present in the neuroendocrine axis. For example, in the female rat, cyclic ovulation ceases (65) and in the monkey there is abolition of the diurnal or inductive variation in corticosterone secretion (96,180). Numerous stimulation and lesion experiments involving different extrahypothalamic sites (e.g., amygdala, preoptic area, hippocampus, and interpeduncular nucleus) confirm that these areas exert an influence on various parameters of adenohypophyseal secretion (29,36,50,65,102,108,109,194). One might assume that these effects arise through transsynaptic modulation of the excitability of tuberoin-

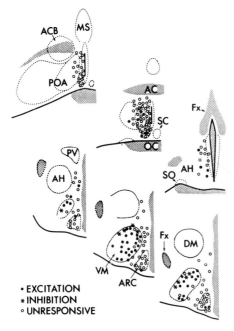

• EXCITATION
* INHIBITION
° UNRESPONSIVE

FIG. 5–6. Summary diagram to illustrate the influence of amygdala stimulation on the activity of tuberoinfundibular neurons.

Symbols superimposed on six coronal sections through the mediobasal hypothalamus and preoptic area depict both the location of tuberoinfundibular neurons and their response to amygdala stimulation. Filled circles indicate cells whose excitability is initially enhanced; asterisks, those whose activity is initially inhibited by amygdala stimulation; open circles, unresponsive cells. Abbreviations as in Fig. 5–1. ACB, nucleus accumbens.

fundibular peptidergic neurons. Preliminary electrophysiological support for this postulate is now available from recent investigations in the rat hypothalamus.

Amygdala

In studies on the electrophysiology of amygdalohypothalamic relationships, prominent excitatory evoked responses have been recorded in the majority of ventromedial nucleus neurons following amygdala stimulation; an equally pronounced inhibition often followed this excitation or was observed as an initial response in a small percentage of cells (132,143). Most tuberoinfundibular neurons located within the hypothalamic ventromedial nucleus display similar short-latency excitatory or inhibitory responses (Fig. 5–6). Few ventromedial nucleus neurons follow orthodromic activation from amygdala at frequencies beyond 30 Hz. This could be attributed to failure at presynaptic levels, but is more likely the result of cumulative postsynaptic inhibition. Very powerful postsynaptic inhibition is a common feature of recordings from hypothalamic neurons, particularly those in the ventromedial nucleus, and can be activated through a variety of pathways. The presence of similar inhibitory periods observed from the same cell after stimulation of more than one site (Fig. 5–3) raises the possibility of a common inhibitory mechanism.

There has been some controversy regarding pathways through which the amygdala exerts its influence on ventromedial hypothalamic neurons. Previous electrophysiological studies in the cat indicate a dual projection from amygdala to ventromedial hypothalamus, originating from the corticomedial and basolateral amygdala and projecting through the stria terminalis and ventral amygdalofugal pathways, respectively (37). However, evidence from recent studies in the rat indicates that only the stria terminalis carries the majority of fibers from the amygdala to the ventromedial hypothalamic nucleus (143). Amygdala-evoked responses within the ventromedial nucleus are virtually abolished after lesions of the stria terminalis (143). Also, activation latencies following stimulation of the amygdala are longer than after stimulation in the stria terminalis. These amygdalohypothalamic fibers in the stria terminalis appear to be principally excitatory in nature. They terminate on dendritic spines of ventromedial nucleus neurons (54), a location usually associated with excitation (63). Furthermore, the majority of ventromedial nucleus neurons demonstrate an initial excitatory response following stimulation in either the stria terminalis or the amygdala (143). The initial inhibitory re-

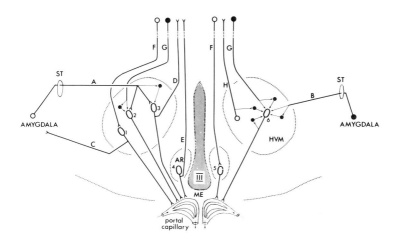

FIG. 5–7. Circuit diagram of mediobasal hypothalamic tuberoinfundibular neurons.

This schematic section through the mediobasal hypothalamus outlines the relative positions of the ventromedial (HVM) and arcuate (AR) nuclei. Tuberoinfundibular neurons are identified by Nos. 1–6 and project directly to the median eminence (ME) portal capillary plexus. The figure illustrates postulated connections of these tuberoinfundibular neurons with the amygdala, medial preoptic, and anterior hypothalamic areas. The heavy continuous lines depict principal connections. Tuberoinfundibular neurons in HVM (Nos. 1–3, 6) receive connections from both the amygdala and more rostral regions, whereas most arcuate tuberoinfundibular neurons (Nos. 4 and 5) are connected only with rostral regions. Afferent extrahypothalamic pathways (A, F) mediating excitatory connections are shown to originate from open circles, whereas inhibitory connections (B, G) are shown to originate from solid circles. The inhibitory pathways may project directly or through afferent collaterals to local inhibitory interneurons (small solid circles in HVM). The fine solid lines indicate intranuclear recurrent and afferent collateral inhibitory pathways. Note that some tuberoinfundibular neurons (e.g., No. 6; see Fig. 5–3) may receive inhibitory connections from several sources: through direct or afferent collateral pathways from amygdala (B) and medial preoptic-anterior hypothalamic area (G); through recurrent collateral pathways from ascending fibers of adjacent HVM neurons (H) or axon collaterals in the tuberoinfundibular tract. Axons of some tuberoinfundibular neurons (Nos. 1, 3, and 4) bifurcate and send fibers to the amygdala (C) and medial preoptic area (D, E). Reproduced from (147).

sponses observed from a smaller number of ventromedial nucleus neurons after stimulation in amygdala or stria terminalis (Fig. 5–4E) could be mediated through a monosynaptic inhibitory pathway from the amygdala (37, 133). However, long inhibitory pathways are unusual in the central nervous system; most postsynaptic inhibition appears to engage local short-axon inhibitory interneurons. In fact, the longer latencies for inhibition than for excitation recorded within the ventromedial nucleus would allow adequate time for activation of an interneuron. Thus, an inhibitory interneuron has been tentatively interposed in the general schema of connections between the amygdala and mediobasal hypothalamic tuberoinfundibular neurons in Fig. 5–7.

The influence of the amygdala on the tuberoinfundibular system is most evident on cells located within the ventromedial nucleus. Tuberoinfundibular neurons in rostral hypothalamic and medial preoptic areas are generally uninfluenced by amygdala stimulation; however, these cells tend to be electrically inactive, and consequently one cannot rule out an inhibitory connection from the amygdala onto these particular tuberoinfundibular cells. The striking lack of effect of the amygdala stimulus on medial preoptic tuberoinfundibular cells contrasts with the generally excitatory effects evoked on adjacent nontuberoinfundibular medial preoptic neurons (L. P. Renaud, *unpublished observations*).

Medial Preoptic-Anterior Hypothalamic Areas

The results of a recent study (147) indicate that electrical stimulation in the medial preoptic or anterior hypothalamic areas influences the excitability of a small number of mediobasal hypothalamic tuberoinfundibular neurons. Short-latency excitations or inhibitions are observed after stimulation of these rostral regions (Fig. 5–3E). The schematic circuit diagram in Fig. 5–7 attempts to define in simple terms some of the possible relationships between the preoptic-anterior hypothalamic area, amygdala, and mediobasal hypothalamic tuberoinfundibular neurons.

Dorsal Hippocampus

Both excitatory and inhibitory responses have been recorded from hypothalamic neurons after dorsal hippocampus stimulation (151). Although the data are preliminary, similar responses have been recorded from tuberoinfundibular neurons located in the periventricular area, the arcuate nucleus, and the dorsal part of the ventromedial nucleus (L. P. Renaud, *unpublished observations*). It is of interest that tuberoinfundibular neurons in these areas are generally unresponsive to amygdala stimulation (Fig. 5–6). This suggests a topographical organization in the afferent projections from amygdala and dorsal hippocampus to the tuberoinfundibular system. Results from certain neuroendocrine experiments do in fact indicate different influences of amygdala and hippocampus on the neuroendocrine axis (36).

Periaqueductal Gray

Preliminary experiments have indicated that a substantial number of neurons in the ventromedial hypothalamic nucleus and arcuate nucleus project to the periaqueductal gray (147,151) or receive afferent projections from that area (151). However, tuberoinfundibular neurons appear generally unresponsive to periaqueductal gray stimulation (H. W. Blume, Q. J. Pittman, and L. P. Renaud, *unpublished observations*). This would suggest the lack of a substantial direct connection between mediobasal hypothalamic tuberoinfundibular neurons and this midbrain region.

In view of the data available from stimulation and lesioning experiments, the connections between extrahypothalamic regions and the tuberoinfundibular system are considered important for the regulation of adenohypophyseal secretion. A more precise interpretation of these connections awaits identification of the peptidergic nature of individual tuberoinfundibular neurons subsequent to their electrophysiological characterization.

NEUROPHARMACOLOGY

In the previous section, electrophysiological aspects of some of the synaptic pathways involving tuberoinfundibular neurons were outlined, but an investigation of the possible synaptic transmitters involved in these pathways has barely begun. Virtually every putative neurotransmitter agent has been implicated in hypothalamic regulation of adenohypophyseal secretion (24,59,60, 72,94,99,106,107,112). It is presumed that these agents act by modifying the excitability of tuberoinfundibular cells through an interaction with specific receptor sites. Microiontophoresis of putative neurotransmitter agents and their antagonists offers one method of testing for specific receptor sites on individual neurons. It is definitely advantageous to supplement this method of study with an electrophysiological characterization of the neuron under examination, as is described in the preceding sections. Hopefully this may lead to identification of neurotransmitters involved in these specific pathways to tuberoinfundibular (and other) hypothalamic neurons.

Monoamines

Moss and his colleagues (115,119) have reported on an extensive study of tuberoinfundibular neurons in the arcuate nucleus. Based on their sensitivity to iontophoretically applied norepinephrine and dopamine, there appear to be two distinct populations of tuberoinfundibular neurons. Tuberoinfundibular

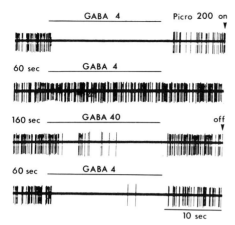

FIG. 5–8. GABA-picrotoxin interaction.

Four oscillograph records illustrate the results of microiontophoresis of GABA and picrotoxin on a neuron in the hypothalamic ventromedial nucleus. In the first trace, application of 4 nA of GABA (*horizontal line*) is associated with a reversible suppression in the glutamate-evoked firing frequency of this neuron. The response is antagonized after application of picrotoxin (200 nA) for 60 sec (second trace). In the third trace, a 10-fold increase in the GABA ejecting current is required to overcome the picrotoxin antagonism. The fourth trace illustrates recovery of the original GABA-evoked suppression, 60 sec after the picrotoxin ejection current is turned off. From Q. J. Pittman, H. W. Blume, B. W. MacKenzie, and L. P. Renaud (*unpublished observations*).

neurons whose activity is increased following application of norepinephrine are usually depressed or uninfluenced by application of dopamine. Conversely, tuberoinfundibular neurons activated by application of dopamine are either depressed or unresponsive to norepinephrine. Unidentified arcuate neurons generally display a different response pattern: some neurons are activated by both norepinephrine and dopamine, or depressed by both, or excited by one and depressed by the other. Preliminary reports using iontophoretic application of receptor blocking agents suggest that pimozide, a dopamine receptor blocker, antagonizes dopamine- but not norepinephrine-induced excitations, whereas phentolamine, an α-adrenergic receptor blocker, antagonizes both dopamine and norepinephrine excitations of arcuate tuberoinfundibular neurons. These results suggest that there are receptor sites on arcuate neurons for both dopamine and norepinephrine, and imply the existence of dopaminergic and adrenergic pathways to these cells. Recent electrophysiological studies on the tuberoinfundibular system using systemic injections of α-methyl-*p*-tyrosine support this contention (158,183,184). There is ample reference in the neuroendocrine literature to the existence of such pathways (53,58,68, 101,102,175), but their precise origin remains to be determined.

Amino Acids

Little is known of the response of identified tuberoinfundibular neurons to amino acids. Only L-glutamate has been tested by microiontophoresis, and its action has been exclusively excitatory (119,144,146). Two other amino acids, gamma-aminobutyric acid (GABA) and glycine are generally considered to be inhibitory neurotransmitters in the central nervous system (98). There is now indirect evidence that GABA may be a neurotransmitter in the recurrent inhibitory pathway to tuberoinfundibular neurons. Intravenous picrotoxin, an effective GABA antagonist (Fig. 5–8, see 34,88,90,98) inter-

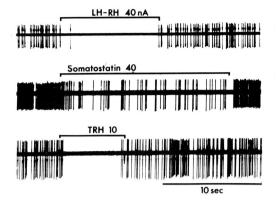

FIG. 5–9. Microiontophoresis of TRH, LRH, and somatostatin.

Three oscillograph records of spike trains illustrate the decrease in spike discharge frequency usually associated with microiontophoresis of three hypothalamic peptides onto different neurons in the hypothalamic ventromedial nucleus. Peptides were applied from adjacent channels of multibarreled micropipettes at relatively low currents (in nanoamperes, indicated by the numbers above the solid horizontal lines). Reproduced from (153).

feres with this recurrent inhibition (138,158,183). Strychnine, a glycine antagonist (33,40,89,98,138), has no influence on this recurrent inhibition (138,158,183).

Applied by microiontophoresis, GABA has a depressant action on the excitability of many hypothalamic neurons; its actions can be reversibly abolished by two antagonists, picrotoxin (Fig. 5–8) and bicuculline (40,138). Glycine also decreases the excitability of hypothalamic neurons, and its action is reversibly antagonized by strychnine (40,138). GABA is generally a more potent depressant agent, and also more likely to be involved in synaptic inhibition in the hypothalamus. The GABA antagonists picrotoxin and bicuculline applied intravenously interfere with synaptic inhibition (138), whereas strychnine is without effect. GABA is present in hypothalamic tissue (155) and hypothalamic nerve terminals (105) and may be part of the hypothalamic control mechanism for release of ACTH (106), LH (131), and prolactin (161).

Peptides

There is some compelling evidence to suggest that hypothalamic releasing factors may function at central synapses. Electrophysiological data indicate extensive axon collaterals in the tuberoinfundibular system, a putative peptidergic neural network. Three hypothalamic peptides (TRH, LRH, and somatostatin) are found within synaptosomes and vesicle-like structures in areas outside of the hypothalamus. These peptides influence animal behavior through a direct action on the central nervous system (120,139). High-affinity binding of TRH has been observed in membrane fractions obtained from certain regions of the central nervous system (27), suggesting the presence of central receptor sites for this peptide.

Microiontophoretic application of TRH, LRH, and somatostatin to neurons in the mediobasal hypothalamus and preoptic area is associated with prominent short-term changes in neuronal excitability (47,85,86,115,116,118,

150,152,153,178). Individual neurons respond to a particular peptide in a specific manner, i.e., the activity can be depressed by one peptide and enhanced or uninfluenced by another (47,115,116,178). The most frequently observed effect is decreased excitability (Fig. 5–9). It is of interest that tuberoinfundibular neurons in the arcuate nucleus are generally unresponsive to both TRH and LRH when compared with adjacent unidentified neurons (115,116). Extrahypothalamic regions such as the cerebral and cerebellar cortices and brainstem also contain peptide-sensitive neurons. However, the percentage of responsive cells is lower in these areas (152,153,178).

In the course of these microiontophoretic studies one is impressed by the high potency of these peptides; the amount required to produce a biological response is a fraction of an fmole/sec (87,178). Therefore, the observed effects are more likely to be physiological rather than pharmacological responses.

COMMENTS

Our knowledge of the tuberoinfundibular system is expanding rapidly in terms of both morphological and physiological definition. In particular, the demonstration of axon collaterals in tuberoinfundibular neurons raises the possibility of peptide release and action as neurotransmitters or neuromodulators at central synapses (5,127,148). According to Dale's hypothesis (35), the same substance(s) liberated into the portal circulation in the median eminence should also be released at these central synapses. Hypothalamic peptides do have potent effects on central neuronal excitability. One could envision these agents as inhibitory neurotransmitters in the monosynaptic pathway proposed to explain recurrent inhibition in the tuberoinfundibular system (see Fig. 5–5, No. 1). However, this is unlikely since tuberoinfundibular neurons are relatively insensitive to TRH and LRH applied by microiontophoresis (115,116). Alternately, an excitatory transmitter action for these peptides would be compatible with the model of a disynaptic recurrent inhibitory pathway (Fig. 5–5, No. 2), since excitation would be required at the initial synapse.

It is important to point out that despite the possible involvement of peptides at central synapses, evidence for their role as neurotransmitter agents is only indirect; the established criteria (176) have yet to be met. Furthermore, arguments based on Dale's hypothesis are predicated on the assumption that the tuberoinfundibular system as defined by electrophysiology is synonymous with the peptidergic tuberoinfundibular system.

It may also be appropriate to consider alternate possibilities to the strict application of Dale's hypothesis. First, different transmitter agents may be transported in different branches of the same tuberoinfundibular neuron. This violates Dale's hypothesis, and has yet to be reported. Second, more than one transmitter may be synthesized and released from the same nerve terminal.

This proposal has received increasing attention (22,26) and would require but a slight modification of Dale's postulate. It might explain why two or more types of vesicles are present in median eminence nerve terminals (170), perhaps an indication of storage sites for peptides and other neurotransmitter agents. If more than one agent is released simultaneously at central synaptic sites, the specificity or affinity of postsynaptic receptors could then determine the appropriate agent for synaptic interaction. Alternately, the peptides may act as neuromodulators at selected synapses working in conjunction with conventional neurotransmitter agents. Perhaps an indication of the latter is the evidence that TRH can enhance acetylcholine-evoked excitation in rat cerebral cortex (186).

In conclusion, the tuberoinfundibular system appears to be more than an isolated collection of hypothalamic neurosecretory cells engaged in the regulation of adenohypophyseal secretion. Its extensive afferent and efferent connections with extrahypothalamic brain regions indicate that it is a true neural network. A study of the cellular neurophysiology and neuropharmacology of this system is fundamental to an understanding of central neuroendocrine mechanisms and the role of peptides in brain.

ACKNOWLEDGMENTS

The authors are grateful to Brian MacKenzie and Robert Nestor for technical assistance, Mrs. M. Walker for typographical aid, Nick Schestakowich for photographic reproductions, and the Canadian Medical Research Council for financial support of the work conducted in this laboratory. L. P. Renaud is the recipient of a Canadian MRC Scholarship, H. W. Blume and Q. J. Pittman are holders of Canadian MRC Fellowships.

REFERENCES

1. Alpert, L. C., Brawer, J. R., Patel, Y. C., and Reichlin, S. (1975): Somatostatinergic neurons in anterior hypothalamus: Immunohistochemical localization. *Endocrinology,* 98:255–258.
2. Amoss, M., Burgus, R., Blackwell, R., Vale, W., Fellows, R., and Guillemin, R. (1971): Purification, amino-acid composition and N-terminus of hypothalamic luteinizing hormone releasing factor (LRF) of ovine origin. *Biochem. Biophys. Res. Commun.,* 44:205–210.
3. Atunes, J. L., Carmel, P. W., Ferin, M., and Zimmerman, E. A. (1976): Paraventricular nucleus: The origin of vasopressin secreting terminals on hypophyseal portal vessels in the monkey. *Endocrinology,* 98:A324.
4. Arnauld, E., Dufy, B., and Vincent, J. D. (1975): Hypothalamic supraoptic neurones: Rates and patterns of action potential firing during water deprivation in the unanaesthetized monkey. *Brain Res.,* 100:315–325.
5. Barker, J. L. (1977): Physiological roles of peptides in the nervous system. In: *Peptides in Neurobiology,* edited by H. Gainer. Plenum Press, New York (*in press*).
6. Barker, J. L., Crayton, J. W., and Nicoll, R. A. (1971): Antidromic and orthodromic responses of paraventricular and supraoptic neurosecretory cells. *Brain Res.,* 33:353–366.
7. Barnea, A., Ben-Jonathan, N., Colston, C., Johnston, J. M., and Porter, J. C.

(1975): Differential sub-cellular compartmentalization of thyrotropin releasing hormone (TRH) and gonadotropin releasing hormone (LRH) in hypothalamic tissue. *Proc. Natl. Acad. Sci. USA*, 72:3153–3157.

8. Barry, J., and Dubois, M. P. (1975): Immunofluorescence study of LRF producing neurons in the cat and the dog. *Neuroendocrinology*, 18:290–298.

9. Barry, J., Dubois, M. P., and Carette, B. (1974): Immunofluorescence study of the preoptico-infundibular LRF neurosecretory pathway in the normal, castrated or testosterone-treated male guinea pig. *Endocrinology*, 95:1415–1423.

10. Ben-Jonathan, N., Oliver, C., Weiner, J., Mical, S., and Porter, J. C. (1977): Dopamine in hypophyseal portal plasma of the rat during the estrous cycle and throughout pregnancy. *Endocrinology*, 100:452–458.

11. Björklund, A., Falck, B., Hromek, F., Owen, C., and West, K. A. (1970): Identification and terminal distribution of the tubero-hypophyseal monoamine system in the rat by means of stereotaxic and microspectrofluorometric techniques. *Brain Res.*, 17:1–23.

12. Björklund, A., Falck, B., Nobin, A., and Stenevi, V. (1974): Organization of the dopamine and noradrenaline innervations of the median eminence—pituitary region in the rat. In: *Neurosecretion—the Final Neuroendocrine Pathway*, edited by F. Knowles and L. Vollrath, pp. 209–222. Springer-Verlag, New York.

13. Björklund, A., and Nobin, A. (1973): Fluorescence histochemical and microspectrofluorometric mapping of dopamine and noradrenaline cell groups in the rat diencephalon. *Brain Res.*, 51:191–205.

14. Blackwell, R. E., and Guillemin, R. (1973): Hypothalamic control of adenohypophyseal secretions. *Annu. Rev. Physiol.*, 35:357–370.

15. Blake, C. A., and Sawyer, C. H. (1974): Effects of hypothalamic deafferentation on the pulsatile rhythm in plasma concentrations of luteinizing hormone in ovariectomized rats. *Endocrinology*, 94:730–736.

16. Blakemore, M. A., Dyer, R. G., and Morris, S. F. (1974): Identification of periventricular cells projecting to the median eminence. *J. Physiol.*, 242:12P–13P.

17. Brazeau, P., Vale, W., Burgus, R., Ling, N., Butcher, M., Rivier, J., and Guillemin, R. (1973): Hypothalamic polypeptide that inhibits secretion of immunoreactive pituitary growth hormone. *Science*, 179:77–79.

18. Brownstein, M. J., Arimura, A., Fernandez-Durango, R., Schally, A. V., Palkovits, M., and Kizer, J. S. (1977): The effect of hypothalamic deafferentation on somatostatin-like activity in the rat brain. *Endocrinology*, 100:246–249.

19. Brownstein, M., Arimura, A., Sato, H., Schally, A. V., and Kizer, J. S. (1975): The regional distribution of somatostatin in the rat brain. *Endocrinology*, 96:1456–1461.

20. Brownstein, M., Arimura, A., Schally, A. V., Palkovits, M., and Kizer, J. S. (1976): The effect of surgical isolation of the hypothalamus on its luteinizing hormone-releasing hormone content. *Endocrinology*, 98:662–665.

21. Brownstein, M. J., Palkovits, M., Saavedra, J. M., and Kizer, J. S. (1976): Distribution of hypothalamic hormones and neurotransmitters within the diencephalon. In: *Frontiers in Neuroendocrinology, Vol. 4*, edited by L. Martini and W. F. Ganong, pp. 1–23. Raven Press, New York.

22. Brownstein, M. J., Saavedra, J. M., Axelrod, J., Zeman, G. H., and Carpenter, D. O. (1974): Coexistence of several putative neurotransmitters in single identified neurons of aplysia. *Proc. Natl. Acad. Sci. USA*, 71:4662–4665.

23. Brownstein, M. J., Utiger, R. D., Palkovits, M., and Kizer, J. S. (1975): Effect of hypothalamic deafferentation on thyrotropin-releasing hormone levels in rat brain. *Proc. Natl. Acad. Sci. USA*, 72:4177–4179.

24. Burden, J., Hillhouse, E. W., and Jones, M. T. (1974): The inhibitory action of GABA and melatonin on the release of corticotrophin-releasing hormone from the rat hypophysiotrophic area in vitro. *J. Physiol.*, 239:116P.

25. Burgus, R., Dunn, T. F., Desiderio, D., Ward, D. N., Vale, E., and Guillemin, R. (1970): Characterization of ovine hypothalamic hypophysiotropic TSH-releasing factor. *Nature*, 226:321–325.

26. Burnstock, G. (1976): Do some nerve cells release more than one transmitter? *Neuroscience*, 1:239–248.

27. Burt, D. R., and Snyder, S. H. (1975): Thyrotropin releasing hormone (TRH)—apparent receptor binding in rat-brain membranes. *Brain Res.*, 93:309–328.
28. Cajal, S. R. (1911): *Histologie du Système Nerveux de l'Homme et des Vertébrés*, Vol. 2. Maloine, Paris.
29. Casady, R. L., and Taylor, A. N. (1976): Effect of electrical stimulation of the hippocampus upon corticosteroid levels in the freely-behaving, non-stressed rat. *Neuroendocrinology*, 20:68–78.
30. Christ, J. F. (1966): Nerve supply, blood supply and cytology of the neurohypophysis. In: *The Pituitary Gland*, edited by G. W. Harris and B. T. Donovan, pp. 62–130. University of California Press, Berkeley.
31. Cross, B. A., Dyball, R. E. J., Dyer, R. G., Jones, C. W., Lincoln, D. W., Morris, J. F., and Pickering, B. T. (1975): Endocrine neurons. *Recent Prog. Horm. Res.*, 31:243–294.
32. Cross, B. A., and Green, J. D. (1959): Activity of single neurons in the hypothalamus: Effect of osmotic and other stimuli. *J. Physiol.*, 148:554–569.
33. Curtis, D. R., Duggan, A. W., and Johnston, G. A. R. (1971): The specificity of strychnine as a glycine antagonist in the mammalian spinal cord. *Exp. Brain Res.*, 12:547–565.
34. Curtis, D. R., and Johnston, G. A. R. (1974): Amino acid transmitters in the mammalian central nervous system. *Ergeb. Physiol.*, 69:97–188.
35. Dale, H. A. (1935): Pharmacology and nerve endings. *Proc. R. Soc. Med.*, 28:318–332.
36. Döcke, F. (1974): Differential effects of amygdaloid and hippocampal lesions on female puberty. *Neuroendocrinology*, 14:345–350.
37. Dreifuss, J. J. (1972): Effects of electrical stimulation of the amygdaloid complex on the ventromedial hypothalamus. In: *The Neurobiology of the Amygdala*, edited by B. E. Eleftheriou, pp. 295–317. Plenum Press, New York.
38. Dreifuss, J. J., Harris, M. C., and Tribollett, E. (1976): Excitation of phasically firing hypothalamic supraoptic neurones by carotid occlusion in rats. *J. Physiol.*, 257:337–354.
39. Dreifuss, J. J., and Kelly, J. S. (1972): Recurrent inhibition of antidromically identified rat supraoptic neurones. *J. Physiol.*, 220:87–103.
40. Dreifuss, J. J., and Matthews, E. K. (1972): Antagonism between strychnine and glycine, and bicuculline and GABA, in the ventromedial hypothalamus. *Brain Res.*, 45:599–603.
41. Dubois, M. P., Barry, J., and Leonardelli, J. (1974): Mise en evidence par immunofluorescence et repartition de la somatostatine (SRIF) dans l'eminence mediane des vertebrés, mammifières, oiseaux, amphibians et poissons. *C. R. Acad. Sci. [D] (Paris)*, 272:1899–1902.
42. Dubois, M. P., and Kolodziejczyk, E. (1975): Centres hypothalamiques du rat sécrétant la somatostatine: répartition des péricaryons en 2 systèmes magno et parvocellulaires (étude immunocytologique). *C. R. Acad. Sci. [D] (Paris)*, 281:1737–1740.
43. Dyball, R. E. J. (1971): Oxytocin and ADH secretion in relation to electrical activity on antidromically identified supraoptic and paraventricular units. *J. Physiol.*, 214:245–256.
44. Dyball, R. E. J., and Koizumi, K. (1969): Electrical activity in the supraoptic and paraventricular nuclei associated with neurohypophyseal hormone release. *J. Physiol.*, 201:711–722.
45. Dyer, R. G. (1973): An electrophysiological dissection of the hypothalamic regions which regulate the pre-ovulatory secretion of luteinizing hormone in the rat. *J. Physiol.*, 234:421–442.
46. Dyer, R. G. (1975): Characteristics of neurones projecting directly to the region of the median eminence. In: *Hypothalamic Hormones*, edited by M. Motta, P. G. Crosignani, and L. Martini, pp. 169–182. Academic Press, London.
47. Dyer, R. G., and Dyball, R. E. J. (1974): Evidence for a direct effect of LRF and TRF on single unit-activity in rostral hypothalamus. *Nature*, 252:486–488.
48. Eccles, J. C. (1964): *The Physiology of Synapses*. Springer-Verlag, Berlin.

49. Elde, R., Hökfelt, T., Johansson, O., Efendić, S., and Luft, R. (1976): Somatostatin containing pathways in the nervous system. *Neurosci. Abstr.,* 2:759.
50. Ellendorf, F., Colombo, J. A., Blake, C. A., Whitmoyer, D. I., and Sawyer, C. H. (1973): Effects of electrical stimulation of the amygdala on gonadotropin release and ovulation in the rat. *Proc. Soc. Exp. Biol. Med.,* 142:417–420.
51. Ellendorf, F., MacLeod, N. K., and Dyer, R. G. (1976): Bipolar neurones in the rostral hypothalamus. *Brain Res.,* 101:549–553.
52. Epelbaum, J., Brazeau, P., Tsang, D., Brawer, J., and Martin, J. B. (1977): Subcellular distribution of radioimmunoassayable somatostatin in rat brain. *Brain Res.,* 126:309–323.
53. Everett, J. W. (1964): Central neural control of reproductive functions of the adenohypophysis. *Physiol. Rev.,* 44:373–431.
54. Field, P. M. (1972): A quantitative ultrastructural analysis of the distribution of amygdaloid fibers in the preoptic area and the ventromedial hypothalamic nucleus. *Exp. Brain Res.,* 14:527–538.
55. Flament-Durand, J. (1971): Ultrastructural aspects of the paraventricular nuclei in the rat. *Z. Zellforsch.,* 116:61–69.
56. Fuxe, K., and Hökfelt, T. (1967): The influence of central catecholamine neurons on the hormone secretion from the anterior and posterior pituitary. In: *Neurosecretion,* edited by F. Stutinsky, pp. 165–175. Springer, Berlin.
57. Fuxe, K., and Hökfelt, T. (1969): Catecholamines in the hypothalamus and the pituitary gland. In: *Frontiers in Neuroendocrinology, 1969,* edited by W. F. Ganong and L. Martini, pp. 47–96. Oxford University Press, London.
58. Gallo, R. V., Johnson, J. H., Goldman, B. D., Whitmoyer, D. I., and Sawyer, C. H. (1971): Effects of electrochemical stimulation of the ventral hippocampus on hypothalamic electrical activity and pituitary gonadotropin secretion in female rats. *Endocrinology,* 89:704–713.
59. Ganong, W. F. (1974): The role of catecholamines and acetylcholine in the regulation of endocrine function. *Life Sci.,* 15:1401–1414.
60. Ganong, W. F. (1975): Brain amines and the control of ACTH and growth hormone. In: *Hypothalamic Hormones,* edited by M. Motta, F. G. Crossignani, and L. Martini, pp. 237–248. Academic Press, New York.
61. Goldsmith, P. C., and Ganong, W. F. (1975): Ultrastructural localization of luteinizing hormone releasing hormone in the median eminence of the rat. *Brain Res.,* 97:181–193.
62. Goldsmith, P. C., and Zimmerman, E. A. (1975): Ultrastructural localization of neurophysin and vasopressin in rat median eminence. *Endocrinology,* 92:A239.
63. Gray, E. G. (1968): Electron microscopy of excitatory and inhibitory synapses; a brief review. *Prog. Brain Res.,* 31:141–155.
64. Green, J. D. (1969): Neural pathways to the hypophysis: Anatomical and functional. In: *The Hypothalamus,* edited by W. Haymaker, E. Anderson, and W. J. H. Nauta, pp. 276–310. Charles C Thomas, Springfield, Ill.
65. Halász, B. (1969): The endocrine effects of isolation of the hypothalamus from the rest of the brain. In: *Frontiers in Neuroendocrinology, 1969,* edited by W. F. Ganong and L. Martini, pp. 307–342. Oxford University Press, London.
66. Halász, B., Köves, K., Réthelyi, M., Bodoky, M., and Koritsánsky, S. (1975): Recent data on neuronal connections between nervous structures involved in the control of the adenohypophysis. In: *Anatomical Endocrinology,* edited by W. E. Stumpf and L. D. Grant, pp. 9–14. S. Karger, Basel.
67. Halász, B., Pupp, L., and Uhlarik, S. (1962): Hypophysiotrophic area in the hypothalamus. *J. Neuroendocrinol.,* 25:147–154.
68. Haller, E. W., and Barraclough, C. A. (1970): Alternations in unit activity of hypothalamic ventromedial nuclei by stimuli which affect gonadotropic hormone secretion. *Exp. Neurol.,* 29:11–120.
69. Harris, G. W. (1955): *Neural Control of Pituitary Gland.* Edward Arnold, London.
70. Harris, M. C., and Sanghera, M. (1974): Projection of medial basal hypothalamic neurones to the preoptic anterior hypothalamic areas and the paraventricular nucleus in the rat. *Brain Res.,* 81:401–411.

71. Haymaker, W. (1969): Hypothalamo-pituitary neural pathways and the circulatory system of the pituitary. In: *The Hypothalamus*, edited by W. Haymaker, E. Anderson, and W. J. H. Nauta, pp. 219–250. Charles C. Thomas, Springfield, Ill.

72. Hillhouse, E. W., Burden, J., and Jones, M. T. (1974): The control of CRF release at the hypothalamic level. In: *Neurosecretion, the Final Common Pathway*, edited by F. Knowles and L. Vollrath, p. 308. Springer-Verlag, New York.

73. Hökfelt, T. (1977): Aminergic and peptidergic brain pathways. In: *The Hypothalamus*, edited by S. Reichlin. Raven Press, New York (*in press*).

74. Hökfelt, T., Efendić, S., Hellerström, C., Johansson, O., Luft, R., and Arimura, A. (1975): Cellular localization of somatostatin in endocrine-like cells and neurons of the rat with special reference to A₁-cells of the pancreatic islets and to the hypothalamus. *Acta Endocrinol. [Suppl. 200] (Kbh.)*, 80:1–40.

75. Hökfelt, T., Efendić, S., Johannson, O., Luft, B., and Arimura, A. (1974): Immunohistochemical localization of somatostatin (growth-hormone release-inhibiting factor) in guinea-pig brain. *Brain Res.*, 80:165–169.

76. Hökfelt, T., Elde, R., Johansson, O., Luft, R., Nilsson, G., and Arimura, A. (1976): Immunohistochemical evidence for separate populations of somatostatin-containing and substance P-containing primary afferent neurons in the rat. *Neurosci.* 1:131–136.

77. Hökfelt, T., and Fuxe, K. (1972): On the morphology and the neuroendocrine role of the hypothalamic catecholamine neurons. In: *Brain-Endocrine Interaction. Median Eminence: Structure and Function*, edited by K. M. Knigge, D. E. Scott, and A. Weindel, pp. 181–223. S. Karger, Basel.

78. Hökfelt, T., Fuxe, K., Goldstein, M., Johansson, O., Park, D., Fraser, H., and Jeffcoate, S. L. (1974): Immunofluorescence mapping of central monoamine and releasing hormone (LRH) systems. In: *Anatomical Neuroendocrinology*, edited by W. E. Stumpf and L. D. Grant, pp. 381–392. S. Karger, Basel.

79. Hökfelt, T., Fuxe, K., Johansson, O., Jeffcoate, S., and White, N. (1975): Distribution of thyrotropin-releasing hormone (TRH) in the central nervous system as revealed with immunohistochemistry. *Eur. J. Pharmacol.*, 34:389–392.

80. Hökfelt, T., Fuxe, K., Johansson, O., Jeffcoate, S. L., and White, N. (1975): Thyrotropin releasing hormone (TRH)-containing nerve terminals in certain brain stem nuclei and in the spinal cord. *Neurosci. Lett.*, 1:133–139.

81. Hökfelt, T., Johansson, O., Fuxe, K., Lofstrom, A., Goldstein, M., Park, D., Ebstein, R., Fraser, H., Jeffcoate, S., Efendić, S., Luft, R. (1977): Mapping and relationship of hypothalamic neurotransmitters and hypothalamic hormones. *Proceedings of the Sixth International Congress of Pharmacol, Vol. 3*. (*in press*).

82. Ishikawa, K., Koisumi, K., and Brooks, C. McC. (1966): Activity of supraoptic nucleus neurons of the hypothalamus. *Neurology (Minneap.)*, 16:101–106.

83. Kalra, S. P. (1976): Tissue levels of luteinizing hormone-releasing hormone in the preoptic area and hypothalamus, and serum concentrations of gonadotropins following anterior hypothalamic deafferentation and estrogen treatment in the female rat. *Endocrinology*, 99:101–107.

84. Kandel, E. R. (1964): Electrical properties of hypothalamic neuroendocrine cells. *J. Gen. Physiol.*, 47:691–717.

85. Kawakami, M., and Sakuma, Y. (1974): Responses of hypothalamic neurons to the microiontophoresis of LH-RH, LH and FSH under various levels of circulating ovarian hormones. *Neuroendocrinology*, 15:290–307.

86. Kawakami, M., and Sakuma, Y. (1976): Electrophysiological evidence for possible participation of periventricular neurons in anterior pituitary regulation. *Brain Res.*, 101:79–94.

87. Kelly, M. J., and Moss, R. M. (1976): Quantitative evaluation and determination of the biological potency of iontophoretically applied luteinizing hormone releasing hormone (LRH). *Neuropharmacology*, 15:325–328.

88. Kelly, J. S., and Renaud, L. P. (1973): On the pharmacology of the γ-aminobutyric acid receptors on the cuneothalamic relay cells of the cat. *Br. J. Pharmacol.*, 48:369–386.

89. Kelly, J. S., and Renaud, L. P. (1973): On the pharmacology of the glycine receptors on the cuneo-thalamic relay cells in the cat. *Br. J. Pharmacol.*, 48:387–395.

90. Kelly, J. S., and Renaud, L. P. (1973): On the pharmacology of the ascending, descending and recurrent postsynaptic inhibition of the cuneo-thalamic relay cells in the cat. *Br. J. Pharmacol.,* 48:396–408.
91. King, J. C., Gerall, A. A., Fishback, J. B., and Elkind, K. E. (1975): Growth hormone-release inhibiting hormone (GH-RIH) pathway of the rat hypothalamus revealed by the unlabeled antibody peroxidase-antiperoxidase method. *Cell Tissue Res.,* 160:423–430.
92. King, J. C., Parsons, J. A., Erlandsen, S. L., and Williams, T. H. (1974): Luteinizing hormone-releasing hormone (LH-RH) pathways of the rat hypothalamus revealed by the unlabeled antibody peroxidase-antiperoxidase method. *Cell Tissue Res.,* 153:211–217.
93. Koizumi, K., and Yamashita, H. (1972): Studies of antidromically identified neurosecretory cells of the hypothalamus by intracellular and extracellular recordings. *J. Physiol.,* 221:683–705.
94. Kordon, C., and Glowinski, J. (1972): Role of hypothalamic monoaminergic neurones in the gonadotrophin release-regulating mechanisms. *Neuropharmacology,* 11:153–162.
95. Kordon, C., Kerdelhue, B., Pattou, E., and Jutisz, M. (1974): Immunocytochemical localization of LH-RH in axons and nerve terminals of the rat median eminence. *Proc. Soc. Exp. Biol. Med.,* 147:122–127.
96. Krey, L. C., Lu, K.-H., Butler, W. R., Hotchkiss, J., Piva, F., and Knobil, E. (1975): Surgical disconnection of the medial basal hypothalamus and pituitary function in the rhesus monkey. II. GH and cortisol secretion. *Endocrinology,* 96:1088–1093.
97. Krieger, D. T., and Zimmerman, E. A. (1977): The nature of CRF and its relationship to vasopressin CRF. In: *Clinical Endocrinology,* edited by M. Besser and L. Martini. Academic Press, New York (*in press*).
98. Krnjević, K. (1974): Chemical nature of synaptic transmission in vertebrates. *Physiol. Rev.,* 54:418–540.
99. Krulich, L., Giachetti, A., Marchlewska-Kos, A., Hefco, E., and Jameson, H. E. (1977): On the role of the central noradrenergic and dopaminergic systems in the regulation of TSH secretion in the rat. *Endocrinology,* 100:496–505.
100. Leonardelli, J., and Dubois, M. P. (1974): Commandes aminergique et cholinergique des cellules hypothalamiques élaboratrices de LH-RH chez le cobaye. *Ann. Endocrinol. (Paris),* 35:639–645.
101. Lichtensteiger, W. (1969): Cyclic variations of catecholamine content in hypothalamic nerve cells during the estrous cycle of the rat, with a concomitant study of the substantia nigra. *J. Pharmacol. Exp. Ther.,* 165:204–215.
102. Lichtensteiger, W., and Keller, A. J. (1974): Tuberoinfundibular dopamine neurons and the secretion of luteinizing hormone and prolactin: Extrahypothalamic influences, interaction with cholinergic systems and the effect of urethane anesthesia. *Brain Res.,* 74:279–303.
103. Lincoln, D. W., and Wakerley, J. B. (1974): Electrophysiological evidence for the activation of supraoptic neurones during the release of oxytocin. *J. Physiol.,* 242:533–554.
104. Makara, G. B., Harris, M. C., and Spyer, K. M. (1972): Identification and distribution of tuberoinfundibular neurones. *Brain Res.,* 40:283–290.
105. Makara, G. B., Rappay, G., and Stark, E. (1975): Autoradiographic localization of ^{3}H-gamma-aminobutyric acid in the medial hypothalamus. *Exp. Brain. Res.,* 22:449–455.
106. Makara, G. B., and Stark, E. (1974): Effect of gamma-aminobutyric acid (GABA) and GABA antagonist drugs on ACTH release. *Neuroendocrinology,* 16:178–190.
107. Makara, G. B., and Stark, E. (1975): Acetylcholine and amino acid neurotransmitters in the regulation of ACTH secretion. In: *Symposium of the International Society for Psychoneuroendocrinology,* pp. 483–494. Akademiai Kiado, Budapest.
108. Martin, J. B. (1972): Plasma growth hormone (GH) response to hypothalamic or extrahypothalamic electrical stimulation. *Endocrinology,* 91:107–115.
109. Martin, J. B., Kontor, J., and Mead, P. (1973): Plasma GH responses to hypothalamic hippocampal and amygdaloid electrical stimulation: Effects of variation

of stimulation parameters and treatment with α-methyl-para-tyrosine (α-MT). *Endocrinology,* 92:1354–1361.

110. Martin, J. B., and Reichlin, S. (1972): Plasma thyrotropin (TSH) responses to hypothalamic electrical stimulation and to injection of synthetic thyrotropin releasing hormone (TRH). *Endocrinology,* 90:1079–1089.
111. Martinez, P. M. (1960): The structure of the pituitary stalk and the innervation of the neurohypophysis in the cat. Luctor et Emergo, Leiden, dissertation. (Quoted from Szentagothai et al., 1968.)
112. McCann, S. M., and Moss, R. L. (1975): Putative neurotransmitters involved in discharging gonadotropin-releasing neurohormones and the action of LH-releasing hormone in the CNS. *Life Sci.,* 16:833–852.
113. Millhouse, O. E. (1973): The organization of the ventromedial hypothalamic nucleus. *Brain Res.,* 55:71–87.
114. Millhouse, O. E. (1973): Certain ventromedial hypothalamic afferents. *Brain Res.,* 55:88–105.
115. Moss, R. L. (1976): Unit responses in preoptic and arcuate neurons related to anterior pituitary function. In: *Frontiers in Neuroendocrinology, Vol. 4,* edited by L. Martini and W. F. Ganong, pp. 95–128. Raven Press, New York.
116. Moss, R. L. (1977): Role of hypophysiotropic neurohormones in mediating neural and behavioral events. *Fed. Proc.,* 36:1978–1983.
117. Moss, R. L., Dyball, R. E. J., and Cross, B. A. (1972): Excitation of antidromically identified neurosecretory cells in the paraventricular nucleus by oxytocin applied iontophoretically. *Exp. Neurol.,* 34:95–102.
118. Moss, R. L., Kelly, M. J., and Dudley, C. A. (1976): Effect of peptide hormones on extracellular electrical activities of preoptic-hypothalamic neurons. *Neurosci. Abstr.,* 2:652.
119. Moss, R. L., Kelly, M., and Riskind, P. (1975): Tuberoinfundibular neurons: Dopaminergic and norepinephrinergic sensitivity. *Brain Res.,* 89:265–277.
120. Moss, R. L., McCann, S. M., and Dudley, C. A. (1975): Releasing hormones and sexual behavior. *Prog. Brain Res.,* 42:37–46.
121. Moss, R. L., Urban, I., and Cross, B. A. (1972): Microelectrophoresis of cholinergic and aminergic drugs on paraventricular neurons. *Am. J. Physiol.,* 223:310–318.
122. Naik, D. V. (1975): Immuno-electron microscopic localization of luteinizing hormone-releasing hormone in the arcuate nuclei and median eminence of the rat. *Cell Tissue Res.,* 157:437–455.
123. Naik, D. V. (1975): Immunoreactive LH-RH neurons in the hypothalamus identified by light and fluorescent microscopy. *Cell Tissue Res.,* 157:423–436.
124. Nair, R. M. G., Barrett, J. F., Bowers, C. Y., and Schally, A. V. (1970): Structure of porcine thyrotropin releasing hormone. *Biochemistry,* 9:1103–1106.
125. Negoro, H., and Holland, R. C. (1972): Inhibition of unit activity in the hypothalamic paraventricular nucleus following antidromic activation. *Brain Res.,* 42: 385–402.
126. Negoro, H., Visessuwan, S., and Holland, R. C. (1973): Inhibition and excitation of units in paraventricular nucleus after stimulation of the septum, amygdala and neurohypophysis. *Brain Res.,* 57:479–483.
127. Nicoll, R. A., and Barker, J. L. (1971): Excitation of supraoptic neurosecretory cells by angiotensin II. *Nature [New Biol.],* 233:172–174.
128. Nicoll, R. A., and Barker, J. L. (1971): The pharmacology of recurrent inhibition in the supraoptic neurosecretory system. *Brain Res.,* 35:501–511.
129. Novin, D., Sundsten, J. W., and Cross, B. A. (1970): Some properties af antidromically activated units in the paraventricular nucleus of the hypothalamus. *Exp. Neurol.,* 26:330–341.
130. Nowakowski, H. (1951): Infundibular and tuber cinereum der Katz. *Dtsch. Z. Nervenheilkd.,* 165:201–339.
131. Ondo, J. G. (1974): Gamma-aminobutyric acid effects on pituitary gonadotropin secretion. *Science,* 186:738–739.
132. Ono, T., and Oomura, Y. (1975): Excitatory control of hypothalamic ventromedial nucleus by basolateral amygdala in rats. *Pharmacol. Biochem. Behav.,* 3: Suppl. I, 37–47.

133. Oomura, Y., Ono, T., and Ooyama, H. (1970): Inhibitory action of the amygdala on the lateral hypothalamic area in rats. *Nature*, 228:1108–1110.
134. Parsons, J. A., Erlansen, S. L., Heggre, O. D., McEvoy, R. C., and Elde, R. P. (1976): Central and peripheral localization of somatostatin immunoenzyme immunocytochemical studies. *J. Histochem. Cytochem.*, 24:872–882.
135. Pelletier, G., Labrie, F., Arimura, A., and Schally, A. V. (1974): Electron microscopic immunohistochemical localization of growth hormone-release inhibiting hormone (somatostatin) in the rat median eminence. *Am. J. Anat.*, 140:445–450.
136. Pelletier, G., Labrie, F., Puviani, R., Arimura, A., and Schally, A. V. (1974): Immunohistochemical localization of luteinizing hormone-releasing hormone in rat median eminence. *Endocrinology*, 95:314–317.
137. Pelletier, G., Leclerc, R., and Dube, D. (1976): Immunohistochemical localization of hypothalamic hormones. *J. Histochem. Cytochem.*, 24:864–871.
138. Pittman, Q. J., Blume, H. W., MacKenzie, B. W., and Renaud, L. P. (1977): GABA, glycine and synaptic inhibition in the hypothalamic ventromedial nucleus of the rat. *Can. Physiol.*, 8:56.
139. Prange, A. J., Jr., Nemeroff, C. B., Lipton, M. S., Breese, G. R., and Wilson, I. C. (1977): Peptides and the central nervous system. In: *Handbook of Psychopharmacology, Section II*, edited by L. L. Iversen, S. D. Iversen, and S. H. Snyder. Plenum Press, New York (*in press*).
140. Ramirez, V. D., Gautron, J. P., Epelbaum, J., Pattou, E., Zamura, A., and Kordon, C. (1975): Distribution of LH-RH in subcellular fractions of the basomedial hypothalamus. *Mol. Cell. Endocrinol.*, 3:339–350.
141. Renaud, L. P. (1975): Electrophysiological evidence to suggest that hypothalamic releasing (inhibiting) peptides may be liberated from nerve terminals in the CNS. *Neurosci. Abstr.*, 1:441.
142. Renaud, L. P. (1976): Electrophysiological evidence for axon collaterals in the tuberoinfundibular system of the rat. *J. Physiol.*, 254:20P–21P.
143. Renaud, L. P. (1976): An electrophysiological study of amygdalohypothalamic projections to the ventromedial nucleus of the rat. *Brain Res.*, 105:45–58.
144. Renaud, L. P. (1976): Tuberoinfundibular neurons in the basomedial hypothalamus of the rat: Electrophysiological evidence for axon collaterals to hypothalamic and extrahypothalamic areas. *Brain Res.*, 105:59–72.
145. Renaud, L. P. (1976): Tuberoinfundibular neurons: Electrophysiological studies on afferent and efferent connections. *Physiologist*, 19:338.
146. Renaud, L. P. (1976): Influence of amygdala stimulation on the activity of identified tuberoinfundibular neurones in the rat hypothalamus. *J. Physiol.*, 260:237–252.
147. Renaud, L. P. (1977): Influence of medial preoptic-anterior hypothalamic area stimulation on the excitability of mediobasal hypothalamic neurones in the rat. *J. Physiol.*, 264:541–564.
148. Renaud, L. P. (1977): TRH, LHRH and somatostatin: Distribution and physiological action in neural tissue. In: *Neuroscience Symposia, Vol. 2*, edited by W. M. Cowan and J. A. Ferrendelli, pp. 265–290. Raven Press, New York (*in press*).
149. Renaud, L. P., and Hopkins, D. A. (1977): Amygdala afferents from the mediobasal hypothalamus: An electrophysiological and neuroanatomical study in the rat. *Brain Res.*, 121:201–213.
150. Renaud, L. P., and Martin, J. B. (1975): Thyrotropin releasing hormone (TRH) —depressant action on central neuronal-activity. *Brain Res.*, 86:150–154.
151. Renaud, L. P., and Martin, J. B. (1975): Electrophysiological studies of connections of hypothalamic ventromedial nucleus neurons in the rat: Evidence for a role in neuroendocrine integration. *Brain Res.*, 93:145–151.
152. Renaud, L. P., Martin, J. B., and Brazeau, P. (1975): Depressant action of TRH, LH-RH and somatostatin on activity of central neurones. *Nature*, 255:233–235.
153. Renaud, L. P., Martin, J. B., and Brazeau, P. (1976): Hypothalamic releasing factors: Physiological evidence for a regulatory action on central neurons and pathways for their distribution in brain. *Pharmacol. Biochem. Behav.*, 5: Suppl. I, 171–178.
154. Rethélyi, M., and Halász, B. (1970): Origin of the nerve endings in the surface

zone of the median eminence of the rat hypothalamus. *Exp. Brain Res.,* 11:145–158.

155. Robinson, N., and Wells, F. (1973): Distribution and localization of sites of gamma aminobutyric acid metabolism in the adult rat brain. *J. Anat.,* 114:365–378.

156. Sawaki, Y. (1977): Retinohypothalamic projection: Electrophysiological evidence for the existence in female rats. *Brain Res.,* 120:336–341.

157. Sawaki, Y., and Yagi, K. (1973): Electrophysiological identification of cell bodies of the tuberoinfundibular neurones in the rat. *J. Physiol.,* 230:75–85.

158. Sawaki, Y., and Yagi, K. (1976): Inhibition and facilitation of antidromically identified tuberoinfundibular neurones following stimulation of the median eminence in the rat. *J. Physiol.,* 260:447–460.

159. Schally, A. V., Arimura, A., Baba, Y., Nair, R. M. G., Matsuo, J., Redding, T. W., Debeljuk, L., and White, W. F. (1971): Isolation and properties of FSH and LH-releasing hormone. *Biochem. Biophys. Res. Commun.,* 43:393–399.

160. Schally, A. V., Arimura, A., and Kastin, A. J. (1973): Hypothalamic regulatory hormones. *Science,* 179:341–350.

161. Schally, A. V., Redding, T. W., Linthicum, G. L., and Dupont, A. (1976): Inhibition of prolactin release *in-vivo* and *in-vitro* by natural hypothalamic and synthetic gamma aminobutyric acid. *Endocrinology,* 98:216A.

162. Sétáló, G., Sándor, V., Schally, A. V., Arimura, A., and Flerkó, B. (1975): GH-RIH containing elements in the rat hypothalamus. *Brain Res.,* 90:352–356.

163. Sétáló, G., Vigh, S., Schally, A. V., Arimura, A., and Flerkó, B. (1975): LH-RH containing neural elements in the rat hypothalamus. *Endocrinology,* 96:135–142.

164. Sétáló, G., Vigh, S., Schally, A. V., Arimura, A., and Flerkó, B. (1976): Immuno-histological study of the origin of LH-RH containing nerve fibers of the rat hypothalamus. *Brain Res.,* 103:597–602.

165. Silverman, A. J. (1976): Distribution of luteinizing hormone-releasing hormone (LHRH) in the guinea pig brain. *Endocrinology,* 99:30–41.

166. Silverman, A. J., Antunes, J., Ferin, M., and Zimmerman, E. A. (1976): Immunocytochemical localization of luteinizing hormone-releasing hormone (LH-RH) in the hypothalamus of the rhesus monkey. *Neurosci. Abstr.,* 2:657.

167. Silverman, A. J., and Zimmerman, E. A. (1975): Ultrastructural immunocytochemical localization of neurophysin and vasopressin in the median eminence and posterior pituitary of the guinea pig. *Cell. Tissue Res.,* 159:291–301.

168. Spatz, H. (1951): Neues über die Verknüpfung von Hypophyse und Hypothalamus. *Acta Neuroveg. (Wein),* 3:1–49.

169. Szentágothai, J. (1964): The parvicellular neurosecretory system. *Prog. Brain Res.,* 5:1–32.

170. Szentágothai, J., Flerkó, B., Mess, B., and Halász, B. (1968): *Hypothalamic Control of the Anterior Pituitary.* Akademiai Kiado, Budapest.

171. Taber, C. A., and Karavolas, H. J. (1975): Subcellular localization of LH releasing activity in the rat hypothalamus. *Endocrinology,* 96:446–452.

172. Tsang, D., Tan, A. T., Brazeau, P., Lal, S., Renaud, L. P., and Martin, J. B. (1975): Subcellular distribution of somatostatin in extrahypothalamic brain tissue. *Neurosci. Abstr.,* 1:450.

173. Wakerley, J. B., and Lincoln, D. W. (1973): The milk ejection reflex of the rat: A 20- to 40-fold acceleration in the firing of paraventricular neurones during oxytocin release. *J. Endocrinol.,* 57:477–493.

174. Wakerley, J. B., Poulain, D. A., Dyball, R. E. J., and Cross, B. A. (1975): Activity of phasic neurosecretory cells during haemorrhage. *Nature,* 258:82–84.

175. Weiner, R. I., Corski, R. A., and Sawyer, C. H. (1972): Hypothalamic catecholamines and pituitary gonadotropic function. In: *Brain Endocrine Interaction. Median Eminence: Structure and Function,* edited by K. M. Knigge, D. E. Scott, and A. Weindl, pp. 236–244. S. Karger, Basel.

176. Werman, R. (1966): A review—criteria for identification of a central nervous system transmitter. *Comp. Biochem. Physiol.,* 18:745–766.

177. Whittaker, V. P. (1969): The synaptosome. In: *Handbook of Neurochemistry, Vol. 2,* edited by A. Lajtha, pp. 327–364. Plenum Press, New York.

178. Wilbur, J. F., Montoya, E., Plotnikoff, N., White, W. F., Genrich, R., Renaud, L., and Martin, J. B. (1976): Gonadotropin-releasing hormone and thyrotropin-releasing hormone: Distribution and effects in the central nervous system. *Recent Prog. Horm. Res.,* 32:117–153.
179. Willoughby, J. O., Terry, L. C., Brazeau, P., and Martin, J. B. (1977): Pulsatile growth hormone, prolactin and thyrotropin secretion in rats with hypothalamic deafferentation. *Brain Res. (in press).*
180. Wilson, M. M., and Critchlow, V. (1975): Absence of a circadian rhythm in persisting corticosterone fluctuations following surgical isolation of the medial basal hypothalamus. *Neuroendocrinology,* 19:185–192.
181. Winokur, A., Davis, R., and Utiger, R. D. (1977): Subcellular distribution of thyrotropin-releasing hormone (TRH) in rat brain and hypothalamus. *Brain Res.,* 120:423–434.
182. Yagi, K., Azuma, T., and Matsuda, K. (1966): Neurosecretory cell: Capable of conducting impulse in rats. *Science,* 154:778–779.
183. Yagi, K., and Sawaki, Y. (1975): Recurrent inhibition and facilitation: Demonstration in the tuberoinfundibular system and effects of strychnine and picrotoxin. *Brain Res.,* 84:155–159.
184. Yagi, K., and Sawaki, Y. (1977): Median preoptic nucleus neurons: Inhibition and facilitation of spontaneous activity following stimulation of the median eminence in female rats. *Brain Res.,* 120:342–346.
185. Yamashita, H., Koizumi, K., and Brooks, C. McC. (1970): Electrophysiological studies of neurosecretory cells in the cat hypothalamus. *Brain Res.,* 20:462–466.
186. Yarbrough, G. G. (1976): TRH potentiates excitatory action of acetylcholine on cerebral cortical neurones. *Nature,* 263:523–524.
187. Yates, F. E., Russell, S. M., and Maran, J. W. (1971): Brain-adenohypophyseal communication in mammals. *Annu. Rev. Physiol.,* 33:393–444.
188. Zimmerman, E. A. (1976): Localization of hypothalamic hormones by immunocytochemical techniques. In: *Frontiers in Neuroendocrinology, Vol. 4,* edited by L. Martini and W. F. Ganong, pp. 25–62. Raven Press, New York.
189. Zimmerman, E. A. (1976): Localization of neurosecretory peptides in neuroendocrine tissues. In: *Subcellular Mechanisms in Reproductive Neuroendocrinology,* edited by F. Naftolin, K. J. Ryan, and J. Davies, pp. 81–108. Elsevier, Amsterdam.
190. Zimmerman, E. A., and Antunes, J. L. (1976): Organization of the hypothalamic-pituitary system: Current concepts from immunohistochemical studies. *J. Histochem. Cytochem.,* 24:807–815.
191. Zimmerman, E. A., Carmel, P. W., Husain, M. K., Ferin, M., Tannenbaum, M., Frantz, A. G., and Robinson, A. G. (1973): Vasopressin and neurophysin: High concentrations in monkey hypophyseal portal blood. *Science,* 192:925–927.
192. Zimmerman, E. A., and Defendini, R. (1977): Anatomy of neurohypophyseal pathways. In: *The Hypothalamus,* edited by S. Reichlin, R. J. Baldessarini, and J. B. Martin. Raven Press, New York *(in press).*
193. Zimmerman, E. A., Hsu, K. C., Ferrin, M., and Kozlowski, G. P. (1974): Localization of gonadotropin-releasing hormone (GH-RH) in the hypothalamus of the mouse by immunoperoxidase technique. *Endocrinology,* 95:1–8.
194. Zolovick, A. J. (1972): Effects of lesions and electrical stimulation of the amygdala on hypothalamic-hypophyseal regulation. In: *The Neurobiology of the Amygdala,* edited by B. E. Eleftheriou, pp. 643–684. Plenum Press, New York.

Frontiers in Neuroendocrinology, Vol. 5,
edited by W. F. Ganong and L. Martini.
Raven Press, New York © 1978.

Chapter 6

Role of Adrenocortical Hormones in the Modulation of Synthesis and Degradation of Enzymes Involved in the Formation of Catecholamines

H. Thoenen and U. Otten

*Department of Pharmacology, Biocenter of the University of Basel,
CH–4056 Basel, Switzerland*

For a long time neurobiological research was dominated by the interest in short-term effects of neuronal activity, particularly in regard to electrical phenomena and the underlying changes in ionic membrane permeability. Since fully differentiated neurons no longer possess the ability to replicate and, further, as regeneration of single elements is limited, it has been concluded that integrated neuronal systems are composed of inert components connected in a rather stable manner. This concept of the structure and function of integrated neuronal systems led to their comparison with those of a computer, and, admittedly, many functions of an integrated neuronal system can be mimicked by a computer. However, there is a basic difference between the function of a computer and that of an integrated neuronal system such as the brain: the latter possesses the ability to change its structure according to functional requirements. The functional capacity of the brain is based not only on the large number of neurons and their numerous synaptic connections but also on the capability of neurons to adapt their long-term connectivity according to functional requirements. This capacity for plastic reactions greatly expands the brain's functional capabilities and is a reflection of changes in the synthesis of specific neuronal macromolecules. These changes may be so extensive that even differences in the morphological feature of neurons become apparent (see 10,17,24,48).

The prerequisite for such plastic adaptation is a relatively rapid rate of synthesis and turnover of neuronal macromolecules. Indeed, it has been shown that the rate of protein synthesis in neurons compares favorably with that of exocrine and endocrine cells (see 40). Moreover, an efficient transport system transfers the macromolecules, predominantly formed in the perikaryon, to the functionally important parts of the nerve terminals (see 29). Investigations over the last few years have shown that neuronal plasticity is of importance for the prolonged adaptation to increased transmitter utilization, for the regulation of ontogenetic processes, and possibly also for the long-term storage of information (see 43,48).

It is evident that the structurally and functionally complex mammalian brain is not a suitable object for studying the detailed mechanisms of plastic interaction of neurons. The relatively simply organized peripheral sympathetic nervous system, especially that of rodents, proved to be a favorable model for such studies. It has been shown under a great variety of experimental conditions, which lead to an enhanced activity of the peripheral sympathetic nervous system, that the increased activity of the preganglionic cholinergic nerves leads to a selective induction of tyrosine hydroxylase (TH) and dopamine β-hydroxylase (DBH) in terminal adrenergic neurons, whereas other enzymes involved in the synthesis or metabolic degradation of the physiological transmitter norepinephrine remain unchanged (3,45,48). That the augmented enzyme levels result from an enhanced enzyme synthesis has been demonstrated indirectly by use of inhibitors of protein synthesis (27,36) and directly by immunological procedures (4,11,18). The first messenger in this transsynaptic enzyme induction is acetylcholine acting via nicotinic receptors (see 49). However, it is not yet known how the changes effected by acetylcholine in the neuronal membrane are transformed into a message capable of regulating the expression of specific genetic information in the cell nucleus. Both in the sympathetic ganglia and in the adrenal medulla it has been shown that an increase in the level of cAMP is not an indispensible prerequisite for the subsequent enhanced synthesis of TH and DBH (see 43,48). Therefore, a role of cAMP as a second messenger in this process is rather improbable unless one assumes discrete changes in specific cell compartments which are difficult to discriminate from the background of the general changes, unrelated to this process. Moreover, recent studies have also shown that the depolarization of the neuronal membrane as such is not the relevant signal for the initiation of the cascade of events leading to the enhanced synthesis of specific enzymes (33,49). The enzyme induction elicited in organ cultures of sympathetic ganglia by potassium depolarization has been shown to result from the release of acetylcholine from the still intact cholinergic nerve terminals (32). In decentralized ganglia potassium and other depolarizing agents such as veratridine and batrachotoxin are without effect, whereas under the same experimental conditions the selective induction of TH and DBH could be initiated with acetylcholine or nicotine. This is in agreement with the observation that the blockade of the fast sodium channels with tetrodotoxin (which abolishes the formation of action potentials) does not interfere with the transsynaptic induction (33,49). However, recent experiments suggest that there might be a causal relationship between the changes in ionic permeability of the neuronal membrane, directly regulated via nicotinic receptors, and the subsequent selective TH and DBH induction. It has been shown that the replacement of sodium by Tris in the culture medium impairs this process whereas the selective enzyme induction mediated by nerve growth factor (NGF) remains unchanged (U. Otten and H. Thoenen, *unpublished observations*).

At a very early stage of the investigation of the transsynaptic enzyme induction, it was shown that the neuronally mediated enzyme induction in the adrenal medulla is still possible in hypophysectomized animals (46). This suggests that an augmented production of adrenocortical steroids via an activation of the pituitary-adrenocortical axis is not a prerequisite for the neuronally mediated process. However, these observations do not enable us to determine if glucocorticoids play a modulatory role in transsynaptic induction. Indeed, subsequent experiments have shown that this is the case. It is the aim of the present chapter to characterize this modulatory role, to delineate the relative importance of the hormonal and neuronal regulation for the synthesis of enzymes involved in catecholamine formation, and to compare the modulatory role of glucocorticoids on neuronally and NGF-mediated selective enzyme induction.

MODULATORY ROLE OF GLUCOCORTICOIDS ON TRANSSYNAPTIC ENZYME INDUCTION

Diurnal Rhythm of Selective Enzyme Inducibility by Short-Term Cold Stress or Systemic Administration of Cholinomimetics

In the course of experiments designed to determine the shortest time of increased preganglionic nerve activity necessary to initiate a significant TH induction, we found that the magnitude of the resulting induction depended on the time of the day at which the animals were exposed to cold (30). A more thorough study revealed that the inducibilities of TH in sympathetic ganglia and adrenal medulla were subjected to reciprocal diurnal rhythms: in the adrenal medulla short-term cold exposure resulted in optimal induction in the morning, in the superior cervical ganglia in the afternoon (Fig. 6–1). Because glucocorticoid production in the adrenal cortex is also subjected to a diurnal rhythm and since large doses of glucocorticoids induce TH in superior cervical ganglia provided the preganglionic fibers are intact (15), we suspected that there might be a causal relationship between the two diurnal rhythms. Indeed, it could be shown that the administration of relatively small doses of glucocorticoids, although not initiating TH induction alone, allowed the initiation of TH induction in sympathetic ganglia by short-term cold stress in either morning or afternoon (30).

The concept of the modulatory role of glucocorticoids was further supported by the observation that the injection of a single dose of 8 μmoles/kg of carbamylcholine in the morning could not initiate TH induction in decentralized rat superior cervical ganglia, whereas the same dose became effective in the afternoon (Fig. 6–2). Further, pretreatment with dexamethasone 1 μmole/kg 1 hr prior to carbamylcholine allowed the induction of TH

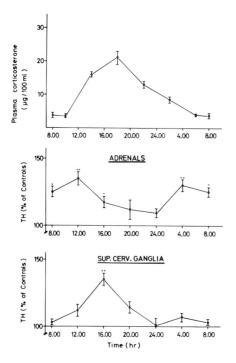

FIG. 6–1. Relationship between the diurnal rhythm of plasma glucocorticoids and TH inducibility by short-term cold stress in rat superior cervical ganglia and adrenals. Well-equilibrated male albino rats of 90–110 g body weight were exposed for 2 hr to 4°C around the clock. The time at which the cold exposure started is indicated on the abscissa. After cold exposure the animals were brought back to the normal environment for 46 hr. Thereafter they were killed and the TH activity determined in adrenals and superior cervical ganglia. Plasma corticosterone levels were determined in a separate group of animals. $*p < 0.05; **p < 0.01$. From Otten and Thoenen (30).

in the morning. It has to be stated very clearly that the diurnal rhythm of the inducibility is observed only under experimental conditions which lead to a short-term increase in the activation of the nicotinic receptors. For instance, no difference between morning and afternoon could be observed after the injection of reserpine. The probable reason for the difference between the

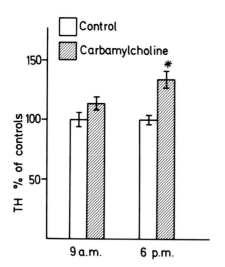

FIG. 6–2. Effect of carbamylcholine on TH activity in superior cervical ganglia of male rats. Carbamylcholine (8 μmoles/kg) was injected s.c. at 9 A.M. or at 6 P.M. TH activity was determined 48 hr later and compared with that of controls killed at the same time of the day. Values are means $\pm$ SEM. $*p < 0.01$.

inducibility by reserpine on the one hand and single injections of carbamyl-choline and short-term cold stress on the other is discussed below together with the question of the reciprocity between sympathetic ganglia and adrenal medulla.

Postnatal Development of the Diurnal Rhythm of TH Inducibility by Short-Term Cold Stress

The concept of a causal relationship between the diurnal rhythm of gluco-corticoid production in the adrenal cortex—reflected also by corresponding changes in the blood—and the diurnal rhythm of TH inducibility by short-term cold stress was strongly supported by investigations concerning TH inducibility by short-term cold stress in the early postnatal period (30). In the adrenal medulla TH induction by short-term cold stress was already possible within the first few postnatal days (Fig. 6–3). Interestingly, this inducibility was not dependent on the time of the day. In contrast, in superior cervical ganglia cold stress neither in the morning nor in the afternoon initiated TH induction until day 15 to 20 when a gradually increasing inducibility in the afternoon became apparent (Fig. 6–3). Concomitant with the appearance of TH inducibility in the afternoon in the superior cervical ganglia, the inducibility in the adrenal medulla was limited in that it became confined to the morning (Fig. 6–4). The appearance of the diurnal rhythm of enzyme inducibility by short-term cold stress is perfectly correlated with the maturation of the pituitary-adrenocortical axis, which is reflected not only by a general increase in ACTH-mediated glucocorticoid production but also by the appearance of a diurnal rhythm (1,39). Pretreatment of 9-day-old animals with doses of dexamethasone which did not initiate changes in TH levels if given alone provided experimental conditions which allowed the initiation of TH

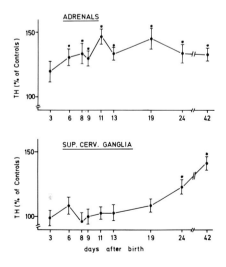

FIG. 6–3. Ontogenetic development of TH inducibility in rat adrenal medulla and superior cervical ganglia by short-term cold stress. At the ages indicated, animals were exposed for 1 hr to 4°C at 9 A.M. (adrenals) or at 4 P.M. (superior cervical ganglia). TH activity in superior cervical ganglia and adrenals was determined 48 hr later. The TH values are expressed in percent of controls and represent the means ± SEM of at least 12 determinations. *p < 0.05. From Otten and Thoenen (30).

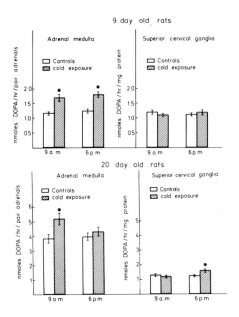

FIG. 6–4. TH induction by cold stress in superior cervical ganglia and adrenal medulla of 9- and 20-day-old rats. Animals were exposed for 1 hr to 4°C at 9 A.M. or at 6 P.M. TH activity in superior cervical ganglia and adrenals was determined 48 hr later and compared with that of controls killed at the same time of the day. The values given represent means ± SEM. *p < 0.01. From Otten and Thoenen (30).

induction by cold stress, both in the morning and in the afternoon (30), demonstrating that the inducibility lacking in the first postnatal weeks was due not to an insufficient development of the ganglionic connectivity but to the not yet functioning pituitary-adrenocortical system.

EFFECT OF GLUCOCORTICOIDS ON ACETYLCHOLINE-MEDIATED SELECTIVE ENZYME INDUCTION IN ORGAN CULTURES OF SYMPATHETIC GANGLIA AND ADRENAL MEDULLA

Selectivity and Concentration Dependence of Enzyme Induction by Glucocorticoids in Superior Cervical Ganglia

The development of organ culture systems allowing investigation of single steps in transsynaptic induction also provided favorable conditions for studying in more detail the modulatory role played by glucocorticoids in this process (31).

For reasons of convenience, most of the experiments reported were performed using the water-soluble synthetic glucocorticoid, dexamethasone. However, similar results were obtained with corticosterone, the major physiological glucocorticoid of the rat. This steroid has to be dissolved in ethanol or another appropriate solvent and is 10 to 30 times less potent than dexamethasone. The latter exhibited a strictly concentration-dependent induction of TH and DBH. The threshold concentration was 10^{-9} M to 10^{-8} M and the maximal effect was achieved at 10^{-7} M. At higher concentrations the effect decreased, and control levels were reached again at 10^{-4} M to 10^{-3} M (Fig. 6–5). In contrast to the response of TH and DBH, the considerably smaller effect on dopa decarboxylase (DDC) did not show the characteristic bell-shaped concentration-response curve; the enzyme levels remained about the same at concentrations between 10^{-7} M and 10^{-3} M. Both the strictly concentration-dependent effect on TH and DBH and the smaller effect on DDC could be abolished by cycloheximide, suggesting that the increased enzyme activity resulted from enhanced protein synthesis. For all enzymes studied, a 4-hr exposure of the ganglia to dexamethasone was sufficient to achieve a maximal effect 24 or 48 hr later (31).

The glucocorticoid-mediated induction of TH and DBH is dependent on intact preganglionic cholinergic nerves. The effect of glucocorticoids on TH and DBH is reduced to a small residual increase if the ganglia used for organ cultures are decentralized 1 to 2 weeks previously *in vivo*. These observations are in agreement with those of Hanbauer et al. (15) made *in vivo*. They showed that the induction of TH effected by high doses of dexamethasone in the rat superior cervical ganglia could be abolished by decentralization.

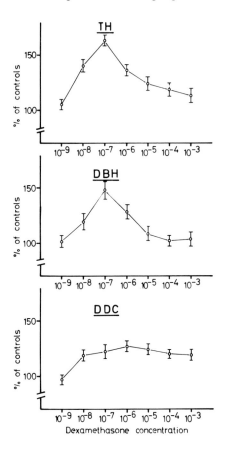

FIG. 6–5. Concentration dependence of effect of dexamethasone on enzyme levels in superior cervical ganglia kept in organ cultures. The ganglia were prepared for organ culture according to the procedures described in detail by Otten and Thoenen (32). Ganglia were exposed for 24 or 48 hr to varying concentrations of dexamethasone. For DBH the exposure to dexamethasone was 24 hr since the maximal effect was reached already at that time. For TH and DDC the exposure time was 48 hr. The values represent the means ± SEM of 8 ganglia.

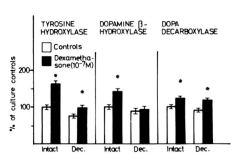

FIG. 6–6. Effect of decentralization on dexamethasone-mediated enzyme induction. Superior cervical ganglia were decentralized 7 days prior to the beginning of the organ culture experiments. Decentralized (Dec.) and intact ganglia were incubated for 4 hr in 0.1 μM dexamethasone, then placed in normal medium for a further 20 or 44 hr. After a total incubation time of 24 or 48 hr the ganglia were homogenized and the activities of DBH (24 hr), TH (48 hr), and DDC (48 hr) were compared with ganglia kept in normal media during the duration of the experiment. The values represent the means $\pm$ SEM of 7 or 8 ganglia. *$p < 0.025$. From Otten and Thoenen (31).

That the essential component of the preganglionic nerves is acetylcholine, most probably leaking out from the gradually degenerating nerve terminals, can be deduced from the observation that ganglionic blocking agents have the same effect as previous decentralization (Fig. 6–6). In contrast to TH and DBH, the response of DDC to glucocorticoids was influenced neither by previous decentralization nor by ganglionic blocking agents. The difference between the effect on TH and DBH on the one hand and DDC on the other, with respect to the degree of induction, the concentration dependence, and the dependence on intact preganglionic cholinergic nerves suggests that glucocorticoids exert a dual effect on sympathetic ganglia. The strictly concentration-dependent bell-shaped response of TH and DBH which depends on the release of acetylcholine from the preganglionic cholinergic nerves represents a very specific action reflecting a potentiation of the neuronally mediated enzyme induction (31). The response of DDC and the residual response of TH and DBH after decentralization or administration of ganglionic blocking agents represent a general nonspecific effect.

Permissive Versus Modulatory Role of Glucocorticoids

Although the response of TH and DBH proved to be strictly concentration dependent, it could not be determined whether glucocorticoids are an absolute prerequisite for acetylcholine-mediated selective induction of TH and DBH or whether they play only a modulatory role. In order to obtain information on this aspect we studied the effect of carbamylcholine on sympathetic ganglia in organ culture from animals which were adrenalectomized 2 weeks before the beginning of the organ culture experiments (31). Carbamylcholine was used in place of acetylcholine since it is not a substrate for acetylcholinesterase. The response of the sympathetic ganglia to a pulse of carbamylcholine still consisted of a statistically significant increase of TH and DBH 48 hr later although the response was considerably smaller than that in the presence of optimal concentrations of dexamethasone (Fig. 6–7). Thus, it can be

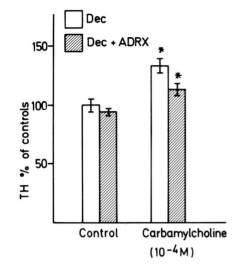

FIG. 6–7. Effect of previous adrenalectomy on carbamylcholine-mediated TH induction in organ cultures of sympathetic ganglia. Superior cervical ganglia of control and adrenalectomized rats were decentralized 7 days prior to the beginning of the organ culture experiments. Decentralized ganglia from intact and adrenalectomized animals were exposed for 4 hr to 0.1 mM carbamylcholine, then kept in normal media for 44 hr. At the end of the incubation period the ganglia were homogenized and the activity of TH was compared with that of ganglia kept in organ culture without carbamylcholine. The values given represent the means ± SEM of 8–10 ganglia. *$p < 0.025$.

concluded that the role of glucocorticoids is modulatory rather than permissive in the process of acetylcholine-mediated transsynaptic regulation of enzyme synthesis in the superior cervical ganglia.

Effect of Glucocorticoids on the Time Necessary to Initiate Selective Enzyme Induction by Carbamylcholine

In the experiments concerning the diurnal rhythm of TH inducibility by cold stress or carbamylcholine, we pointed out that these diurnal rhythms of inducibility were present only under experimental conditions which lead to a short-term activation of the nicotinic receptors of the ganglia. Moreover, a causal relationship between glucocorticoid levels and enzyme inducibility by short-term activation of nicotinic receptors could be detected only when optimal concentrations of glucocorticoids were reached prior to the stimulation of the nicotinic receptors (31,49). This aspect is of particular importance since a major part of experimental conditions leading to an enhanced activity of the peripheral sympathoadrenomedullary system lead also to an activation of the pituitary-adrenocortical system. However, the enhanced production of glucocorticoids starts with a delay of about 30 min (23). Therefore, the question arose whether the effect of glucocorticoids is the same if they are added to the medium together with the cholinomimetics or whether an optimal effect requires a preincubation with glucocorticoids. Moreover, it was essential to know whether glucocorticoids not only influence the maximal response of sympathetic ganglia to cholinomimetics activating nicotinic receptors but whether they also influence the time necessary to achieve a maximal initiation of the inductive process. As shown in Fig. 6–8, maximal induction of TH was

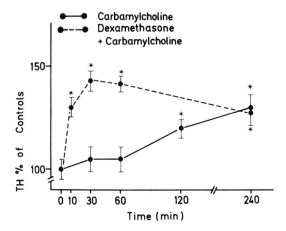

FIG. 6–8. Effect of dexamethasone on the time of exposure to carbamylcholine necessary to initiate maximal TH induction. Superior cervical ganglia were prepared for organ culture as described in Fig. 6–5. For all experiments ganglia were used which had been decentralized *in vivo* 7–10 days before. A first series of ganglia was exposed to carbamylcholine (0.1 mM) alone for varying time periods. For the rest of the incubation time the ganglia were transferred to normal medium until they were homogenized 48 hr after the beginning of the carbamylcholine pulse. A second series of ganglia were preincubated for 2 hr with dexamethasone (0.1 μM) before carbamylcholine was added for varying time periods. *$p < 0.025$.

achieved by incubating the ganglia for at least 4 hr in 10^{-4} M carbamylcholine. In contrast, if the ganglia were preincubated for 2 hr in 10^{-7} M dexamethasone, the exposure time to carbamylcholine could be reduced to 10 min. However, if dexamethasone was added to the culture medium together with carbamylcholine, a 10-min pulse was without detectable inducing effect.

The organ culture experiments described above provide a rational background for the explanation of the diurnal rhythm of TH inducibility by short-term cold stress and single injections of carbamylcholine *in vivo*. Glucocorticoids produce not only an increase in the maximal induction of TH resulting from the activation of nicotinic receptors in postganglionic adrenergic neurons. Even more impressive is the drastic reduction of the exposure time to carbamylcholine necessary for the initiation of the maximal effect. A prerequisite for this effect of glucocorticoids is the preincubation prior to the stimulation of the nicotinic receptors. Therefore, the activation of the pituitary-adrenocortical axis, which also occurs in consequence of short-term cold exposure with a delay of about 30 min (23), comes too late to become effective in creating optimal conditions for TH induction in sympathetic ganglia by a short-lasting enhanced activity of the preganglionic cholinergic nerves.

At present we can only speculate as to the site and mechanism of action of glucocorticoids. The fact that the potentiating effect of glucocorticoids depends on the time of preincubation suggests that a glucocorticoid-receptor complex may be transferred to the cell nucleus when the activation of the nicotinic receptors by carbamylcholine begins. However, it remains to be demonstrated that such specific cytosol receptors exist and that their glucocorticoid complexes are transferred to the nucleus in adrenergic neurons.

The modulatory role in transsynaptic enzyme induction is specific for glucocorticoids since other steroids such as aldosterone, β-estradiol, or testosterone have no effect and progesterone, which binds to glucocorticoid cytosol receptors in other systems without forming an "active" complex (41), also impairs the action of glucocorticoids in this system. If the site of action should be the neuronal membrane, one must assume that the glucocorticoids have a specific site of action influencing, for instance, the activation of nicotinic receptors or the transformation of this activation into a message finally reaching the cell nucleus. A general membrane effect influencing the fluidity of the membrane seems to be rather improbable in view of the lack of effect of other steroids having similar physicochemical properties.

SELECTIVE TH AND DBH INDUCTION BY NERVE GROWTH FACTOR; MODULATORY ROLE OF GLUCOCORTICOIDS

NGF has been shown to be an absolute prerequisite for the normal development of the peripheral sympathetic nervous system and the maintenance of function of the fully differentiated adrenergic neurons (21,22,50). In addition to the impressive promotion of nerve fiber sprouting and the general hypertrophic effect on peripheral adrenergic neurons, a characteristic response to NGF is the selective induction of TH and DBH (44). The similarity of the changes in the enzyme pattern resulting from increased preganglionic nerve activity and administration of NGF suggests that the two different mechanisms merge to a common pathway.

Although the detailed mechanism of action of NGF and that of transsynaptic induction is far from clear, it was of interest to investigate if the influence of glucocorticoids on NGF-mediated enzyme induction was similar to that on transsynaptic enzyme induction. Indeed, in recent experiments it has been shown that glucocorticoids enhance the effect of NGF on selective enzyme induction (Fig. 6–9) and that this enhancement is due to augmented synthesis rather than impaired degradation (34,35). This can be deduced from the observation that the effect of NGF alone and the combined effect of glucocorticoids can be abolished by cycloheximide (34). Moreover, it has been shown that in organ cultures of sympathetic ganglia the incorporation of ³H-leucine into protein selectively precipitated by monospecific antibodies to DBH (and further purified by gel electrophoresis) was enhanced by the combined treatment of NGF and glucocorticoids (U. Otten and C. Gagnon, *unpublished observations*). The addition of glucocorticoids to the incubation medium not only produced an increase in the maximal response to NGF but shifted to the left the concentration-response curve of TH to NGF by a factor of 30 to 50 (Fig. 6–9). As in the case of transsynaptic induction, the

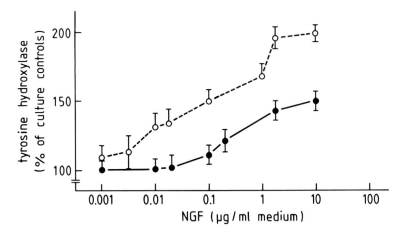

FIG. 6–9. Concentration dependence of NGF-mediated TH increase in cultures of superior cervical ganglia in absence and presence of corticosterone. Superior cervical ganglia were decentralized 8 days prior to the experiment. Ganglia were exposed for 24 hr to varying concentrations of NGF with (O⎯⎯⎯O) or without (●⎯⎯⎯●) corticosterone (5 μM). The ganglia were next washed in phosphate-buffered saline and transferred to normal media for a further 24 hr. They were then homogenized and the TH activity determined. The values given represent means ± SEM of 8 ganglia. From Otten and Thoenen (35).

potentiating effect was highly selective for glucocorticoids since testosterone, β-estradiol, or progesterone had no effect (35).

Even more striking than the shift of the concentration-response curve of NGF by glucocorticoids was the drastic reduction of the time of exposure to NGF necessary to achieve a maximal response (Fig. 6–10). In the absence of glucocorticoids the ganglia had to be exposed for at least 4 hr in order to achieve a maximal elevation of TH 48 hr later. In the presence of 5 μM corticosterone, the time of exposure could be reduced to 10 min. In order to obtain more precise information on how long ganglia in organ culture have to be exposed to NGF in the presence and absence of glucocorticoids, we performed experiments in which the action of NGF was terminated by adding purified monospecific antibodies to the medium (35). Even if the action of NGF was terminated by the addition of antibodies, the difference between NGF alone and NGF plus corticosterone remained impressive. In the presence of glucocorticoids the administration of monospecific NGF antibodies 1 hr after NGF resulted in a reduction of the maximal response by 40%. However, if the same schedule was chosen in the absence of glucocorticoids, TH induction was still completely abolished. In order to obtain a similar reduction of the final response to that with NGF plus glucocorticoids after 1 hr, we had to postpone the addition of the antibodies to at least 4 hr after the addition of NGF (35). The impressive effect of glucocorticoids on the time required for NGF to initiate selective enzyme induction raises the possibility that these findings could provide information on the mechanism and site

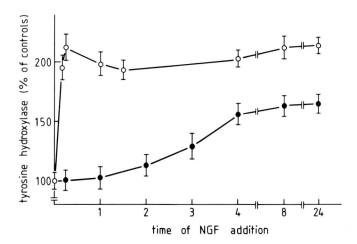

FIG. 6–10. Effect of corticosterone on the time of exposure to NGF necessary to elicit maximal TH increase in cultured superior cervical ganglia. Groups of ganglia were exposed for various time periods to NGF (0.1 μM) (●————●). In other experiments NGF was added for various time periods to ganglia which had been preincubated for 2 hr with corticosterone (5 μM) (○————○). After appropriate exposure times to NGF the ganglia were washed in phosphate-buffered saline and then incubated in control culture medium for the rest of the experiment, i.e., up to 48 hr. The values given represent the means $\pm$ SEM of 8 ganglia. From Otten and Thoenen (35).

of action of NGF. The fact that the NGF reaching the adrenergic cell body by retrograde axonal transport is responsible for the regulation of the synthesis of TH in the perikaryon (37) suggests an intracellular site of action rather than an action via surface receptors triggering from there a cascade of events finally leading to the selective induction of TH and DBH. This interpretation is further supported by recent electron microscopic autoradiographic studies which have demonstrated that NGF which reaches the cell body via retrograde axonal transport is not released to an appreciable extent into the extracellular space (42). This makes an action via surface receptors —even a secondary one—very improbable. However, the observation that corticosterone reduces the exposure time to NGF necessary to initiate maximal TH induction could be thought to challenge the assumption of an intracellular site of action of NGF and favor an initiating mechanism via surface receptors. This seems to be the case for many other polypeptides with hormonal functions (see 19). The interpretation of the results with organ cultures of sympathetic ganglia is complicated by the fact that the penetration of both NGF and monospecific antibodies is relatively slow. Preliminary autoradiographic studies have shown that it takes about 30 min for ^{125}I-labeled NGF antibodies to penetrate to the central part of the ganglia incubated at 37°C. The penetration of ^{125}I-NGF seems to be somewhat faster. In the presence of glucocorticoids the effect of NGF can still be impaired by NGF-antibodies to a considerable extent after 1 hr, which suggests that appreciable amounts of NGF are retained in the extracellular space. In particular, collagen, which is acidic, seems to bind NGF, which is basic, to a considerable extent. The bound material is a slow-release store of NGF which would become available to adrenergic neurons long after the removal of NGF from the medium. Thus, the short exposure time of 10 min necessary to initiate the maximal TH induction by NGF after preincubation of the ganglia with glucocorticoids is to some extent misleading and does not reflect the real exposure time of the adrenergic neurons to NGF. Moreover, recent preliminary electron microscopic autoradiographic studies have shown that glucocorticoids enhance neither the penetration of NGF in the extracellular space of the ganglia nor the uptake of NGF into the ganglia, at least not to an extent which could explain the shift of the concentration-response relationship and the impressive reduction of the time required for initiating maximal selective enzyme induction. Interestingly, either in the absence or presence of glucocorticoids, ^{125}I-NGF could not be localized in the cell nucleus of adrenergic neurons (M. Schwab and H. Thoenen, *unpublished observations*). This is in agreement with the subcellular localization of ^{125}I-NGF and the NGF-horseradish peroxidase coupling product after retrograde axonal transport (42,50). The data make it unlikely that NGF is directly acting on the regulation of the transcription of messenger RNA of TH and DBH or on that of a factor regulating the translation of these enzymes in a specific manner.

The modulatory action of glucocorticoids on the effect of polypeptide hormones does not seem to be unique for NGF. Gospodarowicz et al. (14) have demonstrated that glucocorticoids potentiate the stimulation of DNA synthesis in 3T3 cells by fibroblast growth factor extracted from bovine pituitary glands. On the site and mechanism of action of fibroblast growth factor even less is known than on that of NGF. Moreover, it seems that fibroblast growth factor affects rather general mechanisms of cell function, such as cell growth, whereas NGF selectively regulates the synthesis of two specific enzymes in addition to its general hypertrophic effect.

ROLE PLAYED BY GLUCOCORTICOIDS IN ENZYME SYNTHESIS AND DEGRADATION IN THE ADRENAL MEDULLA; RELATIONSHIP TO PREGANGLIONIC NERVE ACTIVITY

The topographical localization of the mammalian adrenal medulla implies that the chromaffin cells are exposed to excessively high concentrations of glucocorticoids synthesized by the adrenal cortical cells and reaching the medulla via the portal veins (9). The glucocorticoid concentrations in the portal vessels are about two orders of magnitude higher than in the general circulation (38), so any effect of glucocorticoids has to be considered in light of the observation that the adrenergic neurons—which also originate from the neural crest and which have in common many characteristic properties with adrenal medullary cells—show a characteristic bell-shaped concentration-response curve with respect to the induction of TH and DBH by gluco-corticoids (Fig. 6–5).

Phenylethanolamine-N-methyltransferase (PNMT), which catalyzes the conversion of norepinephrine to epinephrine (2,20), was the first enzyme of the adrenal medulla in which the regulatory role of glucocorticoids was investigated (52,53). After hypophysectomy in rats (6), PNMT activity was shown to decay with a half-life of 6 days. This relatively rapid drop in enzyme activity could be prevented or reversed by administration of ACTH or gluco-corticoids (28,53). Since the restoration of the reduced PNMT activity could be prevented by inhibitors of protein synthesis acting at the transcriptional or translational level (53), it was concluded that the restoration of the enzyme levels resulted from a glucocorticoid-mediated induction of enzyme synthesis. It is noteworthy that already in these initial experiments it was not possible to elevate the PNMT activity above control levels by treating sham-operated animals with very high doses of ACTH or glucocorticoids, suggesting that under normal conditions the synthesis of this enzyme occurred at a maximal rate. More recent experiments have provided evidence that the restoration of PNMT levels in hypophysectomized animals does not result from an enhanced synthesis but from a delayed degradation (5,7). Double-labeling studies with pulses of ^{3}H- and ^{14}C-glutamic acid revealed that the incorporation into proteins extracted by affinity columns of monospecific antibodies to PNMT did not differ between sham-operated and hypophysec-tomized animals (5). However, the rate of decay of the labeled PNMT was faster in hypophysectomized than in sham-operated animals. Interestingly, the restoration of PNMT levels in hypophysectomized animals by ACTH depends on intact splanchnic fibers; ACTH is ineffective in restoring PNMT levels of decentralized adrenals in hypophysectomized animals, whereas glucocorticoids were fully effective (5). Thus, it seems that the splanchnic fibers which supply the adrenals play a permissive role in the regulation of the synthesis and/or release of glucocorticoids (5,16). It is not yet established if acetylcholine is the direct or indirect permissive agent as such, or if it is another substance released from the splanchnic fibers. It is not yet known whether the impairment of the degradation of PNMT by glucocorticoids results from a direct protective effect of glucocorticoids on PNMT, from an impairment of the synthesis, or from activation of specific degrading enzymes.

In addition to the regulation of adrenal medullary PNMT levels via gluco-corticoids by impairing enzyme degradation, there is a direct neuronal regulation which affects the synthesis rather than the degradation of PNMT (5,47). The administration of high doses of ACTH or glucocorticoids does not produce an elevation above the control level seen in normal animals (47,53). However, enhanced activity of the preganglionic cholinergic fibers supplying the adrenal medulla elicits augmented synthesis of PNMT resulting in enzyme levels above control (5,47).

A similar dual control by neuronal activity (synthesis) and glucocorticoids (degradation) has been demonstrated for DBH (8,12,25,51). It is not possible to elevate the level of DBH in adrenals above control by administration of ACTH or glucocorticoids in normal animals (8), although a normalization can be achieved by these procedures in hypophysectomized animals. Once again, the effect of ACTH in restoring DBH activity in hypophysectomized rats depends on an intact innervation, whereas the administration of glucocorticoids is also effective in denervated adrenals.

A marked effect of hypophysectomy on adrenal TH levels has also been demonstrated (28). The half-life after hypophysectomy in innervated rat adrenals is 21 days, whereas in denervated adrenals it is 11 days. However, there are marked differences between PNMT and DBH on the one hand and TH on the other. In hypophysectomized rats a restoration of TH was possible only by ACTH but not with doses of glucocorticoids which restored completely the levels of PNMT. On the contrary, administration of high doses of dexamethasone not only did not restore TH activity in hypophysectomized rats but reduced the TH activity in sham-operated animals to those of hypophysectomized animals (28). This suggests that dexamethasone produced a "chemical hypophysectomy." With the information available so far, it is not possible to determine if the synthesis of TH is directly regulated by ACTH or if the concentrations of glucocorticoids necessary to maintain TH at a normal level are higher than those necessary for PNMT and DBH. These concentrations would be reached in the adrenal portal vein blood only after administration of ACTH, stimulating the synthesis of glucocorticoids in the cortex.

The aspects discussed above refer to the regulation of enzyme levels by high concentrations of glucocorticoids in the adrenal medulla, which—at least for DBH and PNMT—affect the rate of degradation rather than the synthesis. These regulatory functions seem to be rather specific for the adrenal medulla, with its peculiar topographical relationship to the adrenal cortex (9). Glucocorticoids also play an important role in the initial stages of transsynaptic induction in adrenals as well as sympathetic ganglia, although the location of the adrenal medulla does not allow an experimental approach as easy and direct as for the sympathetic ganglia. The circadian rhythm of the inducibility of TH by short-term increase in the activity of the preganglionic cholinergic nerves suggests that the optimal time for induction in the adrenal medulla is at the time of lowest glucocorticoid production, whereas in the ganglia the time of the highest production is optimal (30). It appears that at the time of the highest production in the afternoon, the glucocorticoid concentrations in the adrenomedullary venous portal system reach such high levels that a short-term increase in augmented preganglionic activity becomes ineffective. This assumption is in agreement with the observation made in organ cultures of sympathetic ganglia that after reaching an optimal concentration of glucocorticoids (10^{-7} M dexamethasone), a further increase in the concentration diminishes the response until control levels are reached again at 10^{-3} M dexamethasone (Fig. 6–5). In organ culture of the adrenal medulla it has been shown that in the initial stages of transsynaptic enzyme induction, high (10^{-4} M) concentrations of corticosterone completely abolish the subsequent enhanced TH synthesis (13). If the glucocorticoids were added 4 hr after the initiation, the induction was still partially impaired. Six hours after initiation, glucocorticoids were no longer effective, although at this time point a measurable increase in TH and DBH activity was not yet detectable (13). This excludes a nonspecific effect impairing general protein synthesis. The concentrations of glucocorticoids necessary to achieve the effect were rather high (10^{-4} M). However, the highest concentrations reached in the general circulation are 10^{-6} M (1,30). Thus, if one considers the particular topographical localization of the adrenal medulla with respect to the site of corticosterone production (9), the concentrations reached in the portal veins supplying the adrenal medulla (13,30,38) approach those which are inhibitory in organ cultures. This interpretation is further supported by the observation that in the first 2 postnatal weeks, when the glucocorticoid production in the adrenal cortex is generally low and a diurnal rhythm is not yet established (1,39), TH induction in the medulla by short-term cold exposure can be initiated at any time of the day (30). As soon as the glucocorticoid rhythm becomes apparent, the inducibility by short-term cold stress is achieved only during the time of the lowest production.

In previous experiments it has been shown that after rats are injected with high doses of reserpine (16.2 μmoles/kg) TH induction can be abolished by transsection of the splanchnic fibers up to 4 hr after injection (26). A statistically significant reduction is still achieved if the nerves are transsected 6 hr after reserpine administration. However, if the adrenal medullas are put in organ culture 60 min after *in vivo* administration of reserpine, the maximal TH induction is obtained 24 hr later (U. Otten, *unpublished observations*). The major difference between the denervation experiments *in vivo* and the transfer of the medulla into organ culture is the removal of the adrenal medulla from the normal environment which is characterized by high concentrations of corticosterone. High concentrations impair the induction at the initial stages (see above).

CONCLUDING REMARKS

Glucocorticoids play a complex role in the regulation of the synthesis and degradation of enzymes involved in the formation of catecholamines in peripheral adrenergic neurons and adrenal chromaffin cells. Although investigations over the last few years have delineated these effects rather clearly, our understanding of them is still at the descriptive level. The precise site of action and molecular mechanism remain to be established. This is not surprising since the basic mechanisms influenced by glucocorticoids, namely, the transsynaptic neuronal and NGF-mediated selective induction of TH and

DBH, are themselves only partially understood, and many gaps have to be filled before these mechanisms are established at the molecular level. Interestingly, the neuronally mediated induction of TH and DBH has been shown to be enhanced or impaired depending on the concentrations of glucocorticoids present. The impairment is of particular importance in the adrenal medulla which, by reason of its particular topographical relationship to the adrenal cortex, is exposed to glucocorticoid concentrations which are two orders of magnitude higher than those in the general circulation. This difference between the concentrations of glucocorticoids in the general circulation, which bathes peripheral adrenergic neurons, and those in the adrenal medulla is reflected by differences in the modulation of transsynaptic enzyme induction in sympathetic ganglia and adrenal chromaffin cells. Since glucocorticoids influence not only the extent of neuronally mediated enzyme induction but also the time of activation of nicotinic receptors necessary to initiate an optimal induction, the role of glucocorticoids becomes most impressively apparent under experimental conditions which are characterized by an activation of nicotinic receptors for a short time. Thus, the inducibility of TH and DBH in sympathetic ganglia by short-term activation of the preganglionic cholinergic fibers or by a single injection of carbamylcholine is subjected to a diurnal rhythm. A short activation of the nicotinic receptors in ganglia leads to a significant enzyme induction only at the time of the highest glucocorticoid production. In contrast, in the adrenal medulla the glucocorticoid concentrations reached at this time have an inhibitory action. This difference between the adrenal medulla and the sympathetic ganglia is also reflected by the inducibility of TH during the early postnatal period. During the first 2 weeks after birth the rat pituitary-adrenocortical axis is not yet fully developed, the glucocorticoid production is generally low, and there is no diurnal rhythm. During this period adrenal medullary TH is inducible by short-term cold stress at any time of the day. In contrast, the sympathetic ganglia do not respond at all unless the animals are injected with glucocorticoids prior to cold exposure, demonstrating that the absence of induction in this experimental situation is due to a nonfunctioning pituitary-adrenocortical system, rather than to an undeveloped peripheral sympathetic nervous system. As soon as the pituitary-adrenocortical system attains its adult functional pattern, the sympathetic ganglia become responsive at the time of the highest glucocorticoid production and the adrenal medulla at the time of the lowest production. Such a concentration-dependent modulatory role of glucocorticoids, indicated by experiments *in vivo,* has directly been confirmed in organ cultures of rat sympathetic ganglia and adrenal medulla. The concentrations of glucocorticoids necessary to exhibit either enhancing or inhibitory action agree with the concentrations expected *in vivo* in adrenal medulla and sympathetic ganglia under corresponding experimental conditions. Interestingly, the effect of NGF on the selective TH and DBH induction in sympathetic ganglia is enhanced in a manner similar to that of the neuronally mediated induction. Recent experiments have shown that the effects of glucocorticoids are not confined to the modulation of the initial stages of transsynaptic and NGF-mediated enzyme induction. Glucocorticoids also play an important role in the degradation of enzymes involved in the synthesis of norepinephrine and epinephrine; enhanced degradation of DBH and PNMT is observed after hypophysectomy. This enhanced degradation can be inhibited by the administration of ACTH or glucocorticoids. For TH the situation is somewhat different in that the decay of activity after hypophysectomy can be prevented by ACTH but not by glucocorticoids. This leaves the question open as to whether TH levels depend directly on ACTH or whether sufficiently high concentrations of glucocorticoids in the adrenal medulla are reached only by stimulation of glucocorticoid production in the adrenal cortex and not by exogenous administration of glucocorticoids. Moreover, it has been shown that the restoration of DBH and PNMT levels by ACTH depends on an intact nerve supply to the adrenals, suggesting that the regulation of synthesis and/or release of glucocorticoids from the adrenal cortex is dependent on an intact splanchnic innervation.

ACKNOWLEDGMENTS

The authors wish to thank Mrs. N. Scott-Lindsay for her excellent technical assistance and Miss V. Forster for her help in preparation of the manuscript. This work was supported from the Swiss National Foundation for Scientific Research (Grant No. 3.432.74).

REFERENCES

1. Ader, R. (1975): Neonatal stimulation and maturation of the 24-hour adrenocortical rhythm. *Prog. Brain Res.,* 42:333–341.
2. Axelrod, J. (1962): Purification and properties of phenylethanolamine-N-methyl transferase. *J. Biol. Chem.,* 237:1657–1666.
3. Black, I. B., Hendry, I. A., and Iversen, L. L. (1971): Differences in the regulation of tyrosine hydroxylase and dopa decarboxylase in sympathetic ganglia and adrenals. *Nature [New Biol.],* 231:27–29.
4. Chuang, D. M., and Costa, E. (1974): Biosynthesis of tyrosine hydroxylase in rat adrenal medulla after exposure to cold. *Proc. Natl. Acad. Sci. USA,* 71:4570–4574.
5. Ciaranello, R. D. (1977): Regulation of phenylethanolamine *N*-methyltransferase synthesis and degradation. In: *Biochemistry and Function of Monoamine Enzymes,* edited by E. Usdin. Plenum Press, New York (*in press*).
6. Ciaranello, R. D., and Black, I. B. (1971): Kinetics of the glucocorticoid-mediated induction of phenylethanolamine N-methyltransferase in the hypophysectomized rat. *Biochem. Pharmacol.,* 20:3529–3532.
7. Ciaranello, R. D., Dornbusch, J. N., and Barchas, J. D. (1972): Regulation of adrenal phenylethanolamine N-methyltransferase activity in three inbred mouse strains. *Mol. Pharmacol.,* 8:511–520.
8. Ciaranello, R. D., Wooten, G. F., and Axelrod, J. (1976): Regulation of rat adrenal dopamine β-hydroxylase. II. Receptor interaction in the regulation of enzyme synthesis and degradation. *Brain Res.,* 113:349–362.
9. Coupland, R. F. (1975): Blood supply of the adrenal gland. In: *Handbook of*

Physiology, Section 7, edited by H. Blaschko, G. Sayers, and A. D. Smith, pp. 283–294. American Physiological Society, Washington, D.C.

10. Cragg, B. G. (1972): Plasticity of synapses. In: *Structure and Function of Nervous Tissues, Vol. 4,* edited by G. H. Bourne, pp. 1–60. Academic Press, New York.
11. Gagnon, C., Otten, U., and Thoenen, H. (1976): Increased synthesis of dopamine β-hydroxylase in cultured rat adrenal medullae after in vivo administration of reserpine. *J. Neurochem.,* 27:259–265.
12. Gewirtz, G. P., Kvetnansky, R., Weise, V. K., and Kopin, I. J. (1971): Effect of hypophysectomy on adrenal dopamine β-hydroxylase activity in the rat. *Mol. Pharmacol.,* 7:163–168.
13. Goodman, R., Otten, U., and Thoenen, H. (1975): Organ culture of the rat adrenal medulla: A model system for the study of trans-synaptic enzyme induction. *J. Neurochem.,* 25:423–427.
14. Gospodarowicz, D., Rudland, P., Lindstrom, J., and Benirschke, K. (1975): Fibroblast growth factor: Its localization, purification, mode of action, and physiological significance. In: *Advances in Metabolic Disorders, Vol. 8,* edited by R. Lutt and K. Hall, pp. 301–335. Academic Press, New York.
15. Hanbauer, I., Guidotti, A., and Costa, E. (1975): Dexamethasone induces tyrosine hydroxylase in sympathetic ganglia but not in adrenal medulla. *Brain Res.,* 85:527–531.
16. Henry, J. P., Kross, M. E., Stephens, P. M., and Watson, F. M. C. (1976): Evidence that differing psychosocial stimuli lead to adrenal cortical stimulation by autonomic or endocrine pathways. In: *Catecholamines and Stress,* edited by E. Usdin, R. Kyotnansky, and I. J. Kopin, pp. 457–468. Pergamon Press, Oxford.
17. Horn, G., Rose, S. P. R., and Bateson, P. P. G. (1973): Experience and plasticity in the central nervous system. *Science,* 181:506–514.
18. Joh, T. H., Gegliman, C., and Reis, D. J. (1973): Immunochemical demonstration of increased accumulation of tyrosine hydroxylase protein in sympathetic ganglia and adrenal medulla elicited by reserpine. *Proc. Natl. Acad. Sci. USA,* 70:2767–2771.
19. Kahn, C. R. (1976): Membrane receptors for hormones and neurotransmitters. *J. Cell Biol.,* 70:261–286.
20. Kirshner, N., and Goodall, M. (1959): The formation of adrenaline from noradrenaline. *Biochim. Biophys. Acta,* 24:658–659.
21. Levi-Montalcini, R. (1966): The nerve growth factor: Its mode of action on sensory and sympathetic nerve cells. *Harvey Lect.,* 60:217–259.
22. Levi-Montalcini, R., and Angeletti, P. U. (1968): Nerve growth factor. *Physiol. Rev.,* 48:534–569.
23. Maickel, R. P., Westermann, E. O., and Brodie, B. B. (1961): Effects of reserpine and cold exposure on pituitary-adrenocortical function in rats. *J. Pharmacol. Exp. Ther.,* 134:167–175.
24. Mark, R. (1974): *Memory and Nerve Cell Connections.* Oxford University Press, New York.
25. Molinoff, P. B., Brimijoin, S., Weinshilboum, R., and Axelrod, J. (1970): Neuronally-mediated increase in dopamine β-hydroxylase activity. *Proc. Natl. Acad. Sci. USA,* 66:453–458.
26. Mueller, R. A., Otten, U., and Thoenen, H. (1974): The role of cyclic adenosine 3',5'-monophosphate in reserpine-initiated adrenal medullary tyrosine hydroxylase induction. *Mol. Pharmacol.,* 10:855–860.
27. Mueller, R. A., Thoenen, H., and Axelrod, J. (1969): Inhibition of trans-synaptically increased tyrosine hydroxylase activity by cycloheximide and actinomycin D. *Mol. Pharmacol.,* 5:463–469.
28. Mueller, R. A., Thoenen, H., and Axelrod, J. (1970): Effect of pituitary and ACTH on the maintenance of basal tyrosine hydroxylase activity in the rat adrenal gland. *Endocrinology,* 86:751–755.
29. Ochs, S. (1975): Mechanism of axoplasmic transport and its block by pharmacological agents. In: *Proceedings of the 6th International Congress of Pharmacology, Helsinki, Vol. 2,* edited by J. Tuomisto and M. K. Paarsonen, pp. 161–174. Forssan Kirjaparino Oy, Helsinki.

30. Otten, U., and Thoenen, H. (1975): Circadian rhythm of tyrosine hydroxylase induction by short-term cold stress: Modulatory action of glucocorticoids in newborn and adult rats. *Proc. Natl. Acad. Sci. USA*, 72:1415–1419.
31. Otten, U., and Thoenen, H. (1976): Selective induction of tyrosine hydroxylase and dopamine β-hydroxylase in sympathetic ganglia in organ culture: Role of glucocorticoids as modulators. *Mol. Pharmacol.*, 12:353–361.
32. Otten, U., and Thoenen, H. (1976): Mechanism of tyrosine hydroxylase and dopamine β-hydroxylase induction in organ cultures of rat sympathetic ganglia by potassium depolarization and cholinomimetics. *Naunyn-Schmiedebergs Arch. Pharmacol.*, 292:153–159.
33. Otten, U., and Thoenen, H. (1976): Role of membrane depolarization in trans-synaptic induction of tyrosine hydroxylase in organ cultures of sympathetic ganglia. *Neurosci. Lett.*, 2:93–96.
34. Otten, U., and Thoenen, H. (1976): Modulatory role of glucocorticoids on NGF-mediated enzyme induction in organ cultures of sympathetic ganglia. *Brain Res.*, 111:438–441.
35. Otten, U., and Thoenen, H. (1977): Effect of glucocorticoids on NGF-mediated enzyme induction in organ cultures of rat sympathetic ganglia: Enhanced response and reduced time-requirement to initiate enzyme induction. *J. Neurochem.*, 29: 69–75.
36. Otten, U., Paravicini, U., Oesch, F. and Thoenen, H. (1973): Time requirement for the single steps in trans-synaptic induction of tyrosine hydroxylase in the peripheral sympathetic nervous system. *Naunyn-Schmiedebergs Arch. Pharmacol.*, 280:117–127.
37. Paravicini, U., Stöckel, K., and Thoenen, H. (1975): Biological importance of retrograde axonal transport of NGF in adrenergic neurons. *Brain Res.*, 84:279–291.
38. Peytreman, A., Nicholson, W. E., Hardman, J. G., and Liddle, G. W. (1973): Effect of adrenocortitropic hormone on extracellular adenosine 3′,5′-monophosphate in the hypophysectomized rat. *Endocrinology*, 92:1502–1506.
39. Ramaley, J. A. (1974): The changes in basal corticosterone secretion in rats blinded at birth. *Experientia*, 30:827.
40. Richter, D. (1970): Protein metabolism and functional activity. In: *Protein Metabolism of the Nervous System*, edited by A. Lajtha, pp. 241–258. Plenum Press, New York.
41. Samuels, H. H., and Tomkins, G. H. (1970): Relation of steroid structure to enzyme induction in hepatoma tissue culture cells. *J. Mol. Biol.*, 52:57–74.
42. Schwab, M., and Thoenen, H. (1977): Selective trans-synaptic migration of tetanus toxin after retrograde axonal transport in peripheral sympathetic nerves: A comparison with nerve growth factor. *Brain Res.*, 122:459–474.
43. Thoenen, H. (1975): Trans-synaptic regulation of neuronal enzyme synthesis. In: *Handbook of Psychopharmacology, Vol. 3*, edited by L. L. Iversen S. D. Iversen, and S. H. Snyder, pp. 443–475. Plenum Press, New York.
44. Thoenen, H., Angeletti, P. U., Levi-Montalcini, R., and Kettler, R. (1971): Selective induction of tyrosine hydroxylase and dopamine β-hydroxylase in the rat superior cervical ganglia by nerve growth factor. *Proc. Natl. Acad. Sci. USA*, 68:1598–1602.
45. Thoenen, H., Kettler, R., Burkhard, W., and Saner, A. (1971): Neuronally-mediated control of enzymes involved in the synthesis of norepinephrine: Are they regulated as an operational unit? *Naunyn-Schmiedebergs Arch. Pharmacol.*, 270:146–160.
46. Thoenen, H., Mueller, R. A., and Axelrod, J. (1969): Trans-synaptic induction of adrenal tyrosine hydroxylase. *J. Pharmacol. Exp. Ther.*, 169:249–254.
47. Thoenen, H., Mueller, R. A., and Axelrod, J. (1970): Neuronally dependent induction of adrenal phenylethanolamine-N-methyltransferase by 6-hydroxydopamine. *Biochem. Pharmacol.*, 19:669–673.
48. Thoenen, H., and Otten, U. (1976): Molecular events in trans-synaptic regulation of the synthesis of macromolecules. In: *Essays in Neurochemistry and Neuropharmacology, Vol. 1*, edited by M. B. H. Youdim, W. Lovenberg, D. F. Scharman, and J. R. Lagnado, pp. 73–101. John Wiley & Sons.

49. Thoenen, H., and Otten, U. (1977): Trans-synaptic enzyme induction: Ionic requirements and modulatory role of glucocorticoids. In: *Biochemistry and Function of Monoamine Enzymes,* edited by E. Usdin. Plenum Press, New York *(in press)*.
50. Thoenen, H., Schwab, M., and Otten, U. (1977): Nerve growth factor as a mediator of information between effector organs and innervating neurons. In: *Molecular Control of Proliferation and Cytodifferentiation,* edited by J. Papaconstantinou *(in press)*.
51. Weinshilboum, R. M., and Axelrod, J. (1970): Dopamine β-hydroxylase activity in the rat after hypophysectomy. *Endocrinology,* 87:894–899.
52. Wurtman, R. J., and Axelrod, J. (1965): Adrenal synthesis: Control by pituitary gland and adrenal glucocorticoids. *Science,* 150:1464–1465.
53. Wurtman, R. J., and Axelrod, J. (1966): Control of enzymatic synthesis of adrenaline in the adrenal medulla by adrenal cortical steroids. *J. Biol. Chem.,* 241:2301–2305.

Frontiers in Neuroendocrinology, Vol. 5,
edited by W. F. Ganong and L. Martini.
Raven Press, New York © 1978.

Chapter 7

Central Neural Control of Circadian Rhythms

Robert Y. Moore

Department of Neurosciences,
University of California at San Diego,
La Jolla, California 92093

Many functions of living organisms are rhythmic in their occurrence, ranging in periodicity from seconds or less to years. During the past 25 years, however, it has been recognized that one class of rhythms, those whose periodicity is 24 hr, are a ubiquitous feature of living organisms which represent a major component of the adaptation of organisms to their environment. These rhythms, termed "circadian" by Halberg (31), have several specific characteristics. First, they exhibit an extremely regular periodicity of 24 hr which reflects a direct entrainment to the diurnal cycle of light and dark. Alteration of the timing of the cycle of light and dark results in an alteration in the entrainment of the circadian rhythm. Second, they are extremely stable and resist entrainment to a periodicity which varies significantly from 24 hr. Third, they can be endogenously generated and in the absence of the synchronizing stimulus of light and dark, they continue in a "free-running" pattern but with a periodicity which is usually only slightly variant from 24 hr. These rhythms have been the subject of intense experimental investigation, and a number of comprehensive reviews describe our current knowledge of the phenomena (7,32,56). The evidence now available indicates that circadian rhythms are inherent, genetically determined functions of the organism (7,53, 61,62,63) which coordinate the activity of the internal environment of the organism with its external environment in order to achieve maximally effective adaptation. In some organisms, this extends beyond individual adaptation and survival as the phenomenon of reproduction in some species is dependent on intact circadian functions (2,6,57,72).

The focus of this review is the neural control of circadian rhythms in mammals. In the extensive literature on circadian rhythms little attention has been paid to this aspect of their regulation. There appear to be at least two primary components of the central neural control of circadian rhythms. The first relates to the precision with which rhythms are entrained to the diurnal cycle of light and dark. Entrainment indicates that the light-dark cycle is the major environment factor affecting the regulation of circadian rhythms. Since blinding or removal of the synchronizing stimulus of the light-dark cycle results in significant alterations of mammalian circadian rhythms, it is evident that one neural component of circadian rhythm regulation is the visual pathway carrying critical information about environment lighting from the retina to the central nervous system. Second, the inherent nature of circadian rhythms (61–63) and their persistence following removal of visual input (16,51,76) indicate that endogenous central rhythm generating mechanisms exist. The nature and organization of these mechanisms are undoubtedly complex, and we have at present relatively little information concerning them.

There are a number of possible ways in which these mechanisms may be organized, and some potential models have been proposed by Moore-Ede et al. (53). These models (Fig. 7–1) form a useful basis for further discussion. In Model I there is a single driving oscillator which is responsible for actively driving oscillations in a series of passively responding functions. In this model, only in the presence of input from the driving oscillator will the secondary units exhibit oscillating functions. This model leads to several obvious predictions. First, localization and destruction of the driving oscillator should result in loss of all circadian functions. That is, if all secondary oscillating units are responding passively to the driving oscillator, loss of the driving oscillator must result in loss of secondary oscillating functions. Second, phase shifting of the driving oscillator should result in an immediate and equal phase shift in the passive function. That is, if the passive functions are dependent on the driving oscillator entirely, then they must follow it exactly.

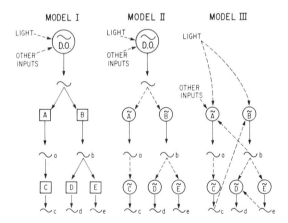

FIG. 7–1. Diagrammatic representation of three alternative models for the mammalian circadian timing system. The symbol ⊘ represents an active cellular unit capable of maintaining a self-sustaining oscillation with its own independent period; □ represents a cellular unit that responds passively to an oscillating driving force; ∼ indicates the output of an oscillating cell unit, which presumably represents neural activity; → is the direction of flow of passive responses to a driving oscillator; and ⟶ indicates entrainment of a self-sustained oscillator by a phase-response mechanism. D.O., driving oscillator. Model I represents a single oscillator system whereas the other models are multioscillator systems organized in a hierarchical (Model II) or nonhierarchical (Model III) manner. Modified and reproduced with permission from Moore-Ede et al. (53).

Third, in Model I destroying the connections between A and C should have no effect on functions d and e, whereas function c should become nonoscillating. That is, since all of the oscillating functions are driven by the driving oscillator, destruction of a limited portion of the connections between the driving oscillator and the secondary, passively driven units should have selective functional consequences. Model II represents a set of oscillators arranged in a hierarchical manner. In this case the driving oscillator will entrain secondary and tertiary oscillators by a phase response mechanism. In this model, removal of the driving oscillator would result in independent oscillation of the secondary oscillators. For example, if the input from the visual system is to the driving oscillator, the independent oscillation of the secondary oscillators should be unrelated to the light-dark cycle, and, consequently, the oscillating functions would not necessarily retain any phase relationship to each other. If, on the other hand, there was visual or other entraining environmental input to the secondary oscillating systems, they could show oscillation in a regular phase relationship to each other. This model allows for the possibility that oscillating functions may readily become dissociated as they are not dependent on a single driving oscillator. Model III represents the situation in which there is no driving oscillator and the oscillating systems are organized in an interacting but nonhierarchical manner. No oscillator functions as a pacemaker, but various inputs would synchronize components of the system which would interact in such a way as to maintain internal synchronization. These are three distinct, independent models, but there is no basis *a priori* for selecting one over the other or for eliminating the possibility that combinations of the three models may be used differently by different mammalian organisms. Indeed, there may be significant interspecies differences in the types of circadian systems which constitute mammalian adaptational mechanisms. In particular, it would seem likely that in higher mammals, such as the anthropoid primates and man, where dissociation of circadian functions is commonplace (3), some combination of Models I and II is likely to occur.

Against this background, it is appropriate to review two questions. The first is the evidence that establishes a visual pathway responsible for the entrainment of circadian rhythms to the environmental cycle of light and dark. The second is the evidence currently available which indicates the localization of a driving oscillator and pertains to the organization of endogenous circadian rhythm generating mechanisms within the context of the models described above.

VISUAL PATHWAYS AND THE ENTRAINMENT OF CIRCADIAN RHYTHMS

The vast majority of work in this area has been done on either the rat or the hamster. The work of Hayhow and his colleagues (33,34) established the modern view of the organization of the rodent visual system. The optic nerve, arising from the ganglion cell layer of the retina, undergoes a nearly complete decussation in the optic chiasm with only a few fibers of the primary optic tract remaining ipsilateral to the eye in which they originated. The accessory optic pathways appear totally crossed. A portion of the accessory optic system, the superior fasciculus, joins the primary optic tract in its course along the diencephalon and terminates partially in a medial terminal nucleus in the rostral midbrain tegmentum. The fibers of the primary optic tract terminate in the lateral geniculate nucleus, both dorsal and ventral divisions, in the pretectal area and in the superior colliculus. A component of the accessory optic pathway, the inferior fasciculus, decussates completely in the optic chiasm and then leaves the primary optic tract to run caudally in the basal portion of the lateral hypothalamic area among the fibers of the medial forebrain bundle. This organization of visual pathways in the rat allowed for a series of ablation experiments to be designed in which either the primary optic tracts, the inferior accessory optic tracts, or all of the visual pathways beyond the optic chiasm could be ablated. There are a number of species differences in the organization of these pathways, and in the hamster visual system there appears to be no inferior fasciculus of the accessory optic system. Hence, all innervation to the primary and accessory optic terminal nuclei traverses the optic tract (20). In other respects, the hamster does not differ significantly from the rat. The paradigm for ablating the components of the optic pathway in the rat has been described on several occasions (47–49,51) and will not be repeated in detail. The visual pathway lesions that can be readily made are, first, ablation of all central retinal projections by section of the optic nerves. Second, primary optic tract section can be achieved by bilateral lesions ablating this pathway as it enters the thalamus. Third, transection of the inferior fasciculus of the accessory optic system can be accomplished by unilateral optic nerve section and transection of the ipsilateral medial forebrain bundle. Since the pathway is completely crossed, the later lesion results in total destruction of inferior accessory optic fibers originating from the eye contralateral to the optic nerve section. Fourth, the two groups of lesions, primary and accessory optic tract lesions, can be combined to destroy all retinal projections extending beyond the level of the optic chiasm.

When we planned our first experiments, it was known that a direct projection from the retina to the hypothalamus was present in some submammalian vertebrates and, indeed, was considered a general component of visual pathways in vertebrates (19). However, attempts to demonstrate retinohypothalamic projections in mammals had met with considerable difficulty, and the literature was inconclusive in that there were papers demonstrating such projections, but without agreement on the sites of their termination, and papers which failed to demonstrate such connections (see Nauta and Haymaker [54] and Moore and Lenn [52] for reviews). Extensive attempts in our hands (45) using conventional neuroanatomical techniques failed to provide substantive evidence for such projections in the rat. On this basis, we reasoned that ablation of all visual pathways beyond the optic chiasm should be equivalent to blinding in its effect on entrainment of a circadian rhythm to the diurnal cycle of light and dark. If ablation of these visual pathways did not alter entrainment of circadian rhythms, that would provide substantial evidence, albeit indirect, for a separate visual pathway, presumably a direct projection from the retina to the hypothalamus. On that basis, experiments were conducted in which the visual pathway lesions noted above were produced and circadian functions analyzed. The two circadian functions analyzed in this laboratory were the circadian rhythm in adrenal corticosterone content (16) and the dramatic circadian rhythm in the pineal enzyme, serotonin N-acetyltransferase, which had been reported by Klein and Weller (39). This is one important component in pineal indolamine metabolism, and other aspects of this metabolism have been reviewed in detail by Wurtman et al. (85). In studies performed in another laboratory, Stephan and Zucker (70) examined activity and drinking rhythms after similar lesions. The results of all of these studies were identical. The observations from our studies are summarized in Table 7–1. For control animals (sham operated) the adrenal corticosterone rhythm showed a peak value at 1900 hr and a trough value at 0700 hr, whereas the pineal serotonin N-acetyltransferase activity showed a peak value at 2400 hr and a trough value at 1300 hr. In both cases these are considered normal entrained circadian rhythms. Bilateral transection of all retinal input to the central nervous system (optic nerve section) resulted in

TABLE 7–1. Effects of primary and accessory optic tract transection on adrenal and pineal circadian rhythms in the rat

Visual pathway transected	Adrenal corticosterone			Pineal serotonin N-acetyltransferase		
	Time of peak value	Time of trough value	Rhythm status	Time of peak value	Time of trough value	Rhythm status
Controls	1900	0700	Entrained	2400	1300	Entrained
Optic nerve	0700	1900	Free-running	Scattered (2400–0700)	1300	Free-running
Primary optic tracts	1900	0700	Entrained	2400	1300	Entrained
Inferior accessory optic tracts	1900	0700	Entrained	2400	1300	Entrained
Combined primary and accessory optic tracts	1900	0700	Entrained	2400	1300	Entrained

Animals were maintained in a light-dark cycle (lights on 0700–1900 hr) and sacrificed at four time points: 0700, 1300, 1900, and 2400 hr, on the 21st day after operation. Adrenals were analyzed for corticosterone content and pineals for activity of the enzyme serotonin N-acetyltransferase. Lesions were verified histologically. Original data in Moore and Eichler (48,49) and Moore and Klein (51).

free-running rhythms in both adrenal corticosterone and pineal serotonin
N-acetyltransferase. In contrast to this, transection of the primary optic
tracts, the inferior accessory optic tracts, or all visual pathways beyond the
optic chiasm did not affect either the amplitude or entrainment of the adrenal
or pineal rhythms. Taken together, these observations strongly suggested that
a separate, and hitherto undescribed, visual pathway was mediating the entrainment of both circadian rhythms to the diurnal cycle of light and dark.
That is, since transection of the optic nerves resulted in loss of entrainment
and transection of all visual pathways beyond the optic chiasm was without
effect on entrainment, there is a strong implication that there is a visual pathway originating in the eye but terminating prior to the origin of the optic
tracts. Even though our extensive attempts to demonstrate a direct retinohypothalamic projection using conventional silver impregnation methods for
degenerating axons had failed (45), studies being performed at the time on
the incorporation of tritiated amino acids injected into the eye into protein
in ganglion cells of the retina and their transport to the terminals of visual
pathways suggested that an autoradiographic analysis might provide further
information (15,26,36,79). On this basis, we injected tritiated amino acids
into the vitreous of the eye and analyzed axonal transport to the terminal
nuclei of the visual system by autoradiography (46,50,52). In these studies,
all of the known central retinal projections described by Hayhow et al
(33,34) in the rat were evident and conformed in distribution to prior descriptions. In addition, however, our attention was directed to the region
immediately adjacent to the optic chiasm for several reasons. First, the
lesions of visual pathways noted above clearly indicated that other pathways
would probably terminate in the vicinity of the chiasm. Second, in large and
conflicting literature on retinohypothalamic projections, there were indica-
tions of a direct projection from the retina to the suprachiasmatic region

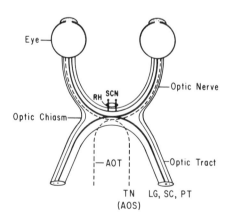

FIG. 7–2. Diagram of the central retinal projections in the rat. The optic nerves arise from the
ganglion cell layer of the retina and enter the
optic chiasm. Three major components arise from
the optic chiasm. The first is the retinohypothalamic projection (RH), which terminates bilaterally
in the suprachiasmatic nuclei (SCN) of the hypothalamus. The second is the primary optic tract,
which provides predominantly crossed and some
uncrossed afferents to the lateral geniculate
(LG) nuclei, the pretectal (PT) area, and the superior colliculus (SC). It also includes components
of the accessory optic system, the superior fasciculus (not shown in diagram), which terminates
in the dorsal, lateral, and medial terminal nuclei
of the accessory optic system. The third component is the accessory optic tract (AOT), which
terminates in the medial terminal nucleus (TN)
of the accessory optic system (AOS). Reproduced
with permission from Moore and Eichler (49).

(8,55,64). Third, data from hypothalamic deafferentation experiments strongly implicated the suprachiasmatic region in the entrainment and regulation of diurnal events (see Halasz [30] for review). Fourth, Critchlow (16) had shown that lesions in the suprachiasmatic area interfered with the female rat constant estrous response to light.

In our initial autoradiographic study on the rat (50,52), labeled axons could be traced from the optic nerve into the chiasm and from the chiasm into the suprachiasmatic nuclei bilaterally. The location of the suprachiasmatic nuclei in the rat is shown in Fig. 7–2. These nuclei lie immediately adjacent to the midline ventral and lateral to the third ventricle and bounded dorsally and laterally by the anterior hypothalamic area and ventrally by the optic chiasm. At their greatest extent the nuclei appear spherical in coronal sections and are approximately 0.6 mm in diameter. They first appear at rostral levels of the optic chiasm and extend to the most caudal extent of the optic chiasm. The total length of the nucleus averages approximately 10,000 neurons (J. N. Riley and R. Y. Moore, *unpublished observations*). In the rat, no retinal axons enter the first 400 μm of the suprachiasmatic nucleus. Caudal to that there is innervation which begins in the ventral portion of the nucleus and

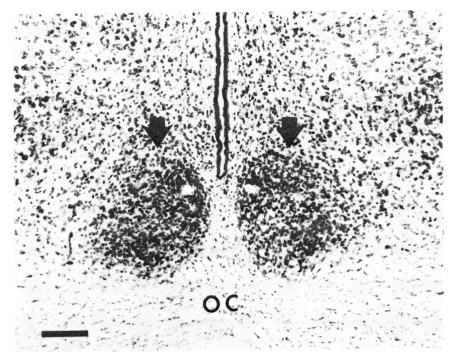

FIG. 7–3. Photomicrograph of a coronal section through the anterior hypothalamic area at the middle of the suprachiasmatic nuclei. Arrows indicate the suprachiasmatic nuclei. OC, optic chiasm. Marker bar = 100 μm.

spreads caudally to extend throughout the entire ventral and lateral portions of the nucleus (Fig. 7–3). This is approximately twice as great on the contralateral side as on the ipsilateral side. The dense innervation continues throughout the extent of the nucleus so that there is retinal innervation of the entire caudal three-fourths of the nucleus. Some labeling is evident in the anterior hypothalamic area immediately adjacent to the suprachiasmatic nucleus, but none has been observed in other hypothalamic nuclei (36,50,52). It is our interpretation at the present time that the small amount of labeling in the anterior hypothalamic area adjacent to the suprachiasmatic nucleus represents innervation of suprachiasmatic nucleus neurons as Golgi impregnations demonstrate that the dendrites of suprachiasmatic nucleus neurons extend beyond the boundaries of the nucleus in its caudal portions (J. N. Riley and R. Y. Moore, *unpublished observations*). Ultrastructural studies of the suprachiasmatic nucleus following section of the optic nerve in the rat (36,52) and in the mouse (84) indicate that retinohypothalamic axons terminate in synaptic contact with small dendrites and dendritic spines of suprachiasmatic nucleus neurons. In the rat, the degenerating axon terminals exhibit both

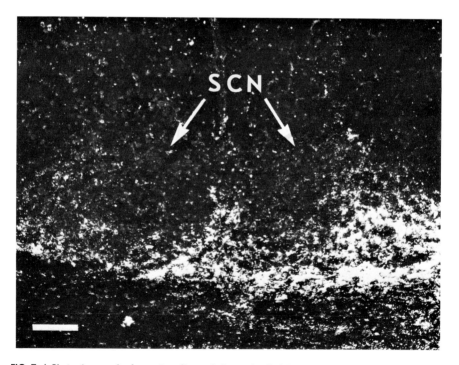

FIG. 7–4. Photomicrograph of an autoradiograph from a level of the anterior hypothalamic area identical to that shown in Fig. 7–3. SCN, suprachiasmatic nuclei. This photograph, taken with dark-field illumination, shows dense labeling of the suprachiasmatic nuclei 1 day after intraocular injection of 30 μCi tritiated proline. The labeling is greater on the contralateral than on the ipsilateral side and is largely confined to the ventral and lateral portions of the nucleus. Marker bar = 100 μm.

typical dark degeneration and the neurofilamentous type of degeneration (36). Although no formal quantitative analysis has been attempted, it is our impression that the retinohypothalamic projection gives rise to approximately 2 to 4% of the terminals in the suprachiasmatic nucleus in the areas in which there is dense innervation. The current view of the organization of the rat visual pathways is shown in Fig. 7–4.

Subsequent studies have been carried out on a large variety of mammalian species including prototherian, metatherian, and eutherian mammals. Within the last group a diverse series of species ranging from representatives of rodents, lagomorphs, insectivores, carnivores, prosimian primates, Old World monkeys, New World monkeys, and great apes has been investigated. The remarkable feature of these studies is the striking uniformity of the retino-hypothalamic projection among mammalian species. The projection has been nearly identical in virtually every species studied. That is, the innervation is predominantly in the caudal portion of the nucleus, is most dense in the ventral and lateral portions of the nucleus, and is bilateral with approximately twice as great an innervation of the contralateral as the ipsilateral supra-chiasmatic nucleus. Thus, it would appear that the retinohypothalamic pro-jection is a constant feature of the mammalian visual system, and, indeed, it appears to be the component of the system which undergoes the least altera-tion in mammalian phylogenetic development. The species in which the retinohypothalamic projection has been demonstrated are listed in Table 7–2.

TABLE 7–2. *The retinohypothalamic tract in mammals: species demonstrated to have a direct projection to the suprachiasmatic nuclei*

Species	Investigator(s)
Prototherian mammals	
Platypus (*Ornithorhyncus anatinns*)	Campbell & Hayhow (9)
Metatherian mammals	
Opossum (*Didelphis virginiana*)	Moore (46); Cavalcante et al. (10)
Eutherian mammals	
Rat (*Rattus norvegicus*)	Moore et al. (50); Moore & Lenn (52); Hendrickson et al. (36); Stanfield & Cowan (69); Mason & Lincoln (43)
Mouse (*Mus musculus*)	Drager (18); Wenisch (84)
Hamster (*Mesocricetus auratus*)	Eichler & Moore (20)
Guinea pig (*Cavia porcellus*)	Hendrickson et al. (36)
Rabbit (*Oryctolagus cuniculus*)	Hendrickson et al. (36)
Ferret (*Mustelo furo*)	Thorpe (80)
Hedgehog (*Hemiechinus auratus*)	Moore (46)
Cat (*Felis domesticus*)	Hendrickson et al. (36); Moore (46)
Tree shrew (*Tupaia glis*)	Moore (46); Conrad & Stumpf (13)
Galago (*Galago senegalensis*)	Moore (46)
Squirrel monkey (*Saimiri sciureus*)	Tigges & O'Steen (82)
Marmoset (*Saguinus oedipus*)	Moore (46)
Macaque monkey (*Macaca mulatta*)	Hendrickson et al. (36); Moore (46)
Chimpanzee (*Pan troglodytes*)	Tigges et al. (81)

THE SUPRACHIASMATIC NUCLEUS

The demonstration of a direct retinohypothalamic projection to the suprachiasmatic nucleus has stimulated a substantial amount of investigation into its organization and connections. This forms a logical basis for consideration of its functional role in circadian rhythm regulation, and the data available are reviewed briefly here.

Neurons

The nerve cells of the suprachiasmatic nucleus are easily identified in the light microscope as a tightly compacted group of small cells (approximately 6 to 12 μm in diameter) lying just above the optic chiasm and lateral to the third ventricle. In the light microscope (Fig. 7–3) neurons exhibit scant cytoplasm and a prominent nucleolus which is usually eccentrically placed near the nuclear membrane. The suprachiasmatic nucleus was first clearly identified by Spiegel and Zweig (68) in several mammalian species and has been described in the rat by Gurdjian (29), Krieg (40), and Szentagothai et al. (78). Ultrastructural studies of the suprachiasmatic nucleus have been carried out in the rat and rabbit by Suburo and Pellegrino de Iraldi (73), Clattenburg et al. (11,12), Güldner and Wolff (28), Güldner (27), and Lenn et al. (41). Suprachiasmatic nucleus neurons typically show nuclear identations. The cytoplasm of the neurons contains the usual organelles, and only two studies (11,12) have shown evidence of neurosecretory activity. The nucleus has been found, however, to contain some cells with immuno-histochemically demonstrable luteinizing hormone releasing hormone (67).

Neuropil

The study of Güldner (27) represents the most extensive analysis of the synaptology of the nucleus. Five types of synapses are distinguished which can be placed into two major groups. The first is represented by two types of asymmetrical Gray type I synapses. These represent approximately a third of the synapses in the nucleus and are located along dendritic shafts and spines, rarely making axosomatic contacts. They contain symmetrical, clear vesicles approximately 450 Å in diameter. Subjunctional bodies are often associated with these synapses, and the occasional "crest" synapses evident in the suprachiasmatic nucleus are included in this classification. It would appear from the work of Moore and Lenn (52), Hendrickson et al. (36), and Wenisch (84) that this classification includes the terminals of retinohypothalamic fibers. There are three types of symmetrical Gray type II synapses which make up approximately two-thirds of the total synaptic contacts in the nucleus. One type makes axodendritic or axosomatic synapses and contains spherical, clear vesicles of approximately 500 Å in diameter. The second type of symmetrical synapse also includes both axodendritic and axosomatic synapses with club-like postsynaptic protrusions within the presynaptic elements. The size of the clear vesicles in these presynaptic elements varies from approximately 400 to 1,000 Å. The third type of symmetrical synapse is comprised of dendrodendritic, dendrosomatic, or somatodendritic synapses occurring, at least partly, in reciprocal arrangements. These represent an intrinsic system within the nucleus. The dendrodendritic synapses have been described in great detail by Güldner and Wolf (28). After three-dimensional reconstruction, dense core vesicles were identified in all of the asymmetrical synapses and most of the symmetrical synapses (27). The synaptology of the nucleus is obviously extremely complex, and the origin of the various synaptic types has not been elucidated.

It should be noted that interesting sex differences have been observed in suprachiasmatic nucleus neurons in the rat. Multivesiculated bodies are much more numerous in the dendrites of female rats than in those of male rat suprachiasmatic nucleus neurons. In addition, Clattenburg et al. (11,12) have demonstrated ultrastructural changes in the neurons of the suprachiasmatic nucleus of the rabbit following endocrine manipulation, including changes that could be associated with secretory activity.

Connections of the Suprachiasmatic Nucleus

Until the demonstration of the termination of retinohypothalamic tract fibers within the suprachiasmatic nucleus (36,50,52), there was little information on either the afferent or efferent projections of the suprachiasmatic nucleus. The work of Fuxe (25) demonstrated the presence of serotonin-containing terminals within the suprachiasmatic nucleus, and this was confirmed by Aghajanian et al. (1) who demonstrated that the origin of these serotonin terminals is from the median raphe. Subsequent studies have shown that the suprachiasmatic nucleus receives descending projections from the anterior hypothalamic area, including the anterior portion of the periventricular nucleus (14,74), and ascending fibers from the tuberal hypothalamic area (Fichera and Moore, *unpublished observations*). In addition, there is a second, indirect visual projection on the suprachiasmatic nucleus. Studies by Swanson et al. (77) and Ribak and Peters (60) have demonstrated a bilateral projection from the ventral lateral geniculate nucleus to the suprachiasmatic nucleus which overlaps the retinohypothalamic projection in both its distribution and its relative density. Two further possible afferent inputs should be considered. First, it is likely that there is a brainstem norepinephrine projection on suprachiasmatic nucleus neurons. Although the nucleus does not contain a significant number of norepinephrine fibers in material prepared by the fluorescence histochemical methods, it is surrounded by a dense capsule of norepinephrine axon terminals (Mosko and Moore, *unpublished observations*). There is evidence from Golgi material that the dendrites of suprachiasmatic nucleus neurons extend outside of the nucleus (40,78) so that they could be in a position to be innervated by the dense capsule of norepinephrine fibers surrounding the nucleus. Second, the medial corticohypothalamic projection arising from the hippocampal formation (59,76) passes immediately adjacent to the suprachiasmatic nucleus and, as with the norepinephrine fibers, could provide an input to suprachiasmatic nucleus neuron dendrites in its passage to the region of the arcuate nucleus. This could be of particular significance in view of the role of the hippocampus as an adrenal corticoid receptor, the suprachiasmatic nucleus in regulation of adrenal rhythms (48), and the site of termination of the medial corticohypothalamic tract in the area in which corticotropin releasing hormone appears to be produced (17).

Efferent Projections

The efferent projections of the suprachiasmatic nucleus neurons were observed in Golgi material to take a dorsal and caudal direction, but it was not possible in such material to trace them to their termination (40,78). In a recent study using the autoradiographic tracing method, however, Swanson and Cowan (75) were able to produce a localized injection of tritiated amino acid into the rat suprachiasmatic nucleus. This gave rise to a projection which could be followed dorsally and caudally in the periventricular area as far as the caudal end of the ventromedial nucleus. The projection passes from the suprachiasmatic nucleus in a dorsal and caudal direction through the ventral periventricular area and arcuate nucleus, throughout the periventricular area and ventrally into the ventral tuberal area. It continues caudally in this position with little label evident in either the dorsomedial or ventromedial nuclei

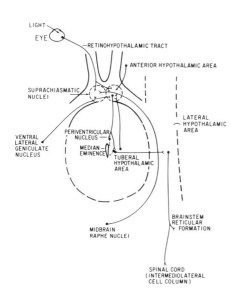

FIG. 7–5. Diagrammatic representation of the connections of the suprachiasmatic nuclei as they are now known. The diagram is of the base of the brain with the suprachiasmatic nuclei designated by dashed lines within the optic chiasm. Afferent input to the suprachiasmatic nuclei has been shown from the eye, the anterior hypothalamic area, the ventral lateral geniculate nucleus, the tuberal hypothalamic area, and the midbrain raphe nuclei. The only efferent projections known are to the periventricular and tuberal hypothalamus. See text for description.

of the hypothalamus. Some label is evident in the arcuate nucleus and in the internal and subependymal layers of the median eminence, but this is sparse in comparison to that in the periventricular and ventral tuberal areas. The ventral tuberal area has been shown in Golgi preparations to have reciprocal connections with the lateral hypothalamic area neurons. These have recently been shown (66) to project directly on both brainstem and the intermedio-lateral cell column of the spinal cord. Thus, the efferent projections of the suprachiasmatic nucleus are organized so that they can affect both hypo-thalamo-pituitary functions and functions dependent on descending projec-tions to the brainstem and spinal cord. A summary of the connections of the suprachiasmatic nucleus, as they are now known, is shown in Fig. 7–5.

THE SUPRACHIASMATIC NUCLEUS AND CIRCADIAN RHYTHMS

The demonstration of a direct retinohypothalamic projection to the supra-chiasmatic nucleus as a feature of the mammalian visual system (see above) and the experimental evidence that it was essential for the entrainment of circadian rhythms (48,51,70) suggested that transection of the retinohypo-thalamic projection would have significant functional consequences. In the rat, however, it is not possible to cut the pathway without destroying the suprachiasmatic nuclei because of the close proximity of the nuclei to the optic chiasm and their very small size. Consequently, Stephan and Zucker (71) and Moore and Eichler (48) in independent experiments examined the effects of suprachiasmatic nucleus ablation on circadian rhythms in the rat. In the study of Stephan and Zucker (71) activity and drinking rhythms were examined, whereas in that of Moore and Eichler (48) the adrenal corticoste-rone rhythm was analyzed. In each case the reasonable expectation would have been that ablation of the nuclei should result in free-running rhythms because of ablation of the retinohypothalamic projection. This was not the effect observed, however, and in both instances the rhythms being studied were found to be abolished by bilateral ablation of the suprachiasmatic nuclei. This occurred independent of damage to the optic chiasm. The inter-pretation, in each case, was that the evidence supported the view that the suprachiasmatic nucleus participated in the central neural regulation of the circadian function under study. These were the first studies to show abolition of circadian rhythms by a highly localized brain lesion. Prior studies by Richter (61) had implicated the hypothalamus in circadian rhythm regulation, but the localization of his lesions was not clearly specified or demonstrated. From the description given it would seem most likely that they ablated the efferent projections of the suprachiasmatic nuclei.

The interpretation of the effects of suprachiasmatic lesions was not un-equivocal, however. Alternative explanations were available and some of these were open to direct experimental attack. In particular, one interpreta-tion was that the lesion was interrupting fibers descending through the suprachiasmatic nucleus region from a rostral site to a caudal hypothalamic region which was critical for rhythm generation. A second interpretation was that the rhythm-generating mechanism was located near the suprachiasmatic nucleus and that this area would project on the suprachiasmatic nuclei to allow coupling with the input from the synchronizing stimulus. Thus, it could be argued that the lesions were not confined to the suprachiasmatic nucleus and that the involvement of adjacent tissue was responsible for the effect. For that reason, in further studies partial hypothalamic deafferentation was performed by making a knife cut rostral to the suprachiasmatic nuclei and caudal to the suprachiasmatic nuclei; in addition, an extensive analysis was undertaken to determine the exact distribution of suprachiasmatic nucleus lesions which were effective in abolishing circadian rhythmicity (Table 7–3). In this study the rhythm in the pineal enzyme, serotonin N-acetyltransferase (39), was used as the indicator of circadian function (51). Hypothalamic deafferentation rostral to the suprachiasmatic nuclei did not affect the circadian rhythm in pineal serotonin N-acetyltransferase, but the rhythm was totally abolished by partial hypothalamic deafferentation with a knife cut caudal to the suprachiasmatic nuclei. The localization of the caudal knife cuts, as verified histologically, indicated that they would totally transect the descend-

TABLE 7–3. *Hypothalamic lesions: effects on circadian rhythms in adrenal corticosterone and pineal serotonin N-acetyltransferase in the rat*

	Rhythm					
	Adrenal corticosterone			Pineal serotonin N-acetyltransferase		
Hypothalamic lesion	Time of peak value	Time of trough value	Rhythm status	Time of peak value	Time of trough value	Rhythm status
Sham deafferentation	1900	0700	Entrained	2400	1300	Entrained
Anterior hypothalamic deafferentation—rostral to optic chiasm	1900	0700	Entrained	2400	1300	Entrained
Anterior hypothalamic deafferentation—caudal to optic chiasm	None	None	Abolished	None	None	Abolished
Anterior hypothalamic area lesion	1900	0700	Entrained	2400	1300	Entrained
Suprachiasmatic nucleus lesion	None	None	Abolished	None	None	Abolished

Animals were maintained in a light-dark cycle (lights on 0700–1900 hr) throughout the study. They were sacrificed on the 21st day after operation at four time points: 0700, 1300, 1900, and 2400 hr. Adrenals were analyzed for corticosterone content and pineals for activity of the enzyme serotonin N-acetyltransferase. Lesions were verified histologically. The partial hypothalamic deafferentations were performed with a modified Halasz knife. Sham deafferentation refers to placing the knife in the exact position where the deafferentation caudal to the chiasm would be made and then withdrawing it. Anterior hypothalamic lesions are lesions destroying components of the anterior hypothalamic area but sparing the suprachiasmatic nucleus. For further details see Moore and Eichler (48) and Moore and Klein (51).

ing projection from the suprachiasmatic nucleus to the periventricular and tuberal hypothalamus (75). In addition, analysis of the electrolytic lesions in the suprachiasmatic area indicated that they could be subdivided into two groups. The first group consisted of lesions which ablated the suprachiasmatic nuclei or at least the caudal three-fourths of the nuclei. These lesions varied in extent; some were small and largely confined to the suprachiasmatic nucleus, but others involved adjacent optic chiasm and anterior hypothalamic area (51). Lesions that did not affect the circadian rhythm in pineal serotonin *N*-acetyltransferase spared, at a minimum, the caudal one-half of the suprachiasmatic nuclei. These lesions were quite variable in both location and extent. Some were unilateral whereas others were bilateral and ablated large amounts of anterior hypothalamic area down to but not including the suprachiasmatic nuclei. Consequently, it was our interpretation that the ablation of the suprachiasmatic nuclei, or their descending projections, was essential to abolition of the circadian rhythm in pineal serotonin *N*-acetyltransferase (51). Similar observations were made for the adrenal corticosterone rhythm, and the results of both studies are summarized in Table 7–3. Subsequently, studies have been carried out in other laboratories which have extended and amplified these observations. These are summarized in Table 7–4. Rusak and Zucker (65) demonstrated that activity rhythms in the hamster are abolished by suprachiasmatic nucleus lesions and that the duration of the effect was as long as 365 days. Ibuka and Kawamura (37) demonstrated that sleep-wake cycles were abolished in the rat over a 63-day period. This study

TABLE 7–4. *Suprachiasmatic nucleus ablation: effects on circadian rhythms in mammals*

Investigator(s)	Animal	Rhythm(s)	Post-lesion rhythm status	Postoperative survival period (days)
Stephan & Zucker (71)	Rat	Activity, drinking	Abolished	120
Moore & Eichler (48)	Rat	Adrenal corticosterone	Abolished	21
Moore & Klein (51)	Rat	Pineal serotonin *N*-acetyltransferase	Abolished	21
Rusak & Zucker (65)	Hamster	Activity	Abolished	365
Ibuka & Kawamura (37)	Rat	Sleep-wake	Abolished	63
Stetson & Watson-Whitmyre (72)	Hamster	Activity, estrous cycling, photoperiodic photosensitivity	Abolished	80–210
Wansley & Holloway (83)	Rat	Learning, temperature	Abolished	20+
Brown-Grant & Raisman (6)	Rat	Estrous cycling, ovulation	Abolished	~100
Raisman & Brown-Grant (58)	Rat	Ovulation, activity, feeding & drinking, serum corticosterone, pineal serotonin *N*-acetyltransferase	Abolished	120–180

is of particular interest in that in any given day the amount of time spent in waking, deep sleep, and paradoxical sleep is entirely normal but there is no circadian rhythmicity. Stetson and Watson-Whitmyer (72) demonstrated that suprachiasmatic nucleus lesions abolished activity rhythms, estrous cycling, and photoperiod sensitivity in the hamster. Wansley and Holloway (83) have shown that the circadian rhythm in temperature in the rat is abolished concomitant with the circadian rhythm in the capacity to perform certain behavioral tasks. Lastly, in an extensive series of experiments, Brown-Grant and Raisman (6,58) have shown loss of ovulation following suprachiasmatic nucleus lesions and have concluded that this can be interpreted only as a loss of circadian function. A further important aspect of their studies is the precise anatomical localization of the critical area for the effect to the suprachiasmatic nuclei. It has been known for a number of years that lesions in the suprachiasmatic nucleus produce gonadal effects in female rats (see Flerko [24], Moore and Eichler [49], and Brown-Grant and Raisman [6] for reviews), but only recently has a distinct "suprachiasmatic syndrome" (6,58) been proposed relating to the nucleus itself.

Thus, there is no circadian rhythm in the rat or hamster which has been studied to the present time that has not been abolished by suprachiasmatic nucleus lesions. It should be emphasized that the effect also appears restricted to ablation of the suprachiasmatic nucleus or its efferent projections. Destruction of regions which project to the suprachiasmatic nucleus, or the projections themselves, have not been demonstrated, thus far, to have similar effects on circadian rhythms. For example, Stephan and Zucker (70) found that lesions of the lateral geniculate body had some effect on entrainment of rhythms but did not affect circadian rhythmicity as such. In addition, a series of studies (4,5,51) has shown that destruction of the midbrain raphe nuclei giving rise to the serotonin innervation of the suprachiasmatic nucleus has no lasting effect on circadian rhythmicity. Lesions destroying the medial forebrain bundle bilaterally (see Moore and Eichler [49] for review) affect a variety of circadian rhythms, but the interpretation of such effects is complex and determined by a number of factors. Among them is the fact that such lesions abolish most descending central sympathetic control and, consequently, rhythms dependent on central sympathetic regulation are lost.

A further interesting correlation between circadian rhythms and the suprachiasmatic nucleus has arisen from developmental studies. The earliest known circadian rhythm to develop in the rat is that in the pineal enzyme, serotonin N-acetyltransferase. This rhythm first becomes evident between 4 and 6 days of age (21,23). The rhythm first appears when the sympathetic innervation of the pineal has arrived (38,42) and the retinohypothalamic projection is reaching the suprachiasmatic nucleus (22,69). The development of the retinohypothalamic projection is not essential, however, for the development of the rhythm, and it appears to develop between the fourth and seventh postnatal day in the rat and in animals blinded at birth and maintained in constant light, indicating that central circadian oscillating mechanisms initiate their function in this early postnatal period (23). This is of particular interest in that it corresponds exactly to the time at which the suprachiasmatic nucleus is undergoing a marked developmental maturation in its neuropil (41).

CONCLUSIONS

The studies that have been discussed in this review appear to allow two general conclusions. The first is that a retinohypothalamic projection is a consistent feature of the vertebrate visual system. In the mammalian visual system it is the least phylogenetically variant of all components of the central retinal projections. As far as is known at present, it terminates exclusively in the suprachiasmatic nucleus, and each suprachiasmatic nucleus receives a bilateral projection from each retina. In addition, there is substantive evidence to indicate that the retinohypothalamic projection is the only component of the central retinal projections which is essential for the entrainment of circadian rhythms to the diurnal cycle of light and dark. Other components of the central visual pathway may participate in this phenomenon, but only the retinohypothalamic projection has been demonstrated to be essential. It could be argued that this demonstration is not entirely compelling as it is one based on negative evidence; i.e., it is based on the evidence that ablation of all other visual pathways has no more than transient effects on entrainment of circadian rhythms in the presence of an intact retinohypothalamic projection. No study has been carried out as yet in which the retinohypothalamic tract has been severed with the remaining visual pathways intact.

The demonstration of the retinohypothalamic projection to the suprachiasmatic nucleus led to experiments which have engendered the second conclusion. In these experiments it was found that ablation of the suprachiasmatic nuclei results in a loss of all circadian rhythms which have been studied (Table 7–3; 49,86). As indicated above, in no experiment carried out to the present has ablation of the suprachiasmatic nuclei failed to abolish a circadian rhythm.

On a general basis, the central mechanisms of circadian rhythm generation would appear to have two distinct but interacting functions. The first is the circadian rhythm in photoperiodic time measurement. There is considerable evidence that a circadian function exists for the measurement of photoperiod (see Menaker [44] for review). This is not only experimentally demonstrable but it is evident from the phenomenon of entrainment. The second component of circadian function is the generation of an oscillating signal. Several models for this phenomenon are presented in the beginning of this chapter. The data presented here do not appear to be consistent with the third of these models (Fig. 7–1). Indeed, data available at present indicate that the suprachiasmatic nucleus, in the animals studied, mediates both circadian functions, and the analysis of these data suggests that they are in better accord with Model I than with Model II. Therefore, in all instances studied thus far, suprachiasmatic lesions have abolished all circadian functions without altering other aspects of the function in question. The sleep-wake data provide a particularly good example of this (37). All components of the sleep-wake cycle were present in normal amount following the suprachiasmatic nucleus lesion; only the circadian rhythmicity was lost. Similarly, in the estrous cycle studies of Brown-Grant and Raisman (6,58) the effect of suprachiasmatic nucleus lesions was to abolish circadian functions and, in that way, abolish the luteinizing hormone surge which normally occurs on the day of proestrous and ovulation. No endocrine functions were altered as such. Nevertheless, Model I with the suprachiasmatic nucleus designated as the driving oscillator should not be accepted without some caution. There is substantial evidence to indicate that most endogenous circadian pacemakers are composed of multiple, hierarchically organized oscillators (3,53,56), and thus far all studies of the suprachiasmatic nucleus syndrome have been carried out on the rat or hamster. Higher mammals, particularly primates, appear to show a greater capacity for dissociation of rhythms, and such species clearly have circadian systems organized much more like those in Model II or a combination of Models I and II. With this reservation, however, one must conclude that the information obtained during the last few years has brought the suprachiasmatic nucleus to consideration as a pivotal component of circadian rhythm-generating functions in mammals. Since these functions serve a major role in the adaptive responsiveness of the organism to its environment, further study of the suprachiasmatic nucleus in its role in circadian rhythm generation will give us important insight into the neural mechanisms which participate in circadian functions. The generation of circadian rhythms is a unique neural function, and further understanding of this function will have significant implications not only for a special aspect of the adaptation of organisms to their environment but also for diseases in which these functions are impaired.

ACKNOWLEDGMENTS

This work has been supported by USPHS Grant NS-12267 from the National Institutes of Health. The author is grateful to a number of collaborators, particularly Drs. Victor B. Eichler, David C. Klein, Michael Felong, and Nicholas J. Lenn for their contributions.

REFERENCES

1. Aghajanian, G. K., Bloom, F. E., and Sheard, M. H. (1969): Electron microscopy of degeneration within the serotonin pathway of rat brain. *Brain Res.*, 13:266–273.
2. Alleva, J. J., Waleski, M. W., and Alleva, F. R. (1971): A biological clock controlling the estrous cycle of the hamster. *Endocrinology*, 88:1368–1379.
3. Aschoff, J., and Wever, R. (1976): Human circadian rhythms: A multioscillator system. *Fed. Proc.*, 35:2326–2332.
4. Balestrery, F. G., and Moberg, G. P. (1976): Effect of midbrain raphe nuclei lesions

on the circadian rhythm of plasma corticosterone in the rat. *Brain Res.,* 118:503–508.

5. Block, M., and Zucker, I. (1976): Circadian rhythms of rat locomotor activity after lesions of the midbrain raphe nuclei. *J. Comp. Physiol.,* 109:235–247.

6. Brown-Grant, K., and Raisman, G. (1977): Abnormalities in reproductive function associated with the destruction of the suprachiasmatic nuclei in female rats. *Proc. Roy. Soc. Lond. [Biol.] (in press).*

7. Bünning, E. (1977): *The Physiological Clock, Ed. 3.* Springer-Verlag, New York.

8. Campbell, C. B. G. (1969): The visual system of insectivores and primates. *Ann. N.Y. Acad. Sci.,* 167:388–403.

9. Campbell, C. B. G., and Hayhow, W. R. (1972): Primary optic pathways in the duckbill platypus *Ornithorhynchus anatinis:* An experimental study. *J. Comp. Neurol.,* 145:195–208.

10. Cavalcante, L. A., Roche-Miranda, C. E., and Lant, R. (1975): Hypothalamic, tectal and accessory optic projections in the opossum. *Brain Res.,* 84:302–307.

11. Clattenburg, R. E., Montemurro, D. G., and Bruni, J. E. (1975): Neurosecretory activity within suprachiasmatic neurons of the female rabbit following castration. *Neuroendocrinology,* 17:211–224.

12. Clattenburg, R. E., Singh, R. P., and Montemurro, D. G. (1972): Post-coital ultrastructural changes in neurons of the suprachiasmatic nucleus of the rabbit. *Z. Zellforsch.,* 125:448–459.

13. Conrad, C. D., and Stumpf, W. E. (1974): Retinal projections traced with thaw-mount autoradiography and multiple injections of tritiated precursor or precursor cocktail. *Cell Tissue Res.,* 155:283–290.

14. Conrad, L. C. A., and Pfaff, D. W. (1976): Efferents from the medial basal forebrain and hypothalamus in the rat. II. An autoradiographic study of the anterior hypothalamus. *J. Comp. Neurol.,* 169:221–261.

15. Cowan, W. M., Gottlieb, D. I., Hendrickson, A. E., Price, J. L., and Woolsey, T. A. (1972): The autoradiographic demonstration of axonal connections in the central nervous system. *Brain Res.,* 37:21–51.

16. Critchlow, V. (1963): The role of light in the neuroendocrine system. In: *Advances in Neuroendocrinology,* edited by V. Nalbandov, pp. 377–401. University of Illinois Press, Urbana.

17. Csernus, V., Lengvari, I., and Halasz, B. (1975): Further studies on ACTH secretion from pituitary grafts in the hypophysiotrophic area. *Neuroendocrinology,* 17:18–26.

18. Drager, U. (1974): Autoradiography of tritiated proline and fucose transported transneuronally from the eye to the visual cortex in pigmented and albino mice. *Brain Res.,* 82:284–292.

19. Ebbesson, S. O. E. (1970): On the organization of central visual pathways in vertebrates. *Brain Behav. Evol.,* 3:178–194.

20. Eichler, V. B., and Moore, R. Y. (1974): The primary and accessory optic systems in the golden hamster, *Mesocricetus auratus. Acta Anat.,* 89:359–371.

21. Ellison, N., Weller, J. L., and Klein, D. C. (1972): Development of a circadian rhythm in the activity of pineal serotonin N-acetyltransferase. *J. Neurochem.,* 19:1335–1341.

22. Felong, M. (1976): The postnatal development of a retinohypothalamic projection in the rat. *Anat. Rec.,* 184:400.

23. Felong, M., and Moore, R. Y. (1976): Development of a circadian rhythm in pineal N-acetyltransferase in the rat. *Neurosci. Abstr.,* 2:670.

24. Flerko, B. (1966): Control of gonadotropin secretion in the female. In: *Neuroendocrinology, Vol. 1,* edited by L. Martini and W. F. Ganong, pp. 613–668. Academic Press, New York.

25. Fuxe, K. (1965): Evidence for the existence of monoamine neurons in the central nervous system. IV. Distribution of monoamine nerve terminals in the central nervous system. *Acta. Physiol. Scand. [Suppl. 274],* 64:39–85.

26. Goldberg, S., and Kotani, M. (1967): The projection of optic nerve fibers in the frog, *Rana Catesbeiana,* as studied by autoradiography. *Anat. Rec.,* 158:325–332.

27. Güldner, F. H. (1976): Synaptology of the rat suprachiasmatic nucleus. *Cell Tissue Res.*, 165:509–544.
28. Güldner, F. H., and Wolff, J. R. (1974): Dendro-dendritic synapses in the suprachiasmatic nucleus of the rat hypothalamus. *J. Neurocytol.*, 3:245–250.
29. Gurdjian, E. S. (1927): The diencephalon of the albino rat. *J. Comp. Neurol.*, 43: 1–114.
30. Halasz, B. (1969): Endocrine effects of isolation of the hypothalamus from the rest of the brain. In: *Frontiers in Neuroendocrinology, 1969,* edited by W. F. Ganong and L. Martini, pp. 307–342. Oxford University Press, New York.
31. Halberg, F. (1960): Temporal coordination of physiologic function. *Cold Spring Harbor Symp. Quant. Biol.*, 25:289–310.
32. Halberg, F. (1968): Chronobiology. *Annu. Rev. Physiol.*, 31:675–725.
33. Hayhow, W. R., Sefton, A., and Webb, C. (1962): Primary optic centers in the rat in relation to the terminal distribution of the crossed and uncrossed optic nerve fibers. *J. Comp. Neurol.*, 118:295–322.
34. Hayhow, W. R., Webb, C., and Jervie, A. (1960): The accessory optic system in the rat. *J. Comp. Neurol.*, 115:187–215.
35. Hendrickson, A. E. (1972): Electron microscopic distribution of axoplasmic transport. *J. Comp. Neurol.*, 144:381–398.
36. Hendrickson, A. E., Wagoner, N., and Cowan, W. M. (1972): An autoradiographic and electron microscopic study of retinohypothalamic connections. *Z. Zellforsch.*, 135:1–26.
37. Ibuka, N., and Kawamura, H. (1975): Loss of circadian rhythm in sleep-wakefulness cycle in the rat by suprachiasmatic nucleus lesions. *Brain Res.*, 96:76–81.
38. Kappers, J. A. (1960): The development, topographical relations and innervation of the epiphysis cerebri in the albino rat. *Z. Zellforsch.*, 52:163–215.
39. Klein, D. C., and Weller, J. L. (1970): Indole metabolism in the pineal gland: A circadian rhythm in N-acetyltransferase. *Science*, 169:1093–1095.
40. Krieg, W. J. S. (1932): The hypothalamus of the albino rat. *J. Comp. Neurol.*, 55:19–89.
41. Lenn, N. J., Beebe, B., and Moore, R. Y. (1977): Postnatal development of the suprachiasmatic hypothalamic nucleus of the rat. *Cell Tissue Res. (in press).*
42. Machado, C. R. S., Wragg, L. E., and Machado, A. B. M. (1968): A histochemical study of the sympathetic innervation and 5-hydroxytryptamine in the developing pineal body of the rat. *Brain Res.*, 8:310–318.
43. Mason, C. A., and Lincoln, D. W. (1976): Visualization of the retinohypothalamic projection in the rat by cobalt precipitation. *Cell Tissue Res.*, 168:117–132.
44. Menaker, M. (1974): Aspects of the physiology of circadian rhythmicity in the vertebrate central nervous system. In: *The Neurosciences—Third Study Program,* edited by F. O. Schmitt and F. G. Worden, pp. 479–489. MIT Press, Cambridge, Mass.
45. Moore, R. Y. (1969): Visual pathways controlling neuroendocrine function. In: *Progress in Endocrinology,* edited by C. Gual and F. I. G. Ebling, pp. 490–494. Excerpta Medica, Amsterdam.
46. Moore, R. Y. (1973): Retinohypothalamic projection in mammals. A comparative study. *Brain Res.*, 49:403–409.
47. Moore, R. Y. (1974): Visual pathways and the central neural control of diurnal rhythms. In: *The Neurosciences—Third Study Program,* edited by F. O. Schmitt and F. G. Worden, pp. 537–542. MIT Press, Cambridge, Mass.
48. Moore, R. Y., and Eichler, V. B. (1972): Loss of a circadian adrenal corticosterone rhythm following suprachiasmatic lesions in the rat. *Brain Res.*, 42:201–206.
49. Moore, R. Y., and Eichler, V. B. (1976): Central neural mechanisms in diurnal rhythm regulation and neuroendocrine responses to light. *Psychoneuroendocrinology*, 1:265–279.
50. Moore, R. Y., Karapas, F., and Lenn, N. J. (1971): A retinohypothalamic projection in the rat. *Anat. Rec.*, 169:382–383.
51. Moore, R. Y., and Klein, D. C. (1974): Visual pathways and the central neural control of a circadian rhythm in pineal serotonin N-acetyltransferase activity. *Brain Res.*, 71:17–33.

52. Moore, R. Y., and Lenn, N. J. (1972): A retinohypothalamic projection in the rat. *J. Comp. Neurol.,* 146:1–14.
53. Moore-Ede, M. C., Schmelzer, W. S., Kass, D. A., and Herd, J. A. (1976): Internal organization of the circadian timing system in multicellular animals. *Fed. Proc.,* 35:2333–2338.
54. Nauta, W. J. H., and Haymaker, W. (1969): Retinohypothalamic connections. In: *The Hypothalamus,* edited by W. Haymaker, E. Anderson, and W. J. H. Nauta, pp. 187–189. Charles C. Thomas, Springfield, Ill.
55. Pate, J. R. (1937): Trans-neural atrophy of the nucleus ovoideus following eye removal in cats. *Anat. Rec.,* 67:39.
56. Pittendrigh, C. S. (1974): Circadian oscillations in cells and the circadian organization of multicellular systems. In: *The Neurosciences—Third Study Program,* edited by F. O. Schmitt and F. G. Worden, pp. 437–458. MIT Press, Cambridge, Mass.
57. Raisman, G. (1970): Some aspects of the neural connections of the hypothalamus In: *The Hypothalamus,* edited by L. Martini, M. Motta, and F. Fraschini, pp. 1–16. Academic Press, New York.
58. Raisman, G., and Brown-Grant, K. (1977): The "suprachiasmatic syndrome": Endocrine and behavioral abnormalities following lesions of the suprachiasmatic nuclei in the female rat. *Proc. Roy. Soc. Lond. [Biol.] (in press).*
59. Raisman, G. W., Cowan, W. M., and Powell, T. P. S. (1965): The extrinsic afferent, commissural and association fibers of the hippocampus. *Brain,* 88:963–996.
60. Ribak, C. E., and Peters, A. (1975): An autoradiographic study of the projections from the lateral geniculate body of the rat. *Brain Res.,* 92:341–368.
61. Richter, C. P. (1967): Sleep and activity: Their relation to the 24 hour clock. *Proc. Assoc. Res. Nerv. Ment. Dis.,* 45:8–27.
62. Richter, C. P. (1968): Inherent twenty-four and lunar clocks of a primate—the squirrel monkey. *Comm. Behav. Biol.,* 1:305–332.
63. Richter, C. P. (1971): Inborn nature of the rat's 24-hour clock. *J. Comp. Physiol. Psychol.,* 75:1–4.
64. Roussy, G., and Mosinger, M. (1935): L'hypothalamus chez l'homme et chez le chien. *Rev. Neurol. (Paris),* 63:1–35.
65. Rusak, B., and Zucker, I. (1975): Biological rhythms and animal behavior. *Annu. Rev. Psychol.,* 26:137–171.
66. Saper, C. B., Loewy, A. D., Swanson, L. W., and Cowan, W. M. (1976): Direct hypothalamus-autonomic connections. *Brain Res.,* 117:305–312.
67. Setalo, G., Vigh, S., Schally, A. V., Arimura, A., and Flerko, B. (1976): Immunohistological study of the origin of LH-RH containing nerve fibers of the rat hypothalamus. *Brain Res.,* 103:597–602.
68. Spiegel, E. A., and Zweig, H. (1917): Zur cytoarchitectonik des tuber cinereum. *Arch. Neurol. Inst. Wien. Univ.,* 22:278–312.
69. Stanfield, B., and Cowan, W. M. (1976): Evidence for a change in the retinohypothalamic projection in the rat following early removal of one eye. *Brain Res.,* 104:129–136.
70. Stephan, F. K., and Zucker, I. (1972): Rat drinking rhythms: Central pathways and endocrine factors mediating responsiveness to environmental illumination. *Physiol. Behav.,* 8:315–326.
71. Stephan, F. K., and Zucker, I. (1972): Circadian rhythms in drinking behavior and locomotor activity of rats are eliminated by hypothalamic lesions. *Proc. Natl. Acad. Sci. USA,* 69:1583–1586.
72. Stetson, M. H., and Watson-Whitmyre, M. (1976): Nucleus suprachiasmaticus: The biological clock in the hamster. *Science,* 191:197–199.
73. Suburo, A. M., and Pellegrino de Iraldi, A. (1969): An ultrastructural study of the rat's suprachiasmatic nucleus. *J. Anat.,* 105:439–446.
74. Swanson, L. W. (1976): An autoradiographic study of the efferent connections of the preoptic region in the rat. *J. Comp. Neurol.,* 167:227–256.
75. Swanson, L. W., and Cowan, W. M. (1975): The efferent connections of the suprachiasmatic nucleus of the hypothalamus. *J. Comp. Neurol.,* 160:1–12.
76. Swanson, L. W., and Cowan, W. M. (1977): An autoradiographic study of the or-

ganization of the efferent connections of the hippocampal formation in the rat. *J. Comp. Neurol.,* 172:49–84.

77. Swanson, L. W., Cowan, W. M., and Jones, E. G. (1974): An autoradiographic study of the efferent connections of the ventral lateral geniculate nucleus in the albino rat and cat. *J. Comp. Neurol.,* 156:143–164.
78. Szentagothai, J., Flerko, B., Mess, B., and Halasz, B. (1968): *Hypothalamic Control of the Anterior Pituitary, Ed. 3,* p. 40. Akademiai Kiado, Budapest.
79. Taylor, A. C., and Weiss, P. (1965): Demonstration of axonal flow by the movement of tritium labeled protein in mature optic nerve fibers. *Proc. Natl. Acad. Sci. U.S.A.,* 54:1521–1527.
80. Thorpe, P. A. (1975): The presence of a retinohypothalamic projection in the ferret. *Brain Res.,* 85:343–346.
81. Tigges, J., Bos, J., and Tigges, M. (1977): An autoradiographic investigation of the subcortical visual system in the chimpanzee. *J. Comp. Neurol.,* 172:367–380.
82. Tigges, J., and O'Steen, W. K. (1974): Termination of retinofugal fibers in the squirrel monkey: A re-investigation using autoradiographic methods. *Brain Res.,* 79:489–495.
83. Wansley, R. A., and Holloway, F. A. (1976): Lesions of the suprachiasmatic nucleus (hypothalamus) alter the normal oscillation of retention performance in the rat. *Neurosci. Abstr.,* 1:522.
84. Wenisch, H. J. C. (1976): Retinohypothalamic projection in the mouse: Electron microscopic and iontophoretic investigations of hypothalamic and optic centers. *Cell Tissue Res.,* 167:547–561.
85. Wurtman, R. J., Axelrod, J., and Kelly, D. E. (1968): *The Pineal.* Academic Press, New York.
86. Zucker, I., Rusak, B., and King, R. G., Jr. (1976): Neural basis for circadian rhythms in rodents. *Adv. Psychobiol.,* 3:35–74.

Frontiers in Neuroendocrinology, Vol. 5,
edited by W. F. Ganong and L. Martini.
Raven Press, New York © 1978.

Chapter 8

Clinical Use of Drugs Modifying the Release of Anterior Pituitary Hormones

Emilio del Pozo and Ioana Lancranjan

*Department of Experimental Therapeutics, Medical and Biological Research Division,
Sandoz Ltd., Basel, Switzerland*

Neuroendocrine mechanisms regulating the secretory patterns of pituitary hormones have been the subject of recent investigation. The results indicate that dopamine is an important factor acting as a biochemical messenger to trigger mechanisms controlling the release of pituitary hormones. Clinical data obtained with L-DOPA, which is transformed into dopamine in the organism, attracted the attention of pharmacologists long before central dopamine-agonist properties of ergot compounds were recognized. The finding that bromocriptine, a derivative of lysergic acid, inhibits the secretion of prolactin (PRL) from the pituitary opened new insights into the pharmacological control of neurosecretory mechanisms. More recently, serotoninergic and adrenergic pathways have also been implicated, indicating the complexity of the mechanisms involved. In addition, the suppressive effect of bromocriptine has been extended to growth hormone (GH) in acromegalic subjects. The purpose of this chapter is to summarize recent knowledge concerning the pharmacological background and clinical use of compounds modifying the secretion of anterior pituitary hormones by acting on neuroendocrine mechanisms. To better understand the clinical application of these drugs, the mechanisms involved in the release of prolactin and growth hormone are briefly reviewed at the beginning of the pertinent sections. The data presented are restricted to humans unless reference to work in experimental animals is required for explanatory purposes.

CONTROL OF PROLACTIN RELEASE

The Role of Dopamine and Releasing and Inhibiting Hormones

The integrative neuronal system releasing prolactin in mammals includes catecholaminergic, serotoninergic, and presumably cholinergic and gabaergic elements. The output of this prolactin regulating system is considered to consist of two hypothalamo-hypophyseotropic messengers, a prolactin releasing hormone (PRH) and a prolactin inhibiting hormone (PIH). The first evidence for the presence of PRH in crude hypothalamic extracts was found by Meites et al. (153). Recently, Dular et al. (57) described PRH activity in extracts of bovine pituitary stalk and median eminence. One of the fractions distinct from thyrotropin releasing hormone (TRH) enhanced the release of prolactin but had no effect on thyrotropin (TSH). Although TRH does not seem to be involved in the physiological control of prolactin release, its administration is followed by a rapid rise in plasma concentrations of this hormone, presumably through direct action on the pituitary. We have failed to find PRH activity in extracted human serum from pregnant women. More recently, Hagen et al. (87) presented preliminary evidence for a PRH in methanol-extracted serum of normal male subjects. Knowing that the pituitary gland is exposed to very high concentrations of estrogens throughout gestation, the possible PRH-like effect of steroids through direct action on the galactotrops should also be considered (4).

Findings from experimental and clinical studies indicate that the pituitary galactotrops are subjected to a predominantly inhibitory influence from the hypothalamus. It has long been known that section of the pituitary stalk increases prolactin secretion in experimental animals (105) and humans (216). This indicates the presence of a PIH at the suprasellar level. Meites et al. (153) found that the rat pituitary continued to secrete prolactin when maintained in culture medium, and Pasteels et al. (165) showed that crude hypothalamic extracts inhibit lactogen secretion *in vitro*. More insight into the mechanisms governing the secretion of PIH by the hypothalamus was obtained after the characterization of the tuberoinfundibular system (88) and its identification as a part of complex pathways regulating the secretion of prolactin by the anterior pituitary (95,96). This system was postulated to act at the level of the median eminence to release PIH, utilizing dopamine (DA) as the neurotransmitter. Any stimulation of the synthesis of DA, e.g., the administration of L-DOPA which is endogenously transformed into DA, was postulated to increase PIH and thus reduce prolactin secretion from the pituitary galactotrops. Mechanisms leading to the opposite effect, namely, a block in DA release, were believed to elevate serum PRL. By reason of its DA dependency, this functional unit has been characterized as the tuberoinfundibular-dopaminergic (TIDA) system (95) (Fig. 8–1). However, evidence is now accumulating that PIH itself is DA.

A number of pharmacological agents, mainly tricyclic neuroleptics, elevate plasma prolactin by altering brain dopamine turnover or by blocking specific dopamine receptors. Similar effects are produced by compounds known to act primarily as tranquilizers, such as reserpine. This subject has been extensively reviewed (74,172). Only chlorpromazine, sulpiride (124), and more recently metoclopramide (104) have found acceptance in the clinical evaluation of pituitary prolactin reserve. Morphine administration has also been found to significantly elevate PRL without altering GH (212). This effect was prevented by apomorphine, a potent DA-receptor agonist, suggesting that

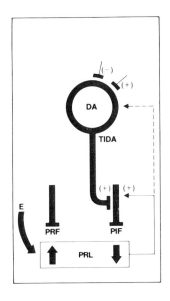

FIG. 8–1. Regulation of prolactin secretion by the tuberoinfundibular-dopamine (TIDA) system. DA, dopamine; PIH, prolactin inhibitory hormone; PRH, prolactin releasing hormone; E, estrogens; (+) and (−) indicate positive or negative influences on the particular pathway. Prolactin self-inhibitory effect via a suprasellar short-loop mechanism is also indicated. From del Pozo et al. (172) with permission.

morphine might act through PIH blockade. Recently, the opioid peptide β-endorphin (β-LPH [61–91]) was reported to stimulate PRL release in rats (187).

Much attention has been devoted recently to the effect of ergot compounds on the dopaminergic system controlling PRL secretion. These drugs possess a tetracyclic ring structure designated as ergoline (6-methyl-ergoline). Three main subgroups can be differentiated (Fig. 8–2):(a) lysergic acid derivatives, such as the ergonovines, ergocornines, methysergide, and bromocriptine (CB 154, Parlodel®), each with a different pharmacological profile; (b) clavine derivatives, such as Lergotril (Lilly 83 636); and (c) compounds characterized as amino-ergolines (Lysuride, Schering). Among these, bromocriptine was selected because of its strong PRL inhibitory action (68). The pharmacological profile included absence of the uterotonic and vascular effects common to other ergots of the same group. This drug was also free of the hallucinogenic properties of LSD, another lysergic acid derivative with strong PRL-inhibiting power.

Some uncertainty exists about the mode of action of compounds acting on the dopaminergic system to inhibit PRL secretion. Although a considerable body of evidence supporting a hypothalamic effect of L-DOPA has been provided in experimental animals and in humans, this compound has been effective in suppressing PRL after pituitary stalk section (56). The fact that in this situation chlorpromazine, which seems to stimulate PRL release via the hypothalamus, was ineffective in releasing PRL points toward a direct action of L-DOPA on the pituitary galactotrops. This is further strengthened by the fact that the PRL-stimulating effect of TRH, thought to act directly on the pituitary, is still preserved. In the case of bromocriptine, stimulation of dopa-

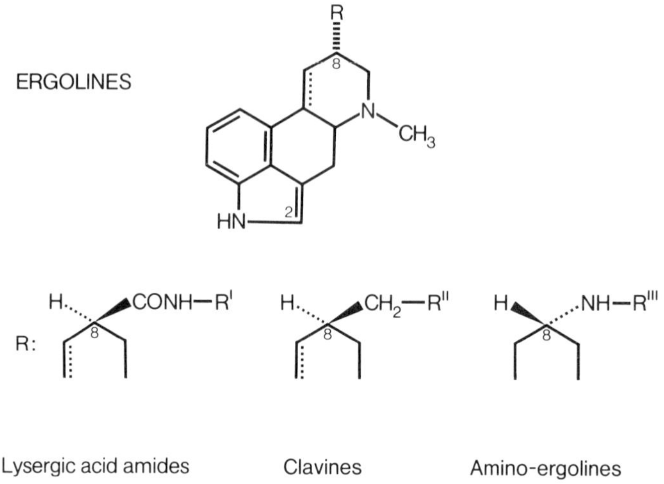

ERGOLINES

R:

Lysergic acid amides   Clavines   Amino-ergolines

FIG. 8–2. Structure of ergoline derivatives. See text.

mine receptors at the level of the CNS can be assumed on the basis of animal and human pharmacological trials (70). A direct action on the pituitary can also be assumed since the effect of TRH on PRL secretion is also abolished by the drug (173). In addition, Flückiger and del Pozo (69) were able to inhibit PRL secretion with bromocriptine in rats with pituitaries implanted under the kidney capsule. These studies and the data on L-DOPA discussed earlier would imply the existence of dopamine receptors on the pituitary cell membrane. Indeed, MacLeod et al. (138) have presented *in vitro* data indicating specific ³H-dopamine binding to pituitary receptors. Thus, bromocriptine would act not only at the level of the hypothalamus but also directly on the pituitary as a dopamine-receptor agonist.

Role of Serotonin

The role of serotonin in humans has been the subject of recent investigations. MacIndoe and Turkington (136) administered intravenously relatively large amounts (5 to 10 g) of L-tryptophan, a serotonin precursor, to normal individuals. They recorded substantial elevations of plasma PRL concentrations 20 to 40 min after initiation of the infusion. Further, Kato et al. (107) showed that the intravenous administration of 200 mg 5-hydroxytryptophan (5-HTP) also enhances PRL secretion. Recently, Lancranjan et al. (119) were successful in elevating plasma PRL subsequent to an intravenous infusion of a new soluble ester of 1-5-HTP (Ro-35940). However, this effect reached statistical significance only in females. In contrast, Smythe et al. (206) and Beck-Peccoz et al. (9) were unable to modify basal plasma PRL when they gave L-tryptophan or 5-HTP orally. It can be assumed that the route of administration had some bearing on the absence of response observed after oral intake.

The effect of serotonin antagonists on PRL secretion has also been investigated. Mendelson et al. (154) reported a significant suppression of sleep-related hyperprolactinemia after oral administration of methysergide, 2 mg every 6 hr to normal individuals. The authors concluded that serotonin is important in modulating PRL secretion. We (*unpublished observations*) have tested the effect of methysergide on resting PRL levels as compared with a nonergot serotonin antagonist, a benzocycloheptathiophene (Pizotifen®, Sandoz). The oral administration of 1 mg methysergide to normal individuals induced a significant fall in plasma PRL, whereas doses up to 2 mg Pizotifen® failed to induce any changes. Furthermore, Pizotifen® was found not to modify the release of PRL during sleep (E. del Pozo, P. Clarenbach, I. Lancranjan, and H. Cramer, *unpublished observations*). The fact that a serotonin antagonist chemically unrelated to ergot did not modify basal PRL secretion suggests that methysergide contains a different PRL-active moiety, presumably dopaminergic in nature.

As a specific serotonin receptor blocking agent, methergoline has been found to lower unstimulated basal PRL in acromegalic subjects (41). The comparison of this drug with other serotonin antagonists and dopaminergic drugs led to the conclusion that the inhibitory effect of methergoline on both hormones was probably due to a dopaminergic mechanism of action rather than to serotonin blockade.

Influence of Adrenergic Pathways

The galactogenic action of some psychostimulant drugs such as amphetamine is not easy to explain. There is indirect evidence that this effect may take place through central activation of norepinephrine synthesis, but dose-related positive and negative influences may also be operative. Pertinent data in humans are lacking. Alpha-adrenergic stimulation with clonidine has been reported not to modify basal PRL secretion (115). Also, β-receptor blockade with pindolol has no effect on pituitary lactotropic function (Lancranjan and del Pozo, *unpublished observations*).

Role of γ-Aminobutyric Acid

Recently, another neurotransmitter, γ-aminobutyric acid (GABA) has been implicated in the regulation of PRL secretion. Studies conducted in rats by Mioduszewski et al. (155) have shown that the infusion of GABA into the lateral ventricle of female rats significantly stimulated PRL release. The response seems to be mediated through the hypothalamus, since the injection of this substance into rats with their pituitaries transplanted to the kidney capsule did not alter serum PRL.

Effect of Cholinergic Blockade

The report by Blake and Sawyer (19) suggesting a cholinergic factor in the suckling-induced rise of PRL in rats was followed by confirmatory reports using different methodological approaches (67,151). Some inconsistencies have been noticed in work concerning the effects of various agonists and antagonists of the cholinergic system (79,84,125), but the available data indicate that anticholinergic drugs inhibit prolactin release. The biological significance of this observation remains uncertain. Thus, atropine blockade in rats is insufficient to interrupt the pseudopregnant state (151), whereas bromocriptine is effective (68). The mechanism of action of atropine remains uncertain although an effect through activation of DA neurons via PIH has been proposed (126). The role of cholinergic pathways in the release of PRL in humans has not yet been ascertained.

PERIPHERAL ACTIONS OF PROLACTIN

PRL and the Adrenals

Although the lactogenic role of PRL has received primary emphasis, receptor-binding studies have shown that other tissues have high binding affinity for PRL (75). Thus, it was shown that adrenals specifically bound 51% of labeled prolactin. In contrast, mammary tissue bound only 20%, and the ovaries only 13%.

Adrenal medullary function is influenced by dopaminergic mechanisms (183). A relationship between galactorrhea and steroid synthesis was first reported about 15 years before PRL was recognized as a separate entity from growth hormone. In this report, Forbes et al. (71) described 15 cases of galactorrhea associated with low FSH, and 13 of the 15 had elevated urinary 17-ketosteroids. Giusti et al. (81) have presented a correlation between the basal plasma PRL and dehydroepiandrosterone sulfate (DHAS), the latter increasing in a parallel manner with rising PRL concentrations in hyperprolactinemic women. These findings and the not uncommon occurrence of hirsutism in such patients are reminiscent of some features found in the polycystic ovary syndrome.

The effect of glucocorticosteroids on the mechanism inducing pituitary release of PRL has also been investigated. Copinschi et al. (46) found that the administration of dexamethasone prior to an insulin tolerance test blunted the response of ACTH and PRL to hypoglycemia. Osterman et al. (164) arrived at the same results but reported large individual variations. It is interesting to note that Re et al. (184) found the PRL response to TRH unchanged after dexamethasone administration, suggesting that the suppressive effect of this compound is mediated by the hypothalamus.

Edwards et al. (60) showed that the administration of bromocriptine in increasing doses up to 7.5 mg daily to healthy volunteers inhibited the rise in plasma aldosterone that normally follows the administration of furosemide, and the authors suggested that PRL may modulate the secretion of aldosterone. However, bromocriptine could have acted directly on the adrenals. Ølgaard et al. (163) were unable to alter plasma aldosterone levels in anephric patients treated with bromocriptine despite a substantial reduction in plasma PRL concentrations. More recently, Marek and Horky (145) administering doses of 10 mg every 6 hr to two patients with primary aldosteronism were unable to modify plasma aldosterone and renin. Electrolytes were also unaffected by therapy. Administration of this drug to a patient with primary hyperaldosteronism by Edwards and Jeffcoate (59) lowered the recumbent plasma aldosterone level and blocked the postural response. del Pozo et al. (171) reported normal aldosterone response to postural changes in three subjects treated chronically with 5 mg bromocriptine daily.

Action of PRL at Mammary Tissue Level

In some animals, secretion can be detected in the mammary alveoli during pregnancy when plasma PRL has not reached lactational level. It can be assumed that during this period the lactogenic effect is being induced by placental hormones and does not originate in the pituitary of the mother animal. In women, there is distension of the alveoli by colostrum during the third trimester of pregnancy, but no actual milk secretion occurs. However, plasma PRL concentrations are in the lactational range before midpregnancy. The mechanism of this secretory block has not been completely elucidated, although there is evidence for an inhibitory action of sex steroids, presumably by rendering the alveolar epithelium insensitive to the action of lactogenic hormones. Copious milk secretion does not appear until 3 to 5 days after childbirth, at about the time sex steroid levels have returned to normal. At this time, PRL concentrations have fallen below predelivery levels. Thus, in the absence of circulating sex steroids, PRL acts on the mammary epithelium to induce milk secretion. The effect has also been recorded in the newborn, leading to the secretion of the so-called witch's milk (94). Later on, lactation continues in the mother despite normal basal PRL, probably due to the stimulating effect of suckling (217). However, a certain basal PRL concentration is required in humans for milk secretion to continue. This may also indicate that little PRL is required for the maintenance of peripheral receptors once they have been induced (22).

Action of PRL on the Gonads

McNatty et al. (152) first reported that high concentrations of PRL depressed progesterone secretion by cultured human granulosa cells, but the

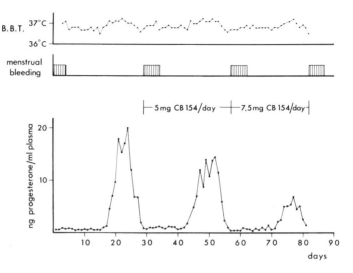

FIG. 8–3. Effect of increasing doses of bromocriptine (CB 154) on progesterone synthesis in a normally menstruating woman. From Schulz et al. (198) with permission.

neutralization of this lactogen with rabbit antiserum also caused a significant decrease in progesterone production. These findings suggest a permissive role of PRL in the maintenance of granulosa cell function, whereas exposure to excessive concentrations blocks progesterone synthesis. The inhibitory effect has been demonstrated by Delvoye et al. (53) and by Robyn et al. (188) by increasing basal PRL in normally menstruating women with sulpiride, a galactogenic drug. The clinical equivalent, shortening the postovulatory period in hyperprolactinemic women exhibiting regular menstrual cycles is discussed in the next section.

The permissive effect of PRL on granulosa cell function is more difficult to demonstrate (55). The administration of 3 mg bromocriptine daily to normally menstruating females failed to alter the sequence of hormonal changes leading to ovulation and normal formation of the corpus luteum (174). It was subsequently shown by Schulz et al. (198,199) that a gradual dose increase to 7.5 mg daily induced a reduction of plasma progesterone as well as a decrease in PRL secretion during the luteal phase of the cycle (Fig. 8–3).

A testicular action of PRL in man has not been demonstrated, although a relationship between this lactogen and testosterone has been proposed (193). Endogenous hyperprolactinemia induces secondary hypogonadism and subfertility (see below).

Action of PRL on the Gonadostat

Hyperprolactinemia is generally associated with amenorrhea. That this effect of PRL is exerted at a suprasellar level is demonstrated by the normal to exaggerated LH response found after LRH administration (177,211). Bohnet et al. (20) were first to show that the hyperprolactinemia induced with TRH in normal women disturbed the cyclic release of LH. Hyperprolactinemia is generally characterized by absence of the LH surges that are essential for cycles to occur (23). Normal cycles are readily restored by the administration of bromocriptine (21).

Renal Actions of PRL

Although a considerable body of evidence suggests a role for PRL in the regulation of renal function in other species, no definite renal effects have been established in humans. Changes in PRL secretory rates with changes in plasma osmolarity, reported by Buckman et al. (30,32) and Buckman and Peake (31), could not be confirmed by Adler et al. (1), Baumann and Loriaux (7), and Baumann et al. (8). By suppressing endogenous PRL with bromocriptine, del Pozo and Ohnhaus (175) failed to demonstrate a regulatory effect of this lactogen in renal physiology.

MECHANISM OF CYCLIC DISTURBANCES INDUCED BY PRL

In women, galactorrhea may be found in the presence of ovulatory cycles and normal plasma PRL, but increasing plasma concentrations of this hormone are accompanied by cyclic disturbances ranging from irregular menstrual bleeding or inappropriate luteal function to anovulatory periods and cessation of menses. The mechanisms by which PRL exerts its antiovulatory effect are still far from clear. In many cases there is a previous history of oligomenorrhea preceding cyclic arrest. Discontinuation of bromocriptine treatment in women with previous amenorrhea-galactorrhea can be followed by reappearance of milk secretion and a phase of deficient luteinization or anovulation with one or two vaginal bleedings before menses stop completely (201). Furthermore, bromocriptine administration in a dose insufficient to completely normalize plasma PRL levels in a previously amenorrheic woman was able to induce menses, but luteal progestagen production was obviously deficient (178). Thus, it can be assumed that a certain degree of hyperprolactinemia interferes with ovarian function. Women with anovulatory cycles or short luteal phases seldom have plasma PRL levels above 50 ng/ml. Values above 50 ng/ml are almost invariably associated with amenorrhea. This type of ovarian failure can be partially compensated by basal estrogen secretion adequate to prevent reactive hypergonadotropinemia, since LH and FSH are not always elevated (209). Another explanation could be a suppressive effect of PRL at the level of the "gonadostat" in the hypothalamus. The effect is not exerted on the pituitary gland, since injected LRH produces an increase in LH secretion (226). Suprasellar blockade could be the cause of the lack of LH surges (21,23) in hyperprolactinemic amenorrhea. As noted above, treatment with bromocriptine restores the normal secretory rhythm. However, there are some differences in timing between the effect of this drug on PRL secretion and resumption of ovulation (209).

A psychogenic component in hyperprolactinemia has recently come to light. Zacur et al. (224) recorded abnormal psychometric scores in two hyperprolactinemic women. Restoration of normal basal plasma PRL with bromocriptine was followed by normalization of psychological function at the time regular menstrual periods resumed.

CLINICAL APPLICATION OF DRUGS INHIBITING PRL SECRETION

Inappropriate PRL secretion can lead in the nonpregnant individual to a series of clinical and biochemical effects as a result of the different central and peripheral actions outlined in the preceding section (Table 8–1). These manifestations are naturally reflected in a number of clinical conditions, the description of which is outside the scope of this review.

TABLE 8–1. *Effects of inappropriately increased prolactin secretion*

Females	
Clinical	Failure to enter menarche
	Galactorrhea with ovulatory cycles
	Premenstrual edema formation?
	Meno-metrorrhagia
	Short luteal phase
	Anovulatory cycles
	Amenorrhea[a]
Biochemical	Elevated plasma PRL concentrations[b]
	Lack of sleep-related PRL elevations
	Absence of LH-pulsatility
	Low basal estrogens[c]
	Elevated androgenic steroids
	Positive pituitary and ovarian response to exogenous stimulation
	Clomiphene resistance
Males	
Clinical	Failure to enter puberty
	Galactorrhea
	Lack of PRL elevations during sleep
	Oligo-aspermia
	Signs of androgen failure
	Elevated plasma PRL concentrations[b]
Biochemical	Low androgen production
	Positive pituitary and testicular response to exogenous stimulation

[a] Not necessarily associated with galactorrhea.
[b] Exceptions are not rare (see text).
[c] Normal basal estrogens with normal or even elevated FSH are common.

Treatment with L-DOPA

The management of hyperprolactinemia was unsatisfactory before drugs suppressing PRL secretion became available. After Malarkey et al. (142) found variable responses to the acute administration of L-DOPA, Turkington (215), Zarate et al. (225), and Ayalon et al. (5) reported restoration of menses in a number of women with galactorrhea-amenorrhea treated with this compound. Ovulation was supported by the occurrence of pregnancy in some instances.

Clinical Use of Ergot Derivatives

Clinical trials with bromocriptine in humans have amply confirmed the antigalactic properties of this compound demonstrated in animal experimentation. After bromocriptine was found to effectively inhibit basal plasma PRL in normal female volunteers, the administration of the drug to postpartum women was shown to suppress milk letdown (29,189,218). The effect of this therapy on a group of seven women who did not wish to breastfeed their infants is presented in Fig. 8–4. The studies were then extended to established lactation when basal PRL had already reached the normal range (29,174). In this situation as well, a rapid fall in plasma PRL was observed and lactation ceased, demonstrating the importance of PRL in the maintenance of milk secretion in humans. Soon after the first trials with

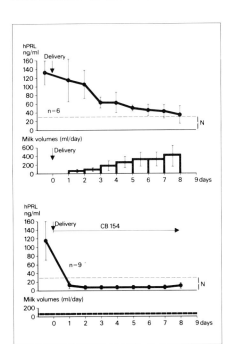

FIG. 8–4. Response to bromocriptine (CB 154) in 9 postpartum women (*lower panel*) compared to 6 untreated lactating mothers (*upper panel*). There is a rapid fall in plasma prolactin (hPRL) in the treated group and milk secretion is inhibited. From Brun del Re et al. (29) with permission.

bromocriptine were initiated in nonpuerperal galactorrhea-amenorrhea, it was reported that, in addition to suppression of lactation, bromocriptine rapidly restored menses and fertility (13,134,177,190) in a variety of conditions ranging from puberal retardation to idiopathic or tumoral galactorrhea. A typical response pattern is presented in Fig. 8–5. A 26-year-old nuliparous woman reported amenorrhea of 12 months' duration after discontinuation of an oral contraceptive. Galactorrhea had not been noticed by the patient, but milk could be easily obtained from both breasts on slight pressure. Onset of treatment with bromocriptine (2.5 mg twice a day) was followed by restoration of menstrual cycles and normal ovulatory mechanisms.

Between 10 and 27% of amenorrheic women exhibit hyperprolactinemia without galactorrhea (21,73,166). These patients also respond to bromocriptine with resumption of ovulatory periods. The lack of effect of PRL on mammary tissue in these cases is unexplained.

The effect of PRL on ovarian function is attracting considerable attention. Wenner (221) was first to suggest a relationship between infertility due to short luteal phase and PRL. Later, del Pozo et al. (176) reported that short luteal phase and low progesterone secretion may be associated with elevated plasma PRL concentrations in some infertile women. Indeed, three out of four women in whom PRL was suppressed with bromocriptine became pregnant, two of them on the first treatment cycle (178). Seppälä et al. (201) were able to follow the sequence of events leading first to inappropriate luteal function and later to amenorrhea when bromocriptine treatment was discontinued in two women with a previous history of galactorrhea-amenorrhea. Also, Corenblum et al. (48) observed restoration of menses but a short hyperthermic phase in two women with the galactorrhea-amenorrhea syndrome

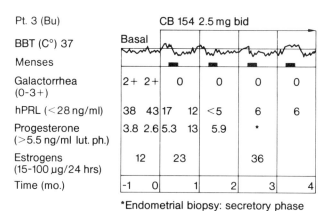

*Endometrial biopsy: secretory phase

FIG. 8–5. Restoration of ovulatory cycles by bromocriptine (CB 154) in a woman with galactorrhea-amenorrhea following discontinuation of an oral contraceptive. From del Pozo et al. (177) with permission of the editors. Normal values for hPRL, progesterone, and estrogens are shown in parentheses. An arbitrary scale of 1+ to 3+ is used to express the degree of galactorrhea.

treated with clomiphene alone or associated with mestranol. Treatment with bromocriptine was followed by normal ovulatory cycles, and pregnancy was reported in one of them. Up to now the authors have treated 10 cases, 6 of which have conceived (179). The response pattern in one case is presented in Fig. 8–6.

An effect of PRL suppression on adrenal steroid synthesis could be expected after the induction of PRL-secreting tumors in rats accompanied by remarkable adrenal hyperplasia (78). Bigazzi (*personal communication*) observed in 1973 normalization of elevated urinary DHAS following bromocriptine therapy in a woman with galactorrhea. More recently, Edwards and Jeffcoate (59) have shown that increased adrenal androgen production in hyperprolactinemia can be normalized by either glucocorticoids or bromocriptine therapy. Bassi et al. (6) have reported increased plasma DHAS in 10 cases of hyperprolactinemic amenorrhea. Other steroids measured were normal in the diseased group. Treatment with bromocriptine normalized DHAS excretion in three patients. These findings reinforce data presented in the previous section supporting a humoral link between prolactin and synthesis of androgenic precursors by the adrenal. It is noteworthy that this treatment was also effective in reducing basal PRL to the normal range. These findings indicate not only a stimulatory effect of PRL on the synthesis of androgen precursors, presumably at the level of the adrenals, but also a common site of action on the CNS to block the release of PRL and probably ACTH, as has been suggested by Copinschi et al. (46).

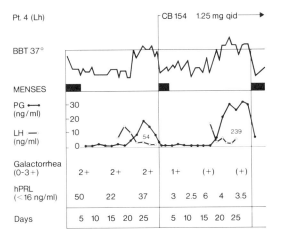

FIG. 8–6. Restoration of normal luteal function by bromocriptine (CB 154) in an infertile woman exhibiting moderately elevated plasma prolactin (hPRL) and deficient progesterone (PG) synthesis. From del Pozo et al. (179) with permission.

Effect of Bromocriptine on Reproduction

Results of bromocriptine therapy in 197 infertile women are presented in Table 8–2. Reestablishment of menses, presence of ovulation, and high incidence of pregnancy were recorded in hyperprolactinemic amenorrhea. The pregnancy rate in the normoprolactinemic group was more modest. This emphasizes the role of this lactogen in the blockade of ovulation, when present in elevated concentrations. In addition, treatment with bromocriptine in 48 normally menstruating but infertile women through deficient luteal function prolonged the duration of the hyperthermic phase in 42 (88%), and 10 (21%) conceived.

Some galactorrhea patients may require increases in bromocriptine dosage in order to restore cyclic activity despite adequate PRL suppression (172). Therefore, one could speculate that two different central mechanisms are affected by this drug. The observation that some normoprolactinemic women with secondary amenorrhea may resume menses (202,213) or be converted to clomiphene responsiveness through the administration of bromocriptine also supports this conclusion.

Male hyperprolactinemia is a less common condition as judged by the available data. PRL-induced delay in the onset of puberty has been observed in male subjects. Cumulative data reveal elevated plasma PRL in all 18 cases observed by the authors and collected from the literature (47,72,211). Galactorrhea was present in 13 and diverse degrees of gynecomastia in 11. Libido was decreased and androgens were low. Although some degree of potency was present in some of them, their wives had failed to conceive. Treatment with an average dose of 5 mg bromocriptine lowered PRL in all cases and suppressed galactorrhea. Signs of hypoandrogenism regressed, and there was a return of libido. Three of their wives became pregnant.

More difficult to assess is the relationship between oligoazoospermia and PRL in normoprolactinemic individuals without other signs of endocrine abnormality. All 12 oligospermic patients screened by the authors had normal plasma PRL, but Roulier et al. (191) found elevated levels in 4 out of 51 cases. More recently, Saidi et al. (196) reported improvement in androgenization and sperm counts in oligospermic subjects treated with bromocriptine,

TABLE 8–2. *Effect of bromocriptine therapy in 197 infertile women*

	No.	Restored menses	Proven ovulation	Pregnancies
Amenorrhea with hyperprolactinemia	127	114 (90%)	103 (81%)	69 (54%)
Amenorrhea with normoprolactinemia	70	38 (54%)	21 (28%)	4 (5%)

although a clear relationship between gonadal status and plasma lactogen concentration was not established.

At the time of submitting this manuscript, information was available on 268 completed pregnancies in which bromocriptine had been administered in the early weeks (R. Griffith, P. Braun, and I. Turkalj, *unpublished observations*). Forty-three of these pregnancies resulted in abortion (31 spontaneous, 10 induced) and 2 extrauterine pregnancies occurred. A frequency of spontaneous abortions of 11.6% is well within the average incidence in women conceiving without therapy, and compares favorably with that encountered in women rendered fertile by other means such as clomiphene or gonadotropin therapy. Also the twin pregnancy rate of 2.2% is not above that seen in the normal population, reflecting absence of ovarian hyperstimulation.

The possible role of this drug in the endocrine system of the fetus has also been studied. Data are available from three women receiving daily doses of 5, 10, and 35 mg, respectively, throughout pregnancy. PRL and GH were measured in the serum of mothers and newborns, and also in amniotic fluid. Bromocriptine suppressed plasma PRL in both mothers and newborns, but did not modify it in the amniotic fluid. GH contents of these physiologic fluids were not altered by treatment. After delivery the infants exhibited a gradual increase in plasma PRL for 2 days, with a subsequent decline 3 to 7 days after birth. In untreated newborns, plasma PRL is high at birth and declines on days 3 through 7. The secretion of GH in the neonates was not modified by bromocriptine, and inhibition of PRL throughout gestation seemed to have no influence on other possible effects of this hormone such as fetal growth.

Effects of Other Ergot Derivatives on PRL

Ergometrine (ergonovine) is a compound with uterotonic properties that is in current use in obstetric practice. Shane and Naftolin (204) recorded a slight but significant decrease in plasma PRL after a single intravenous administration of 0.2 mg ergonovine maleate to postpartum women. The authors concluded that repetitive doses may have an inhibitory effect on lactation, but no pertinent studies have been reported as yet. Lawrence and Hagen (121) have reported reestablishment of menses in four women with ergonovine maleate 0.2 mg three times daily. Ovulatory cycles could be confirmed in three of the four by the occurrence of pregnancy. Attempts to suppress lactation in humans with methylergometrine (methylergonovine, Methergine®, Sandoz) have shown contradictory results (85,203). Weiss et al. (220) administered 0.2 mg of this compound intramuscularly to a group of postpartum women. The normal short-lived PRL increase observed in the immediate postpartum was used as a parameter. The injection of methylergonovine significantly ($p < 0.002$) reduced the magnitude of this elevation when compared with women receiving only saline. Studies reported by Perez-

Lopez et al. (167) have demonstrated a PRL-inhibitory effect of methyl-ergonovine after intravenous administration of 0.2 mg to women on the third postpartum day. The same treatment was also effective in acutely reducing basal plasma PRL in normal individuals. This suppressive action was also found by del Pozo et al. (172) in normal volunteers. Canales et al. (35) extended their investigations with the same compound to the first postpartum week. Ten women received 0.2 mg orally three times daily, which is the routinely recommended dose to facilitate uterine involution in the postpartum. The authors recorded a significant fall in basal plasma PRL in comparison with an untreated group, but milk letdown occurred in seven cases and in the other three a progressive decrease of milk secretion was observed. There was no mention of the effect of the drug on milk volumes. del Pozo et al. (170) were unable to find changes in plasma PRL or milk volumes in a group of postpartum women treated with oral methylergometrine, 0.2 mg three times daily for 7 days. Milk volumes collected increased in a linear pattern corresponding to the control women. Further studies by this group have helped to explain inconsistencies between these two reports. In post-partum women, sequential blood sampling after oral administration of 0.2 mg methylergonovine three times daily showed a short-lived depression of plasma PRL following ingestion of the drug. Treatment did not modify the nocturnal pattern of PRL secretion, and fasted blood samples obtained in the morning yielded plasma PRL concentrations normal for the postpartum period. This would explain the normal course of lactation observed in women receiving this medication. Much higher doses would be required to maintain continuous PRL inhibition.

Lergotrile is an ergoline of the clavine type. After its PRL-inhibitory prop-erties were demonstrated in experimental animals, studies in humans showed that doses of 2 to 6 mg effectively reduced serum PRL levels and delayed

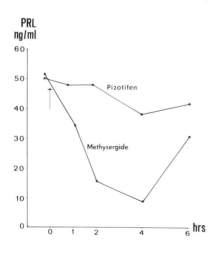

FIG. 8–7. Effect of 3 mg methysergide in a case of hyperprolactinemia as compared with 2 mg Pizotifen®, a nonergot serotonin antagonist.

the onset of perphenazine-induced hyperprolactinemia (123). Lergotrile has also been found effective in suppressing nonpuerperal galactorrhea (43).

The different pharmacologic profiles of ergot and nonergot serotonin antagonists become obvious in the biological test. Figure 8–7 presents the PRL response pattern to acute methysergide and Pizotifen® administration in a case of galactorrhea-amenorrhea. Pizotifen®, a nonergot antiserotoninergic agent, did not modify the basal PRL secretion rate, whereas methysergide induced a marked fall.

Extraendocrine Implications of Treatment with Bromocriptine

The inhibitory effect of bromocriptine also finds clinical application in conditions not primarily related to endocrinological disturbances. Thus, Peters and Breckwoldt (*unpublished observations*) were able to prevent further development of mastitis in 18 nursing mothers simply by reducing mammary engorgement with bromocriptine. Furthermore, the reversibility of bromocriptine action following short-term treatment permits resumption of normal lactation when desired (Brun del Re and del Pozo, *unpublished observations*).

The possible involvement of PRL in fibrous transformation of the breast, a common diagnosis in middle-aged women, has been the subject of clinical work. Schulz et al. (197) administered a course of bromocriptine to 15 women with severe mastodynia due to degenerative fibrosis of the breast. In 10 of them pain subsided completely, 3 showed some improvement, and 2 were resistant to therapy. The authors concluded that PRL may play an important role in the maintenance of mastodynia accompanying fibrosis of breast, whereas the basic disease does not seem to be influenced by treatment (227).

The effect of PRL suppression on cyclic edema and on the premenstrual syndrome has been variable. It seems that a selective group of patients can be improved mainly by alleviating premenstrual mastodynia and reducing excessive weight gain.

Interaction Between Phenothiazines and Bromocriptine

As mentioned previously, TRH and phenothiazines such as chlorpromazine increase prolactin secretion in normal individuals. Bromocriptine, 2.5 mg, administered prior to the test injection, effectively suppresses this effect of both compounds. Knowing that phenothiazines on repeated administration can also cause a sustained release of prolactin, we undertook a study with bromocriptine in a group of 22 psychiatric patients receiving chronically 100 mg chlorpromazine or more daily. Average basal prolactin levels were significantly ($p < 0.001$) elevated (28 ± 2.6 ng/ml; normal = 11.1 ± 1.3 ng/ml). Bromocriptine, 3 mg daily, which effectively inhibits prolactin (174) in normal untreated subjects, failed to modify basal prolactin levels or the response to a standard dose of TRH (200 μg). A gradual dosage increase to 2.5 mg three times daily was necessary before basal plasma prolactin was normalized and the peak response to TRH reduced from 198 ± 9.8 (SE) ng/ml to 24.4 ± 3.3 (SE) ng/ml. Results were interpreted as reflecting competitive drug antagonism (69).

CONTROL OF GROWTH HORMONE SECRETION

The increasing clinical use of drugs modulating growth hormone (GH) secretion has occurred during the last few years due to the accumulated data on brain regulation of GH secretion. Martin and co-workers (146–149) Müller (158), Ganong (80,132), Frohman (76,77), and Reichlin (185,186), in their reviews concerning the control of GH secretion, pointed out the role of neurotransmitters and the anatomic specificity of neural control of GH release. Secretion is controlled by growth hormone releasing hormone (GRH), the structure of which is still unknown, and growth hormone release inhibiting hormone (GIH), somatostatin, which has been isolated and chemically identified. Secretion of these hypothalamic hormones is modulated by neurotransmitters released by noradrenergic, dopaminergic, and serotoninergic neurons from different nuclei of the brain. Up to now the main drugs which have been tested for clinical application are drugs which interfere with the balance of neurotransmitters, most of them having complex actions involving more than one system.

Most authors agree that norepinephrine, dopamine, and serotonin have a stimulatory role on GH secretion in humans. In experimental animals, Martin et al. (149) showed that inhibitors of catecholamine or serotonin synthesis and α- and β-adrenergic receptor blockade do not affect the GH response to hypothalamic stimulation. On the other hand, the rise in GH plasma levels after amygdaloid or hippocampal stimulation is blocked by inhibitors of catecholamine and serotonin synthesis and by α-receptor blockade. Thus, monoamines are involved as neurotransmitters in the mediation of signals from the extrahypothalamic regions to the hypothalamic nuclei.

Noradrenergic Components

In animals the noradrenergic control of GH release has been reviewed by Müller (158) and Martin (146,147). New data confirm the noradrenergic control of GH secretion in rats and monkeys. Ruch et al. (194) showed that clonidine, a centrally acting α-adrenoceptor stimulating drug, induced a prompt and long-lasting release of growth hormone after i.v. or intraventricular administration in rats. This effect could be prevented by phentolamine administration. The study pointed out that the central α-adrenergic system is an important mechanism in GH modulation in the rat. Similar conclusions for rhesus monkeys were presented by Chambers and Brown (37) and Marantz et al. (144). In humans, L-DOPA, the precursor of both dopamine and norepinephrine (NE), has been found to increase GH secretion in healthy subjects and in patients with Parkinson's disease (24). Phentolamine, an α-adrenoceptor blocking agent, inhibits GH secretion stimulated by L-DOPA (106) as well as by hypoglycemia (17), arginine (102), vasopressin (93), and exercise (180). The stimulatory effect of β-blocking agents on GH released by hypoglycemia (98), epinephrine (18), L-DOPA (50), and glucagon (156) is believed to be due to unopposed α-adrenoceptor activity. Clonidine also releases GH in humans (115). Similar results were found by Lancranjan and Marbach (118) who tested the effect of another central α-receptor agonist, BS 100–141 (Sandoz) (Fig. 8–8). Significant GH release was observed 90 to 180 min after oral administration of 2 mg in young, normal male volunteers. In a randomized crossover study, a significant increase of GH secretion was found after single oral doses of 2 and 4 mg BS 100–141 and 0.30 mg clonidine. Tolerance developed quickly, since long-term administration of BS 100–141 failed to maintain high GH plasma levels. There are contradictory results concerning the effect of the administration of β-blockers on GH secretion. Imura et al. (97) reported that intravenous propranolol alone raised plasma GH levels, but an increase was not found

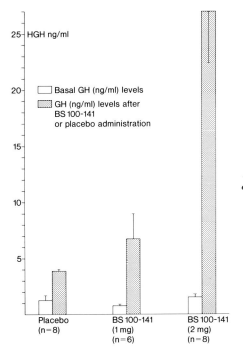

FIG. 8–8. Enhancement of GH secretion by an α-stimulator (BS 100–141) in normal individuals.

by Blackard and Hubbell (18). In order to increase our knowledge about the effect of β-receptor blockers on GH secretion, we have studied the effect of another β-blocker, pindolol, on GH secretion (I. Lancranjan and E. del Pozo, *unpublished observations*). A crossover study with two different doses (5 and 10 mg) was performed in six healthy, young male volunteers. No statistical difference between the placebo and pindolol responses was found.

Dopaminergic Control of GH Secretion

There are still contradictory data on dopaminergic control of GH release in rats (45,131,147,158,194), and no effect could be observed in rhesus monkeys after apomorphine, a specific dopaminergic agonist (37). Marantz et al. (144) also pointed out that in the monkey dopaminergic mechanisms are not involved in GH regulation. They showed that GH secretion stimulated with amphetamine could not be blocked by large doses of pimozide, a dopamine receptor blocker. Bromocriptine does not influence GH secretion *in vitro* and *in vivo* in mice, rats, cows, and goats (91,206,223). Moreover, using clonal cell cultures originating from rat pituitary tumors (GH_3), Tashjian and Hoyt (208) did not observe any effect of bromocriptine on GH secretion and synthesis.

The effect of other ergots on GH secretion has also been investigated. MacLeod and Lehmeyer (139), using male rat pituitaries *in vitro,* observed no effect with ergotamine (4 and 40 μM) on GH secretion, but they reported an inhibitory effect of 10 μM ergocornine and 10 μM ergocriptine on GH synthesis and release. Moreover, Quadri and Meites (182), using rats inoculated with the Mt TW 15 pituitary tumor, found during long-term treatment with 2 mg/kg/day that ergocornine prevented the growth of the tumor and reduced the level of serum GH.

The question of DA control of GH secretion in humans was raised by Lal et al. (112–114), who showed that, contrary to results obtained in monkeys, subemetic doses of apomorphine significantly increased GH secretion. These results were confirmed by Brown et al. (26,27) and by Maany et al. (135). Nilsson's (162) study showing that the GH rise after the administration of apomorphine was not suppressible by glucose indicates that apomorphine activates dopaminergic receptors in the hypothalamus or in the anterior pituitary. More recently, Camanni et al. (33) and Tolis et al. (214) reported that a single dose of bromocriptine was able to release GH in normal men. Studies performed in our laboratory (171) confirmed this but showed that long-term administration of the drug failed to maintain high GH plasma levels (Fig. 8–9). Further indirect proof for DA control of GH secretion came from the study by Schwinn et al. (200) showing that pimozide, a DA receptor blocker, significantly reduced GH released by exercise in normal and diabetic subjects and by arginine in diabetics. New evidence of the role of DA in modulating GH release in humans was reported by Brown and

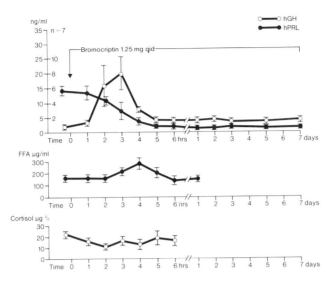

FIG. 8–9. The stimulatory action of bromocriptine (CB 154) on GH in normal persons is short-lived despite continuous treatment. Concomitant elevation of FFA indicates release of biologically active GH. From del Pozo et al. (171) with permission.

Williams (28). They showed that methylphenidate, a drug that releases catecholamines, principally dopamine, and which may also directly stimulate dopamine receptors, significantly increased GH secretion in healthy male volunteers. On the other hand, Massara et al. (150) and Verde et al. (219) failed to stimulate GH secretion in normal subjects by infusing DA. It is known that this neurotransmitter does not cross the blood-brain barrier, but it is also known that the median eminence lies outside this barrier. Consequently, DA control of GH secretion in human physiology does not occur at the level of the median eminence or the pituitary. In summary, the available data provide some evidence that DA might play a role in GH control in humans. However, there are few experimental findings to support this. Moreover, studies in humans are based on the effect of drugs which cannot be considered as specifically and selectively acting on a given system. Therefore, more research will be required before arriving at a definite conclusion.

Serotonin Control of GH Secretion

Even though many conflicting results have been reported (131,158), increasing evidence of serotoninergic control of GH secretion has accumulated over the past few years. Reports of the role of the serotoninergic system on GH secretion in animals are conflicting (131,158,205). Stimulatory effects on GH secretion of serotonin (5-HT) administered intraventricularly in urethane-anesthetized rats (44,45) and of 5-hydroxytryptophan (5-HTP) in nonanesthetized rats (205) are in agreement with the hypothesis that

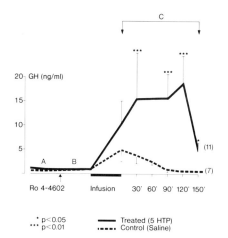

FIG. 8–10. Stimulatory effect of 5-HTP on GH release (explanation in text). From Lancranjan et al. (120) with permission.

serotonin is involved in GH control. However, this hypothesis is not accepted by others (131,158). Stimulation of the raphe nucleus, the site of the cell bodies of the serotoninergic neurons in the brain, was shown to inhibit GH secretion during stimulation, with a significant postinhibitory rebound (147). In rhesus monkeys 5-HTP increased GH secretion and also induced lethargic behavior lasting 2 to 3 hr (37). Similar effects were reported by Jacoby et al. (101) who were able to detect in their treated animals EEG activity similar to that in stage 3–4 of sleep. The first direct evidence of serotoninergic control of GH secretion in humans was the effect of oral administration of 5-HTP on GH release reported by Imura et al. (99). The rise in GH induced by 5-HTP was blocked by administration of glucose (99), and by cyproheptadine, a 5-HT receptor blocker (161). A slight effect of L-tryptophan (150 mg/kg oral administration) on GH release was reported by Müller et al. (159), but Handwerger et al. (90) found no effect after an oral dose of 200 mg 5-HTP. Recently, Lancranjan et al. (119,120) infused 200 mg of a new soluble ester of L-5-HTP (Ro 03–5940) to subjects pretreated with benserazide, which inhibits peripheral decarboxylation, and found a significant increase in GH release 30 to 120 min after the end of the infusion. The treatment with benserazide facilitated central penetration and action of 5-HTP, and GH plasma levels reached high values (Fig. 8–10). There is additional indirect evidence in support of serotoninergic control of GH secretion in humans. Bivens et al. (16) showed that cyproheptadine (4 mg × 8 oral doses) and methysergide (2 mg × 8 oral doses) produced, respectively, a 59% and 35% reduction in the amount of GH released by insulin-induced hypoglycemia. Smythe and Lazarus (207), also using high doses of cyproheptadine, were able to reduce the amount of GH released by insulin and exercise. Similar results were obtained (I. Lancranjan and E. Ohnhaus, *unpublished observations*) with 1 mg × 8 oral doses per 2 days of Pizotifen®, another serotonin receptor antagonist. A lower dose of this drug (1.5 mg/day for 12 days) produced a significant decrease in the GH response to arginine but had no effect on GH release in response to insulin-induced hypoglycemia (Fig. 8–4). A significant reduction in the amount of GH released by insulin was obtained after oral melatonin (1 g) and also after L-DOPA by Smythe and Lazarus (207). The authors view these results as evidence of their hypothesis that neural regulation of GH secretion is controlled only via serotonin receptors and, moreover, that compounds such as L-DOPA and bromocriptine interact with serotonin receptors due to structural similarities between DA, 5-HT, and ergoline ring systems. Suppression by cyproheptadine of GH during sleep was recently reported by Chihara et al. (38). The unpublished observation of del Pozo and co-workers that Pizotifen® (1.5 mg/day for 12 days) is able to reduce GH nocturnal peaks is in agreement with the above results. On the other hand, the enhancement of sleep-related GH secretion by methysergide and a significant reduction of insulin-stimulated GH release (2 mg × 8 doses/2 days) were shown by Mendelson et al. (154). These conflicting data and conclusions on the role of the serotoninergic system on sleep-related GH secretion are due to the complex human pharmacology of these drugs. Neither of them has a pure antiserotoninergic effect. Cyproheptadine also has anticholinergic and antihistaminergic properties which may potentiate the inhibitory antiserotoninergic effect on sleep-related GH release. Furthermore, methysergide, an ergot derivative with antiserotoninergic activity may enhance GH release like other ergots (e.g., bromocriptine). Moreover, Malarkey and Mendel (143) showed that parachlorophenylalanine, a tryptophan hydroxylase inhibitor, failed to inhibit the nocturnal GH peak in patients with Duchenne muscular dystrophy. Since chlorpromazine, diphenylhydantoin, phenobarbital, phentolamine, and propranolol as well as glucose administration (133) do not suppress sleep-related GH secretion, one is tempted to consider that the sleep-induced GH peak is related neither to catecholamines nor to glucoreceptor control.

Histamine and GABA Control of GH Secretion

Studies by Pontiroli et al. (169) have failed to confirm previous work by the same group (168) suggesting a role of histamine as a neurotransmitter in the modulation of GH secretion. These results are in agreement with unreported data by Lancranjan and del Pozo recorded in our laboratory. These investigators were unable to modify insulin-stimulated GH release by pretreatment with clemastine, an antihistaminic agent.

Recently Invitti et al. (100) showed that baclofen, a GABA derivative (30 mg/day for 4 days), blunted the GH response to insulin-induced hypoglycemia. Consequently, it has been suggested that GABA plays a physiologic role in GH secretion. Further studies are required to confirm this interesting hypothesis.

CLINICAL APPLICATION OF DRUG-INDUCED CHANGES IN GH SECRETION

Effect of Dopaminergic Drugs

Some interesting clinical applications of drug-induced GH modulation have been developed. During the last few years particular attention was paid to dopaminergic drugs, due to their unexpected therapeutic effects in acromegalic patients. Liuzzi et al. (128) opened the field by showing an inhibitory effect of L-DOPA on GH release in acromegalic patients. The paradoxical decrease in GH release recorded in this condition with apomorphine (39), and subsequently confirmed by Dunn et al. (58), raised the possibility that dopaminergic drugs might be used as therapeutic tools in acromegaly. A single dose of 2.5 mg bromocriptine significantly decreased plasma GH levels for 4 to 5 hr in seven tested acromegalic patients (127). Camanni et al. (34) also pointed out that in contrast to its effect in normal subjects, a single dose of 2.5 mg bromocriptine inhibited GH secretion in acromegaly. Moreover, a stable and significant reduction of GH levels during long-term treatment with bromocriptine has also been shown by Chiodini et al. (40) and Liuzzi et al. (131) (Fig. 8–11), using doses up to 10 mg/day, and by Thorner et al. (210), using doses up to 40 mg/day. Chiodini et al. (40) reported that there is a correlation between the effect of a single dose and the efficacy of long-term treatment with bromocriptine in acromegalic patients. It has been reported that some acromegalic patients [15 of 29 in a study by Liuzzi et al. (130)] responded to both TRH and dopaminergic drugs. Consequently, it was suggested that there is a correlation between TRH-induced and dopamine-induced GH secretion in most acromegalics. Liuzzi et al.

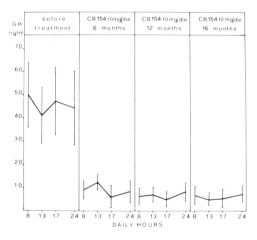

FIG. 8–11. Sustained inhibitory effect of bromocriptine (CB 154) in acromegalic subjects. From Liuzzi et al. (131) with permission.

(130) and Köbberling et al. (108) reported that a combined test with TRH-and DA-like drugs is the best tool for selecting the responders to the long-term therapy with bromocriptine. In order to find the most active dopaminergic drug for acromegalic patients, Camanni et al. (34) performed a thorough screening of bromocriptine, L-DOPA, Piribedil®, amantadine, and D 154 in 28 acromegalic patients. Only L-DOPA (500 mg p.o.), Piribedil® (100 mg p.o.), and bromocriptine (2.5 mg p.o.) significantly reduced plasma GH levels. The long-lasting action of bromocriptine (more than 4 hr) and its more frequent and consistent effect on acromegalic GH plasma levels pointed out that this dopaminergic drug is the best therapeutic tool in the medical treatment of acromegaly. Thorner et al. (210) also reported suppression of GH secretion in 11 acromegalic patients during long-term treatment (11 weeks) with bromocriptine up to 40 mg/day. The authors pointed out that progressively increasing doses were well tolerated and increased the number of successful results. Better glucose tolerance and reduction in hydroxyproline excretion, as well as considerable clinical improvement, were reported. In 12 of 21 acromegalic patients, clinical, hormonal, and metabolic improvement was reported by Sachdev et al. (195) after bromocriptine treatment with doses up to 40 mg/day. The optimum dose was 20 mg. The drug was fully effective in 19% and partially effective in 71% of cases. A dose-dependent suppression of GH secretion was also found by Benker et al. (10,11), who reported that 9 of 14 patients showed decreased GH levels and clinical improvement. Results of a study in 61 patients reported by Bricaire (25) showed good results in 33 cases treated with mean doses of 10 mg bromocriptine daily. In agreement with Liuzzi et al. (130), Bricaire found that a test with 2.5 mg bromocriptine prior to long-term therapy allowed a rough prediction of the later results of the therapy. Many other recent studies have shown the efficacy of bromocriptine in acromegaly, but the most complete and interesting study was reported by Besser et al. (14). Clinical and metabolic improvement was obtained in 82% of 66 treated patients. Moreover, diabetes mellitus, a complication of acromegaly, was completely relieved in 16 of 21 cases and was significantly improved in 5 other patients during bromocriptine therapy. Relief of diabetes in acromegalics treated with this drug was also reported by other authors (3,158,195). Besides the reduction of plasma GH levels, a significant fall in the glucagon response to arginine was found by Fedele et al. (64). The effect of bromocriptine on glucagon secretion might be an additional explanation for improvement of diabetes in acromegaly. Clinical relief is not dependent on the absolute GH levels achieved during bromocriptine treatment; in some cases even a relatively slight reduction of plasma GH was followed by clinical improvement. It could be that total immunoreactive GH does not correspond with the amount of biologically active hormone present. Besser et al. (14) reported a preferential reduction of GH monomer, the biologic active form of GH during bromocriptine therapy. The effect on GH is accompanied by prolactin suppression

in all instances (14,40,210). The clinical benefit appears clear in cases of acromegaly associated with hyperprolactinemia and galactorrhea and/or amenorrhea or male impotency or infertility (14). Restoration of fertility in both men and women and disappearance of galactorrhea were reported. As a consequence of long-term treatment of acromegalic patients with bromocriptine, Besser et al. (14) observed improvement in the visual field in some instances. This suggests a direct inhibitory effect of the drug on tumor growth. Recently, Delitala et al. (51) reported that a single dose of pyridoxine (300 mg i.v.) significantly decreased GH release in 5 acromegalic patients. The effect was identical to that after L-DOPA administration. It was concluded that pyridoxine accelerated L-DOPA conversion to dopamine and made more dopamine available. However, the effect of long-term pyridoxine administration in acromegaly has not been studied.

Effect of Drugs Which Influence Adrenergic Control of GH Secretion

Nakagawa and Mashimo (160) reported the suppressibility of GH levels in acromegaly with phentolamine, presenting evidence that in some acromegalics GH secretion may be under normal hypothalamic control. Similar data were reported by Cryer and Daughaday (49) who showed that phentolamine significantly decreased GH secretion in 7 of 10 patients, and, moreover, that phentolamine and isoproterenol decreased GH secretion in 8 of 10 tested patients. They suggested that an alpha-adrenergic mechanism contributed to the sustained hypersecretion of GH in acromegaly. On the basis of these data and the report (222) that the plasma GH level was more responsive to oral glucose and insulin-induced hypoglycemia in acromegalics with a smaller sellar area, the question arises: Is acromegaly a disorder with different stages, the initial one being the stage when pituitary secretion is still controlled by hypothalamic inputs, or is it a syndrome with different pathogenic pathways?

Serotonin Antagonists and Acromegaly

Feldman et al. (65), Chiodini et al. (41), and Delitala et al. (52) reported the first studies showing the positive effect of serotonin antagonist durgs in acromegaly. One may assume that the overstimulation of GH secretion, due to either the overproduction of GRH (83) or the underproduction of GIH (12), might be mediated by an increased central serotonin turnover. Furthermore, Feldman et al. (66) reported high serum serotonin and high GH levels in carcinoid tumors. In this particular situation, as with acromegaly, GH secretion was not suppressed by glucose administration. The effect of cyproheptadine and methysergide on GH secretion was tested in six acromegalic patients by Feldman et al. (65). Decreased GH plasma levels were shown after cyproheptadine administration (4 mg × 8 doses) in four of six patients and after methysergide (2 mg × 8 doses) in one of four cases investigated.

Chiodini et al. (41) reported that a single dose of 4 mg methergoline inhibited GH and PRL secretion in acromegalic patients. The inhibitory effect on GH and PRL was comparable to that obtained by a single dose of 2.5 mg bromocriptine but less sustained. Cyproheptadine, phentolamine, and pimozide did not significantly influence GH levels in their acromegalic patients. The authors concluded that methergoline inhibition of GH and PRL release in this disease is most probably due to the dopaminergic effect of the drug (see above). Positive results were reported by Delitala et al. (52) in six acromegalic patients treated with single oral doses of 4 mg methergoline, but they noticed with this drug the same long-lasting effect previously reported with bromocriptine. In three cases treated over 6 days (2 mg × 4 times/day) the marked decrease of GH and PRL levels persisted throughout the whole period of treatment. These positive results reported for methergoline, an ergoline derivative, and methysergide, a derivative of lysergic acid, in acromegalic patients suggest that in addition to their antiserotoninergic properties, the effect of both drugs on PRL and GH secretion is at least partially due to their ergot structure. Their dopamine-receptor agonist effects are probably involved as well. The strong inhibitory effect of cyproheptadine in acromegaly (65), not yet proved during long-term treatment, might be more specifically antiserotoninergic, even though the drug also has antihistaminic and anticholinergic effects.

Other Drugs Tested in Acromegaly

Other pharmacological agents that have been reported to decrease plasma GH levels are chlorpromazine (2,109), medroxyprogesterone acetate (122) and releasing hormones (61–63). Recent reports indicate that chlorpromazine (54) and medroxyprogesterone acetate (103,129,140) are not useful therapeutic tools in acromegaly. Pertinent reviews on the effects of somatostatin have been published by Hall et al. (89), Mortimer et al. (157), Prange-Hansen et al. (181), Besser et al. (12,14), Dunn et al. (58), and Christensen et al. (42).

HYPOTHESIS CONCERNING THE PHYSIOPATHOLOGY OF ACROMEGALY AND THE THERAPEUTIC MECHANISM OF ACTION OF DOPAMINERGIC DRUGS

Syndrome or Disease Resulting from Disturbed Neural Control of GH Secretion or GIH/GRH Imbalance

Based on human pharmacological data, sustained α-adrenergic or serotoninergic stimulation may lead to oversecretion of GH, as a first stage of acromegaly. Cryer and Daughaday (49) showed that some acromegalic patients respond in a normal way, decreasing GH secretion after the administration of α-blocking and β-stimulating drugs. The inhibitory effect of anti-serotoninergic drugs such as cyproheptadine, methysergide, and methergoline in some acromegalic patients has already been mentioned. Consequently, we may presume that patients responding normally to inhibition of α-adrenergic and serotoninergic systems might represent one stage or form of acromegaly. Characteristic of this stage is the possibility of modulating GH secretion by stimulating or inhibiting agents such as glucose load, insulin-induced hypoglycemia, and dexamethasone.

A second stage, or another form of acromegaly, might be a functional disconnection between the central nervous system and the pituitary leading to GIH/GRH imbalance. In such cases abnormal responses to common inhibitory or stimulatory tests for GH secretion could occur. Liuzzi et al. (131) supported the idea that DA-stimulating drugs might inhibit both GRH and GIH structures in normal subjects. Thus, in normal controls, dopaminergic drugs may stimulate GH secretion by depressing the GIH centers. In the so-called responder acromegalics, the high circulating levels of GH might be due to a defect in GIH secretion and to overproduction of GRH. Dopaminergic drugs block GIH, inhibiting the GRH overproduction. The functional disconnection between the central nervous system and pituitary might also explain the nonspecific GH-releasing effect of TRH (61) and of LRH (62,192) observed in these cases. We may also assume that a primary imbalanced GRH-increased secretion, due to either an insufficiency of GIH (12) or initially to an abnormally high secretion of GRH (83) overstimulates somatotrop cells and releases a large amount of GH. The overstimulation of somatotrop cells might induce the development of a somatotrop cell tumor, secreting large amounts of GH in an uncontrolled fashion.

Syndrome or Disease Induced by Pituitary Tumors with Modified Somatotrop Receptors

One may agree with Faglia et al. (61,62) and Gomez-Pan et al. (82) that in some functioning pituitary tumors, an alteration of the cellular membrane may exist with the development of receptors responding to nonspecific polypeptides. Furthermore, it can be proposed that dopaminergic drugs occupy the abnormal receptors which are responsive to nonspecific releasing hormones, providing in this way an explanation for the paradoxical effect observed with such drugs in some acromegalics. The high frequency of chromophobe adenomas in acromegaly is well known. Moreover, if chromophobes represent degranulated somatotrop and lactotrop cells (86), one may suppose that in some cases acromegaly is due to the development of tumors with abnormally modified lactotrop cells secreting both GH and PRL and being controlled by factors that normally stimulate or inhibit them. Massara et al. (150) and Verde et al. (219) showed that dopamine infusion failed to stimulate GH secretion in normal subjects but was effective in reducing GH levels in acromegalic subjects. It is known that DA does not cross the blood-brain barrier and that DA is not a direct stimulus at the pituitary level (15,137). Furthermore, sites in the CNS are responsible for dopamine modulation of GH secretion in normal subjects. The inhibitory effect on GH release of DA infused in acromegalic patients argues again for modified receptors on the somatotrops. A further argument for this assumption is the inhibitory effect of L-DOPA on GH released by rat tumor cells (141). Thus, it seems likely that the inhibitory effect of dopaminergic drugs is due to their direct effect on receptors sensitive to dopamine located in the membrane of somatotropic cells of acromegalic patients. Probably a smaller number of such receptors, or the presence of not strictly specific receptors for dopamine in the membrane of somatotrop cells, explains why a larger dose of bromocriptine is required to treat acromegalic patients compared to the smaller doses required in patients with PRL-secreting tumors.

CLINICAL APPLICATION OF ACTH INHIBITION BY ANTISEROTONINERGIC AND DOPAMINERGIC AGENTS

Cavagnini et al. (36) reported that a 4-day treatment with 10 mg daily of methergoline blunted the ACTH response to insulin hypoglycemia in normal subjects. This was accompanied by a moderate but significant fall in plasma cortisol. In contrast, this drug failed to affect the ACTH response to lysine-vasopressin. Based on these data and on experience collected in patients, investigators proposed a physiological stimulating effect of serotonin on ACTH secretion. Lamberts and Birkenhäger (117) investigated the influence of bromocriptine on pituitary-dependent Cushing's disease after this drug had failed to modify plasma ACTH under basal conditions and after stimulation with lysine vasopressin. Four out of seven subjects responded to a single oral dose of 2.5 mg bromocriptine with a significant fall in basal plasma ACTH at different intervals after administration of the drug. The authors concluded that dopaminergic mechanisms may have a bearing in the pathogenesis of Cushing's disease. Benker et al. (10) have also reported a significant fall in plasma ACTH in Nelson's and Cushing's syndromes after administration of 2.5 mg bromocriptine in an acute trial. Lambert and Birkenhäger (116) also recorded a marked drop in plasma PRL and ACTH concentrations in a subject with Nelson's syndrome receiving 5 mg bromocriptine. It is interesting to note that Alcañiz et al. (*unpublished observations*) observed not only a fall in ACTH but also clearance of abnormal pigmentation on such a patient on long-term bromocriptine treatment. The effect of serotoninergic blockade on Cushing's disease has been the subject of recent investigation. Krieger et al. (110) and Krieger and Luria (111) have reported that cyproheptadine reverses the clinical and biochemical picture of Cushing's disease and also improves Nelson's syndrome. In this context it is relevant to note that patients with pituitary Cushing's disease may also show abnormal PRL control (92) indicating the presence of common releasing mechanisms for both hormones, as suggested by Copinschi et al. (47).

REFERENCES

1. Adler, R. A., Noel, G. L., Wartofsky, L., and Frantz, A. G. (1975): Failure of oral water loading and intravenous hypotonic saline to suppress plasma prolactin in man. *J. Clin. Endocrinol. Metab.*, 41:383–389.
2. Alford, F. P., Baker, H. W. G., Burger, H. G., Cameron, D. P., and Keogh, E. J. (1974): The secretion rate of human growth hormone. II. Acromegaly, effect of chlorpromazine treatment. *J. Clin. Endocrinol. Metab.*, 38:309–312.
3. Althoff, P. H., Neubauer, M., Handzel, M., and Schöffling, K. (1975): Untersuchungen zum Einfluss von Somatostatin und Bromocriptin (CB 154) auf die Wachstumshormonsekretion bei Akromegalen. *Verh. Dtsch. Ges. Inn. Med.*, 81: 1515–1520.
4. Aubert, M. L., Grumbach, M. M., and Kaplan, S. L. (1974): The ontogenesis of human fetal hormones. III. Prolactin. *J. Clin. Invest.*, 56:155–164.
5. Ayalon, D., Peyser, M. R., Toaff, R., Cordova, T., Harell, A., Franchimont, P., and Lindner, H. R. (1974): Effect of L-dopa on galactopoiesis and gonadotropin levels in the inappropriate lactating syndrome. *Obstet. Gynecol.*, 44:159–170.
6. Bassi, F., Giusti, G., Vorsi, L., Cattaneo, S., Giannotti, P., Forti, G., Pazzagli, M., Vigiani, C., and Serio, M. (1977): Plasma androgens in women with hyperprolactinemic amenorrhea. *Clin. Endocrinol.*, 6:5–10.
7. Baumann, G., and Loriaux, D. L. (1976): Failure of endogenous prolactin to alter renal salt and water excretion and adrenal function in man. *J. Clin. Endocrinol. Metab.*, 43:643–649.
8. Baumann, G., Marynick, S. P., Winters, S. J., and Loriaux, D. L. (1977): The effect of osmotic stimuli on prolactin secretion and renal water excretion in normal men and in chronic hyperprolactinemia. *J. Clin. Endocrinol. Metab.*, 44:199–202.
9. Beck-Peccoz, P., Ferrari, C., Rondena, M., Paracchi, A., and Faglia, G. (1976): Failure of oral 5-hydroxytryptophan administration to affect prolactin secretion in man. *Horm. Res.*, 7:303–307.
10. Benker, G., Hackenberg, K., Hamburger, B., and Reinwein, D. (1976): Effects of growth hormone release-inhibiting hormone and bromocryptine (CB 154) in states of abnormal pituitary-adrenal function. *Clin. Endocrinol.*, 5:187–190.
11. Benker, G., Zäh, W., Hackenberg, K., Hamburger, B., Günnewig, H., and Reinwein, D. (1976): Long-term treatment of acromegaly with bromocriptine: Postprandial HGH levels and response to TRH and glucose administration. *Horm. Metab. Res.*, 8:291–295.
12. Besser, G. M., Mortimer, C. H., NcNeilly, A. S., Thorner, M. O., Batistoni, G. A., Bloom, S. R., Kastrup, K. W., Hanssen, K. F., Hall, R., Coy, D. H., Kastin, A. J., and Schally, A. V. (1974): Long-term infusion of growth hormone release inhibiting hormone in acromegaly: Effects on pituitary and pancreatic hormones. *Br. Med. J.*, 4:622–627.
13. Besser, G. M., Parke, L., Edwards, C. R. W., Forsyth, I. A., and McNeilly, A. S. (1972): Galactorrhea: Successful treatment with reduction of plasma prolactin levels by Brom-ergocryptine. *Br. Med. J.*, 3:669–672.
14. Besser, G. M., Thorner, M. O., Wass, J. A. H., and Mortimer, C. H. (1976): Therapeutic use of bromocriptine and growth hormone release-inhibiting hormone (GHRIH, somatostatin). Abstracts of the Sixth International Seminar on Reproductive and Sexual Endocrinology, Brussels.
15. Birge, C. A., Jacobs, L. S., Hammer, C. T., and Daughaday, W. H. (1970): Catecholamine inhibition of prolactin secretion by isolated rat adenohypophysis. *Endocrinology*, 86:120–130.
16. Bivens, C. H., Lebovitz, H. E., and Feldman, J. M. (1973): Inhibition of hypoglycemia-induced growth hormone secretion by the serotonin antagonists cyproheptadine and methysergide. *N. Engl. J. Med.*, 289:236–239.
17. Blackard, W. G., and Heidingsfelder, S. A. (1968): Adrenergic receptor control mechanism for growth hormone secretion. *J. Clin. Invest.*, 47:1407–1414.
18. Blackard, W. G., and Hubbell, G. J. (1974): Stimulatory effect of exogenous catecholamines on plasma hGH concentrations in presence of beta adrenergic blockade. *Metabolism*, 19:547–552.

19. Blake, C. A., and Sawyer, C. H. (1972): Nicotine blocks the suckling-induced rise in circulating prolactin in lactating rats. *Science,* 177:619–621.
20. Bohnet, H. G., Dahlen, H. G., and Schneider, H. P. G. (1974): Hyperprolactinemia and pulsatile LH fluctuation. *Acta Endocrinol. (Kbh.) [Suppl.],* 184:109.
21. Bohnet, H. G., Dahlen, H. G., Wuttke, W., and Schneider, H. P. G. (1976): Hyperprolactinemic anovulatory syndrome. *J. Clin. Endocrinol. Metab.,* 42:132–143.
22. Bohnet, H. G., and Friesen, H. G. (1976): Effects of prolactin and growth hormone on prolactin and LH receptors on the dwarf mouse. *J. Reprod. Fertil.,* 48:307–311.
23. Boyar, R. M., Kapen, S., Finkelstein, J. W., Perlow, M., Sassin, J. F., Fukushima, D. K., Weitzman, E. D., and Hellman, L. (1974): Hypothalamic-pituitary function in diverse hyperprolactinemic states. *J. Clin. Invest.,* 53:1588–1598.
24. Boyd, A. E., III, Lebovitz, H. E., and Pfeiffer, J. B. (1970): Stimulation of human growth hormone secretion by L-dopa. *N. Engl. J. Med.,* 283:1425–1429.
25. Bricaire, H. (1976): A propos des résultats obtenus en France par le CB 154 dans le traitement de l'acromégalie. *Ann. Endocrinol. (Paris),* 37:305–308.
26. Brown, G. M., and Chambers, J. W. (1974): Neurotransmitter regulation of growth hormone and ACTH release. *J. Pharmacol. (Paris) [Suppl.],* 2:12.
27. Brown, W. A., von Woert, M. H., and Ambani, L. M. (1973): Effect of apomorphine on growth hormone release in humans. *J. Clin. Endocrinol. Metab.,* 37:463–465.
28. Brown, W. A., and Williams, B. W. (1976): Methylphenidate increases serum growth hormone concentrations. *J. Clin. Endocrinol. Metab.,* 43:937–939.
29. Brun del Re, R., del Pozo, E., de Grandi, P., Friesen, H., Hinselmann, M., and Wyss, H. (1973): Prolactin inhibition and suppression of puerperal lactation by a Br-ergocryptine (CB 154). A comparison with estrogen. *Obstet. Gynecol.,* 41:884–890.
30. Buckman, M. T., Kaminsky, N., Conway, M., and Peake, G. T. (1973): Utility of L-dopa and water loading in evaluation of hyperprolactinemia. *J. Clin. Endocrinol. Metab.,* 36:911–919.
31. Buckman, M. T., and Peake, G. T. (1973): Osmolar control of prolactin secretion in man. *Science,* 181:755–757.
32. Buckman, M. T., Peake, G. T., and Robertson, G. (1976): Hyperprolactinemia influences renal function in man. *Metabolism,* 25:509–516.
33. Camanni, F., Massara, F., Belforte, L., and Molinatti, G. M. (1975): Changes in plasma growth hormone levels in normal and acromegalic subjects following administration of 2-bromo-α-ergocryptine. *J. Clin. Endocrinol. Metab.,* 40:363–366.
34. Camanni, F., Massara, F., Fassio, V., Molinatti, G. M., and Müller, E. E. (1975): Effect of five dopaminergic drugs on plasma growth hormone levels in acromegalic subjects. *Neuroendocrinology,* 19:227–240.
35. Canales, E., Garrido, J. T., Zárate, A., Mason, M., and Soria, J. (1976): Effect of ergonovine on prolactin secretion and milk let-down. *Obstet. Gynecol.,* 48:228–229.
36. Cavagnini, F., Raggi, U., Micossi, P., di Landro, A., and Invitti, C. (1976): Effect of an antiserotoninergic drug, metergoline, on the ACTH and cortisol response to insulin hypoglycemia and lysine-vasopressin in man. *J. Clin. Endocrinol. Metab.,* 43:306–312.
37. Chambers, J. W., and Brown, G. M. (1976): Neurotransmitter regulation of growth hormone and ACTH in the rhesus monkey: Effect of biogenic amines. *Endocrinology,* 98:420–428.
38. Chihara, K., Kato, Y., Maeda, K., Matsukura, S., and Imura, H. (1976): Suppression by cyproheptadine of human growth hormone and cortisol secretion during sleep. *J. Clin. Invest.,* 57:1393–1402.
39. Chiodini, P. G., Liuzzi, A., Botalla, L., Cremascoli, G., and Silvestrini, F. (1974): Inhibitory effect of dopaminergic stimulation on GH release in acromegaly. *J. Clin. Endocrinol. Metab.,* 38:200–206.
40. Chiodini, P. G., Liuzzi, A., Botalla, L., Oppizzi, G., Müller, E. E., and Silvestrini, F. (1975): Stable reduction of plasma growth hormone (hGH) levels during chronic administration of 2-Br-α-ergocryptine (CB 154) in acromegalic patients. *J. Clin. Endocrinol. Metab.,* 40:705–708.
41. Chiodini, P. G., Liuzzi, A., Müller, E. E., Botalla, L., Cremascoli, G., Oppizzi, G.,

Verde, G., and Silvestrini, F. (1976): Inhibitory effect of an ergoline derivative, methergoline, on growth hormone and prolactin levels in acromegalic patients. *J. Clin. Endocrinol. Metab.,* 43:356–363.

42. Christensen, S. E., Nerup, J., Hansen, A. P., and Lundbaek, K. (1976): Effects of somatostatin on basal levels of plasma growth hormone and insulin in acromegalics: Dose-response studies and attempted total growth hormone suppression. *J. Clin. Endocrinol. Metab.,* 42:839–845.

43. Cleary, R. E., Crabtree, R., and Lemberger, L. (1975): The effect of lergotrile on galactorrhea and gonadotropin secretion. *J. Clin. Endocrinol. Metab.,* 40:830–833.

44. Collu, R., Fraschini, F., and Martini, L. (1973): Role of indolamines and catecholamines on the control of gonadotrophin and growth hormone secretion. *Prog. Brain Res.,* 39:297–299.

45. Collu, R., Fraschini, F., Visconti, P., and Martini, L. (1972): Adrenergic and serotoninergic control of growth hormone secretion in adult male rats. *Endocrinology,* 90:1231–1237.

46. Copinschi, G., L'Hermite, M., Leclercq, R., Golstein, J., Vanhaelst, L., Virasoro, E., and Robyn, C. (1975): Effects of glucocorticoids on pituitary hormonal responses to hypoglycemia. Inhibition of prolactin release. *J. Clin. Endocrinol. Metab.,* 40:442–449.

47. Copinschi, G., L'Hermite, M., Pasteels, J. L., and Robyn, C. (1971): 2-Bromo-α-ergocryptine (CB 154) inhibition of prolactin secretion and galactorrhea in a case of pituitary tumour. *Horm. Antag. Gynecol. Invest.,* 2:128–129.

48. Corenblum, B., Pairaudeau, N., and Shewchuk, A. B. (1976): Prolactin hypersecretion and short luteal phase defects. *Obstet. Gynecol.,* 47:486–488.

49. Cryer, P. E., and Daughaday, W. H. (1974): Adrenergic modulation of growth hormone secretion in acromegaly: Suppression during phentolamine and phentolamine-isoproterenol administration. *J. Clin. Endocrinol. Metab.,* 39:658–663.

50. Delitala, G., Masala, A., Alagna, S., and Devilla, L. (1974): Propanolol-levodopa as a test of growth hormone reserve in children with growth retardation. *IRCS Med. Sci.,* 2:1724.

51. Delitala, G., Masala, A., Alagna, S., and Devilla, L. (1976): Effect of pyridoxine on human hypophyseal trophic hormone release: A possible stimulation of hypothalamic dopaminergic pathway. *J. Clin. Endocrinol. Metab.,* 42:603–606.

52. Delitala, G., Masala, A., Alagna, S., Devilla, L., and Lotti, G. (1976): Growth hormone and prolactin release in acromegalic patients following metergoline administration. *J. Clin. Endocrinol. Metab.,* 43:1382–1386.

53. Delvoye, P., Taubert, H.-D., Jürgensen, O., L'Hermite, M., Delogne, J., and Robyn, C. (1974): Influence of circulating prolactin increased by a psychotropic drug on gonadotropin and progesterone secretion. *Acta Endocrinol. (Kbh.) [Suppl.],* 184:110.

54. Demond, R. G., Brammer, S. P., Atkinson, R. L., Howard, W. J., and Earll, J. M. (1973): Chlorpromazine treatment and growth hormone secretory response in acromegaly. *J. Clin. Endocrinol. Metab.,* 36:1189–1195.

55. Denamur, R., Martinet, J., and Short, R. V. (1973): Pituitary control of the ovine corpus luteum. *J. Reprod. Fertil.,* 32:207–220.

56. Diefenbach, W. P., Carmel, P. W., Frantz, A., and Ferin, M. (1976): Suppression of prolactin secretion by L-dopa in the stalk-sectioned rhesus monkey. *J. Clin. Endocrinol. Metab.,* 43:638–642.

57. Dular, R., LaBella, R., Vivian, S., and Eddie, L. (1974): Purifiication of prolactin-releasing and inhibiting factors from beef. *Endocrinology,* 94:563–567.

58. Dunn, P. J., Donald, R. A., and Espiner, E. A. (1976): A comparison of the effect of levodopa and somatostatin on the plasma levels of growth hormone, insulin, glucagon and prolactin in acromegaly. *Clin. Endocrinol.,* 5:167–174.

59. Edwards, C. R. W., and Jeffcoate, W. J. (1976): Bromocriptine and the adrenal cortex. In: *Pharmacological and Clinical Aspects of Bromocriptine (Parlodel),* edited by R. I. S. Bayliss, P. Turner, and W. P. Maclay, pp. 43–51. MCS Consultants, Tunbridge Wells, Kent.

60. Edwards, C. R. W., Thorner, M. O., Miall, P. A., Al-Dujaili, E. A. S., Hanker, J. P.,

and Besser, G. M. (1975): Inhibition of the plasma-aldosterone response to frusemide by bromocriptine. *Lancet,* 2:903–904.
61. Faglia, G., Beck-Peccoz, P., Ferrari, C., Travaglini, P., Ambrosi, B., and Spada, A. (1973): Plasma growth hormone response to thyrotropin-releasing hormone in patients with active acromegaly. *J. Clin. Endocrinol. Metab.,* 36:1259–1262.
62. Faglia, G., Beck-Peccoz, P., Travaglini, P., Paracchi, A., Spada, A., and Lewin, A. (1973): Elevations in plasma growth hormone concentration after luteinizing hormone-releasing hormone (LRH) in patients with active acromegaly. *J. Clin. Endocrinol. Metab.,* 37:338–340.
63. Faglia, G., Paracchi, A., Ferrari, C., Beck-Peccoz, P., Ambrosi, B., Travaglini, P., Spada, A., and Oliver, C. (1976): Influence of L-prolyl-L-leucyl-glycine amide on growth hormone secretion in normal and acromegalic subjects. *J. Clin. Endocrinol. Metab.,* 42:991–994.
64. Fedele, D., Molinari, M., Valerio, A., Muggeo, A., Tiengo, A., and Crepaldi, G. (1976): Growth hormone, insulin and glucagon secretion in acromegaly following treatment with 2-bromo-ergocryptine (CB 154). Abstracts of the Meeting of the European Association for the Study of Diabetes, Helsinki.
65. Feldman, J. M., Plonk, J. W., and Bivens, C. H. (1976): Inhibitory effect of serotonin antagonists on growth hormone release in acromegalic patients. *Clin. Endocrinol.,* 5:71–78.
66. Feldman, J. M., Plonk, J. W., Bivens, C. H., Lebovitz, H. E., and Handwerger, S. (1975): Growth hormone and prolactin secretion in the carcinoid syndrome. *Am. J. Med. Sci.,* 269:333–347.
67. Ferry, J. D., McLean, B. K., and Nikitovitch-Winer, M. B. (1974): Tobacco-smoke inhalation delays suckling-induced prolactin release in the rat. *Proc. Soc. Exp. Biol. Med.,* 147:110–113.
68. Flückiger, E. (1972): Drugs and the control of prolactin secretion. In: *Prolactin and Carcinogenesis,* edited by A. R. Boyns and K. Griffiths, pp. 162–171. Alpha Omega Alpha Publishing, Cardiff, Wales.
69. Flückiger, E., and del Pozo, E. (1977): Influence on the endocrine system. In: *Ergot Alkaloids and Similar Compounds, Handbook of Experimental Pharmacology,* edited by B. Berde and H. O. Shild. Springer-Verlag, Berlin *(in press).*
70. Flückiger, E., Marko, M., Doepfner, W., and Niederer, W. (1976): Effects of ergot alkaloids on the hypothalamo-pituitary axis. *Postgrad. Med. J. (Suppl.),* 52:57–61.
71. Forbes, A. P., Henneman, P. H., Griswold, G. C., and Albright, F. (1954): Syndrome characterized by galactorrhea, amenorrhea and low urinary FSH: Comparison with acromegaly and normal lactation. *J. Clin. Endocrinol. Metab.,* 14:265–271.
72. Fossati, P., Strauch, G., and Tourniaire, J. (1976): Etude de l'activité de la bromocriptine dans les états d'hyperprolactinémie. *Nouv. Presse Med.,* 5:1687–1690.
73. Franks, S., Jacobs, H. S., and Nabarro, I. D. N. (1975): Studies on prolactin secretion in pituitary disease. *J. Endocrinol.,* 67:55P.
74. Frantz, A. G. (1973): The regulation of prolactin secretion in humans. In: *Frontiers in Neuroendocrinology, 1973,* edited by W. F. Ganong and L. Martini, pp. 337–374. Oxford University Press, New York.
75. Friesen, H. G., Tolis, G., Shiu, R., and Hwang, P. (1973): Studies on human prolactin: Chemistry, radioreceptor assay and clinical significance. In: *Human Prolactin,* edited by J. L. Pasteels and C. Robyn, pp. 11–23. Excerpta Medica, Amsterdam.
76. Frohman, L. A., Bernardis, L. L., and Kant, K. J. (1968): Hypothalamic stimulation of GH secretion. *Science,* 162:580–582.
77. Frohman, L. A., and Stachura, M. E. (1975): Neuropharmacologic control of neuroendocrine function in man. *Metabolism,* 24:211–234.
78. Furth, J., Gadsden, E. L., Clifton, K. H., and Anderson, E. (1956): Autonomous mammotropic pituitary tumors in mice. Their somatotropic features and responsiveness to estrogens. *Cancer Res.,* 16:600–607.
79. Gala, R. R., Subramanian, G., Peters, J. A., and Jaques, S. (1976): Influence of

cholinergic receptor blockade on drug-induced prolactin release in the monkey. *Horm. Res.,* 7:118–128.

80. Ganong, W. F. (1975): Brain amines and the control of ACTH and growth hormone secretion. In: *Hypothalamic Hormones,* edited by M. Motta, P. G. Crosignani, and L. Martini, pp. 237–248. Academic Press, New York.

81. Giusti, G., Bassi, F., Borsi, L., Cattaneo, S., Giannotti, P., Lanza, L., Pazzagli, M., Vigiani, C., and Serio, M. (1977): Effects of prolactin on the human adrenal cortex: Plasma dehydroepiandrosterone sulphate in women affected by amenorrhea with hyperprolactinemia. In: *Prolactin and Human Reproduction,* edited by P. G. Crosignani, pp. 239–244. Academic Press, New York.

82. Gomez-Pan, A., Tunbridge, W. M. G., Hall, R., Besser, G. M., Coy, D. H., Schally, A. V., and Kastin, A. J. (1975): Hypothalamic hormone interaction in acromegaly. *Clin. Endocrinol.,* 4:455–460.

83. Gonzales-Barcena, D., Kastin, A. J., Coy, D. H., Glick, S., Schalch, D., Lee, L. A., Arzac, P., and Schally, A. V. (1974): Unaltered plasma GH levels in acromegalics and normal men and women after administration of [Pyro] Glu-Ser-Gly-NH₂, a proposed GH-releasing hormone. *J. Clin. Endocrinol. Metab.,* 38:1134–1136.

84. Grandison, L., Gelato, M., and Meites, J. (1974): Inhibition of prolactin secretion by cholinergic drugs. *Proc. Soc. Exp. Biol. Med.,* 145:1236–1239.

85. Guilhem, P., Pontonnier, A., Monrozies, M., Bardenat, M., and Merle-Beral, A. (1967): Essai de blocage de la galactogénèse par la méthylergobasine. *Bull. Fed. Gynecol. Obstet. Fr.,* 19:277–279.

86. Guyda, H., Robert, F., Colle, E., and Hardy, J. (1973): Histologic ultrastructural, and hormonal characterization of a pituitary tumor secreting both hGH and prolactin. *J. Clin. Endocrinol. Metab.,* 36:531–547.

87. Hagen, T. C., Guansing, A. R., and Sill, A. J. (1976): Preliminary evidence for a human prolactin releasing factor. *Neuroendocrinology,* 21:255–261.

88. Halasz, B., and Pupp, L. (1965): Hormone secretion of the anterior pituitary gland after physical interruption of all nervous pathways to the hypophysiotropic area. *Endocrinology,* 77:553–562.

89. Hall, R., Besser, G. M., Schally, A. V., Coy, D. H., Evered, D., Goldie, D. J., Kastin, A. J., McNeilly, A. S., Mortimer, C. H., Phenekos, C., Tunbridge, W. M. G., and Weightman, D. (1973): Action of growth hormone release inhibiting hormone in healthy men and in acromegaly. *Lancet,* 2:581–586.

90. Handwerger, S., Plonk, J. W., Lebovitz, H. E., Bivens, C. H., and Feldman, J. M. (1975): Failure of 5-hydroxytryptophan to stimulate prolactin and growth hormone secretion in man. *Horm. Metab. Res.,* 7:214–216.

91. Hart, I. C. (1973): Effect of 2-Br-α-ergocryptine on milk yield and the level of PRL and GH in the blood of the goat at milking. *J. Endocrinol.,* 57:179–180.

92. Hashimoto, K. (1975): The pituitary ACTH, GH, LH, FSH, TSH, and prolactin reserves in patients with Cushing's syndrome. *Endocrinol. Jpn.,* 22:67–77.

93. Heidingsfelder, S. A., and Blackard, W. G. (1968): Adrenergic control mechanism for vasopressin-induced plasma growth hormone response. *Metabolism,* 17:1019–1024.

94. Hiba, J., del Pozo, E., Genazzani, A., Pusterla, E., Lancranjan, I., Sidiropoulos, D., and Gunti, J. (1977): Mechanism of milk secretion in the newborn. *J. Clin. Endocrinol. Metab.,* 44:973–976.

95. Hökfelt, T., and Fuxe, K. (1972): On the morphology and the neuroendocrine role of the hypothalamic catecholamine neurons. In: *Brain-Endocrine Interaction. Median Eminence: Structure and Function,* edited by K. M. Knigge, D. E. Scott, and A. Weindl, pp. 181–223. S. Karger, Basel.

96. Hökfelt, T., and Fuxe, K. (1972): Effects of prolactin and ergot alkaloids on the tubero-infundibular dopamine (DA) neurons. *Neuroendocrinology,* 98:100–122.

97. Imura, H., Kato, Y., Ikeda, M., Morimoto, M., and Yawata, M. (1971): Effect of adrenergic-blocking or stimulating agents on plasma growth hormone, immunoreactive insulin, and blood free fatty acid level in man. *J. Clin. Invest.,* 50:1069–1079.

98. Imura, H., Nakai, Y., Kato, Y., Yoshimoto, T., and Moridera, K. (1974): Pro-

pranolol-insulin stimulation test in the diagnosis of growth hormone deficiency. *Horm. Metab. Res.,* 6:343–346.

99. Imura, H., Nakai, Y., and Yoshimi, T. (1973): Effect of 5-hydroxytryptophan (5-HTP) on growth hormone and ACTH release in man. *J. Clin. Endocrinol. Metab.,* 36:204–206.

100. Invitti, C., Cavagnini, F., di Landro, A., and Pinto, M. (1976): Inhibiting effect of a GABA derivative, baclofen, on growth hormone and cortisol response to insulin hypoglycemia in man. Abstracts of the Vth International Congress of Endocrinology, Hamburg.

101. Jacoby, J. H., Greenstein, M., Sassin, J. F., and Weitzmann, E. D. (1974): The effect of monoamine precursors on the release of growth hormone in the rhesus monkey. *Neuroendocrinology,* 14:95–102.

102. Johnson, S. E., Norman, N., and Sjaastad, O. (1974): Decreased arginine-induced HGH response during L-dopa therapy in parkinsonian patients. *Acta Endocrinol. (Kbh.),* 77:686.

103. Josefsberg, Z., Laron, Z., Mathias, S. H., and Keret, R. (1974): Long-term administration of medroxy-progesterone acetate (MPA) to acromegalic patients. *Clin. Endocrinol.,* 3:195–202.

104. Judd, S. J., Lazarus, L., and Smythe, G. (1976): Prolactin secretion by metoclopramide in man. *J. Clin. Endocrinol. Metab.,* 43:313–317.

105. Kanematsu, S., and Sawyer, C. H. (1973): Elevation of plasma prolactin after hypophyseal stalk section in the rat. *Endocrinology,* 93:238–241.

106. Kansai, P. C., Buse, J., Talbert, O. R., and Buse, M. G. (1972): The effect of L-dopa on plasma growth hormone, insulin, and thyroxine. *J. Clin. Endocrinol. Metab.,* 34:99–105.

107. Kato, Y., Nakai, Y., Imura, H., Chihara, K., and Ohgo, S. (1974): Effect of 5-hydroxytryptophan (5-HTP) on plasma prolactin levels in man. *J. Clin. Endocrinol. Metab.,* 38:695–697.

108. Köbberling, J., Schwinn, G., and Dirks, H. (1975): Die Behandlung der Akromegalie mit Bromocriptin. *Dtsch. Med. Wochenschr.,* 100:1540–1542.

109. Kolodny, H. D., Sherman, L., Singh, A., Kim, S., and Benjamin, F. (1971): Acromegaly treated with chlorpromazine—a case study. *N. Engl. J. Med.,* 284:819–822.

110. Krieger, D. T., Amorosa, L., and Linick, F. (1975): Cyproheptadine induced remission of Cushing's disease. *N. Engl. J. Med.,* 293:893–896.

111. Krieger, D. T., and Luria, M. (1976): Effectiveness of cyproheptadine in decreasing plasma ACTH concentrations in Nelson's syndrome. *J. Clin. Endocrinol. Metab.,* 43:1179–1182.

112. Lal, S., de la Vega, C. E., Sourkes, T. L., and Friesen, H. G. (1972): Effect of apomorphine on human growth hormone secretion. *Lancet,* II:661.

113. Lal, S., de la Vega, C. E., Sourkes, T. L., and Friesen, H. G. (1973): Effect of apomorphine on growth hormone, prolactin, luteinizing hormone and follicle-stimulating hormone levels in human serum. *J. Clin. Endocrinol. Metab.,* 37:719–724.

114. Lal, S., Martin, J. B., de la Vega, C. E., and Friesen, H. G. (1975): Comparison of the effect of apomorphine and L-Dopa on serum growth hormone levels in normal men. *Clin. Endocrinol.,* 4:277–285.

115. Lal, S., Tolis, G., Martin, J. B., Brown, G. M., and Guyda, H. (1975): Effect of clonidine on growth hormone, prolactin, luteinizing hormone, follicle-stimulating hormone, and thyroid-stimulating hormone in the serum of normal men. *J. Clin. Endocrinol. Metab.,* 41:827–832.

116. Lamberts, S. W. J., and Birkenhäger, J. C. (1976): Bromocriptine in Nelson's syndrome and Cushing's disease. *Lancet,* 2:811.

117. Lamberts, S. W. J., and Birkenhäger, J. C. (1976): Effect of bromocriptine in pituitary-dependent Cushing's syndrome. *J. Endocrinol.,* 70:315–316.

118. Lancranjan, I., and Marbach, P. (1977): New evidence for growth hormone modulation by the alpha-adrenergic system in man. *Metabolism (in press).*

119. Lancranjan, I., Wirz-Justice, A., Pühringer, W., and del Pozo, E. (1976): The effect of a new soluble ester of 1-5 HTP on growth hormone and prolactin re-

lease in healthy subjects. Abstracts of the VIIth International Congress of the Society of Psychoneuroendocrinology, Strasbourg.

120. Lancranjan, I., Wirz-Justice, A., Pühringer, W., and del Pozo, E. (1977): Effect of 1–5 hydroxytryptophan infusion on growth hormone and prolactin secretion in man. *J. Clin. Endocrinol. Metab.,* 45:588–593.

121. Lawrence, A. M., and Hagen, T. C. (1972): Ergonovine therapy on nonpuerperal galactorrhea. *N. Engl. J. Med.,* 287:150.

122. Lawrence, A. M., and Kirstens, J. (1970): Progestins in the medical management of active acromegaly. *J. Clin. Endocrinol. Metab.,* 30:646–652.

123. Lemberger, L., Crabtree, R., Clemens, J., Dyke, R. W., and Woodburn, R. T. (1974): The inhibitory effect of an ergoline derivative (lergotrile, compound 83636) on prolactin secretion in man. *J. Clin. Endocrinol. Metab.,* 39:579–584.

124. L'Hermite, M., Delvoye, P., Nokin, J., Vekemans, M., and Robyn, C. (1972): Human prolactin secretion, as studied by radioimmunoassay: Some aspects of its regulation. In: *Prolactin and Carcinogenesis,* edited by A. R. Boyns and K. Griffiths, pp. 81–97. Alpha Omega Alpha Publishing, Cardiff, Wales.

125. Libertun, C., and McCann, S. M. (1974): Further evidence for cholinergic control of gonadotropin and prolactin secretion. *Proc. Soc. Exp. Biol. Med.,* 147:498–504.

126. Lichtensteiger, W., and Keller, P. J. (1974): Tubero-infundibular dopamine neurons and the secretion of luteinizing hormones and prolactin extrahypothalamic influences, interaction with cholinergic systems and the effect of urethane anesthesia. *Brain. Res.,* 74:279–303.

127. Liuzzi, A., Chiodini, P. G., Botalla, L., Cremascoli, G., Müller, E. E., and Silvestrini, F. (1974): Decreased plasma growth hormone (GH) levels in acromegalics following CB 154 (2-Br-α-ergocryptine) administration. *J. Clin. Endocrinol. Metab.,* 38:910–912.

128. Liuzzi, A., Chiodini, P. G., Botalla, L., Cremascoli, G., and Silvestrini, F. (1972): Inhibitory effect of L-dopa on GH release in acromegalic patients. *J. Clin. Endocrinol. Metab.,* 35:941–943.

129. Liuzzi, A., Chiodini, P. G., Botalla, L., and Silvestrini, F. (1972): Influence de l'acétate de médroxyprogestérone (MPA) sur le taux plasmatique de la STH chez douze malades atteints d'acromégalie. *Ann. Endocrinol. (Paris),* 33:426–430.

130. Liuzzi, A., Chiodini, P. G., Botalla, L., Silvestrini, F., and Müller, E. E. (1974): Growth hormone (GH)-releasing activity of TRH and GH-lowering effect of dopaminergic drugs in acromegaly: Homogeneity in the two responses. *J. Clin. Endocrinol. Metab.,* 39:871–876.

131. Liuzzi, A., Panerai, A. E., Chiodini, P. G., Secchi, C., Cocchi, D., Botalla, L., Silvestrini, F., and Müller, E. E. (1975): Neuroendocrine control of growth hormone secretion: Experimental and clinical studies. In: *Growth Hormone and Related Peptides,* edited by E. Pecile and E. E. Müller, pp. 236–251. Excerpta Medica, Amsterdam.

132. Lovinger, R. D., Connors, M. H., Kaplan, S. L., Ganong, W. F., and Grumbach, M. M. (1974): Effect of L-dihydroxyphenylalanine (L-dopa), anesthesia and surgical stress on the secretion of growth hormone in the dog. *Endocrinology,* 95:1317–1321.

133. Lucke, C., and Glick, S. M. (1971): Experimental modification of the sleep-induced peak of growth hormone secretion. *J. Clin. Endocrinol. Metab.,* 32:729–736.

134. Lutterbeck, P. M., Pryor, S., Varga, L., and Wenner, R. (1971): Treatment of non-puerperal galactorrhea with an ergot alkaloid. *Br. Med. J.,* 3:228–229.

135. Maany, I., Frantz, A., and Mendels, J. (1975): Apomorphine: Effects on growth hormone. *J. Clin. Endocrinol. Metab.,* 40:162–163.

136. MacIndoe, J. H., and Turkington, R. W. (1973): Stimulation of human prolactin secretion by intravenous infusion of l-tryptophan. *J. Clin. Invest.,* 52:1972–1978.

137. MacLeod, R. M. (1969): Influence of norepinephrine and catecholamine depleting agents on the synthesis and release of prolactin and growth hormone. *Endocrinology,* 85:916–923.

138. MacLeod, R. M., Kimura, H., and Login, I. (1976): Inhibition of prolactin secretion by dopamine and piribedil (ET-495). In: *Growth Hormone and Related*

Peptides, edited by A. Pecile and E. E. Müller, pp. 443–453. Excerpta Medica, Amsterdam.

139. MacLeod, R. M., and Lehmeyer, J. E. (1972): Regulation of the synthesis and release of prolactin. In: *Lactogenic Hormones*, edited by G. E. W. Wolstenholme and J. Knight, pp. 53–76. Churchill-Livingstone, Edinburgh.

140. Malarkey, W. B., and Daughaday, W. H. (1971): Variable response of plasma in acromegalic patients treated with medroxy progesterone acetate. *J. Clin. Endocrinol. Metab.*, 30:632–638.

141. Malarkey, W. B., and Daughaday, W. H. (1972): The influence of L-dopa and adrenergic blockade on growth hormone and prolactin secretion in the MSt TW 15 tumor-bearing rat. *Endocrinology*, 91:1314–1317.

142. Malarkey, W. B., Jacobs, L. S., and Daughaday, W. H. (1971): Levodopa suppression of prolactin in nonpuerperal galactorrhea. *N. Engl. J. Med.*, 285:1160–1163.

143. Malarkey, W. B., and Mendell, J. R. (1976): Failure of a serotonin inhibitor to effect nocturnal GH and prolactin secretion in patients with Duchenne muscular dystrophy. *J. Clin. Endocrinol. Metab.*, 43:889–892.

144. Marantz, R., Sachar, E. J., Weitzman, E., and Sassin, J. (1976): Cortisol and GH response to D- and L-amphetamine in monkeys. *Endocrinology*, 99:459–465.

145. Marek, J., and Horky, K. (1976): Bromocriptine and plasma-aldosterone. *Lancet*, 2:1409.

146. Martin, J. B. (1973): Neural regulation of growth-hormone secretion: Medical progress report. *N. Engl. J. Med.*, 288:1384–1393.

147. Martin, J. B. (1976): Brain regulation of growth hormone secretion. In: *Frontiers in Neuroendocrinology, Vol. 4*, edited by L. Martini and W. F. Ganong, pp. 129–168. Raven Press, New York.

148. Martin, J. B., and Jackson, M. D. (1975): Neural regulation of pituitary TSH and GH secretion. In: *Anatomical Neuroendocrinology, International Conference on Neurobiology of CNS-Hormone Interactions, Chapel Hill 1974*, edited by W. Stumpf and L. Grant, pp. 343–353. S. Karger, Basel.

149. Martin, J. B., Tannenbaum, G., Willoughby, J. O., Renaud, L. P., and Brazeau, P. (1975): Functions of the central nervous system in regulation of pituitary GH secretion. In: *Hypothalamic Hormones*, edited by M. Motta, P. G. Crosignani, and L. Martini, pp. 217–235. Academic Press, New York.

150. Massara, F., Camanni, F., Belforte, L., and Molinatti, G. M. (1976): Dopamine-induced inhibition of prolactin and growth hormone secretion in acromegaly. *Lancet*, 1:485.

151. McLean, B. K., and Nikitovitch-Winer, M. B. (1975): Cholinergic control of the nocturnal prolactin surge in the pseudopregnant rat. *Endocrinology*, 97:763–770.

152. McNatty, K. P., Sawers, R. S., and McNeilly, A. S. (1974): A possible role for prolactin in control of steroid secretion by the human graafian follicle. *Nature*, 250:653–655.

153. Meites, J., Nicoll, C. S., and Talwalker, P. K. (1963): The central nervous system and the secretion and release of prolactin. In: *Advances in Neuroendocrinology*, edited by A. V. Nalbandov, pp. 238–277. University of Illinois Press, Urbana, Ill.

154. Mendelson, W. B., Jacobs, L. S., Reichman, J. D., Othmer, E., Cryer, P. E., Trivedi, B., and Daughaday, W. H. (1975): Methysergide. Suppression of sleep-related prolactin secretion and enhancement of sleep-related growth hormone secretion. *J. Clin. Invest.*, 56:690–697.

155. Mioduszewski, R., Grandison, L., and Meites, J. (1976): Stimulation of prolactin release in rats by GABA. *Proc. Soc. Exp. Biol. Med.*, 151:44–46.

156. Mitchell, M. L., Suvunrungsi, P., and Sawin, C. T. (1971): Effect of propranolol on the response of serum growth hormone to glucagon. *J. Clin. Endocrinol. Metab.*, 32:470–475.

157. Mortimer, C. H., Tunbridge, W. M. G., Carr, D., Yeomans, L., Lind, T., Coy, D. H., Bloom, S. R., Kastin, A., Mallinson, C. N., Besser, G. M., Schally, A. V., and Hall, R. (1974): Effects of growth hormone release-inhibiting hormone on circulating glucagon, insulin, and growth hormone in normal, diabetic, acromegalic and hypopituitary patients. *Lancet*, 1:697.

158. Müller, E. E. (1973): Nervous control of growth hormone secretion. *Neuroendocrinology*, 11:338–369.
159. Müller, E. E., Brambilla, F., Cavagnini, F., Peracchi, M., and Panerai, A. (1974): Slight effect of l-tryptophan on growth hormone release in normal human subjects. *J. Clin. Endocrinol. Metab.*, 39:1–5.
160. Nakagawa, K., and Mashimo, K. (1973): Suppressibility of plasma growth hormone levels in acromegaly with dexamethasone and phentolamine. *J. Clin. Endocrinol. Metab.*, 37:238–246.
161. Nakai, Y., Imura, H., Sakurai, H., Kurahachi, H., and Yoshimi, T., (1974): Effect of cyproheptadine on human growth hormone secretion. *J. Clin. Endocrinol. Metab.*, 38:446–449.
162. Nilsson, K. O. (1975): Lack of effect of hyperglycemia on apomorphine induced growth hormone release in normal man. *Acta Endocrinol. (Kbh.)*, 80:230–236.
163. Ølgaard, K., Hagen, C., Madsen, S., and Hummer, L. (1976): Aldosterone and prolactin. *Lancet*, 2:959.
164. Osterman, P. O., Fagius, J., and Wide, L. (1977): Prolactin levels in the insulin tolerance test with and without pretreatment with dexamethasone. *Acta. Endocrinol. (Kbh.)*, 84:237–245.
165. Pasteels, J. L., Brauman, H., and Brauman, J. (1963): Etude comparée de la sécretion de l'hormone somatotrope par l'hypophyse humaine in vitro, et de son activité lactogénique. *C. R. Acad. Sci. [D] (Paris)*, 256:2031–2033.
166. Pepperell, R. J., Evans, J. H., Brown, J. B., Healy, D., and Burger, H. G. (1977): Serum prolactin levels and the value of bromocriptine in the treatment of anovulatory infertility. *Br. J. Obstet. Gynecol.*, 84:58–66.
167. Perez-Lopez, F. R., Delvoye, P., Denayer, P., L'Hermite, M., Roncero, M. C., and Robyn, C. (1975): Effect of methylergobasine maleate on serum gonadotropin and prolactin in humans. *Acta Endocrinol. (Kbh.)*, 79:644–657.
168. Pontiroli, A. E., Viberti, G. C., Tognetti, A., and Pozza, G. (1975): Inhibitory effect of meclastine, a specific antihistamine agent, on human growth hormone (hGH) secretion. *Acta Endocrinol. (Kbh.) [Suppl.]*, 199:289.
169. Pontiroli, A. E., Viberti, G. C., Vicari, A., and Pozza, G. (1976): Effect of the antihistaminic agents meclastine and dexchlorpheniramine in the response of human growth hormone to arginine infusion and insulin hypoglycemia. *J. Clin. Endocrinol. Metab.*, 43:582–586.
170. del Pozo, E., Brun del Re, R., and Hinselmann, M. (1975): Lack of effect of methyl-ergonovine on postpartum lactation. *Am. J. Obstet. Gynecol.*, 123:845–846.
171. del Pozo, E., Darragh, A., Lancranjan, I., Ebeling, D., Burmeister, P., Bühler, F., Marbach, P., and Braun, P. (1977): Effect of bromocriptine on the endocrine system and fetal development. *Clin. Endocrinol. (in press)*.
172. del Pozo, E., Flückiger, E., and Lancranjan, I. (1976): Endogenous control of prolactin release and its modification by drugs. In: *Basic Applications and Clinical Uses of Hypothalamic Hormones*, edited by A. Charro Salgdado, R. Fernández Durango, and J. G. Löpez del Campo, pp. 137–150. Excerpta Medica, Amsterdam.
173. del Pozo, E., Friesen, H., and Burmeister, P. (1973): Endocrine profile of a specific prolactin inhibitor: Br-ergocryptine (CB 154). A preliminary report. *Schweiz. Med. Wochenschr.*, 103:847–848.
174. del Pozo, E., Goldstein, M., Friesen, H., Brun del Re, R., and Eppenberger, U. (1975): Lack of action of prolactin suppression on the regulation of the human menstrual cycle. *Am. J. Obstet. Gynecol.*, 123:719–723.
175. del Pozo, E., and Ohnhaus, E. E. (1976): Lack of effect of acute prolactin suppression on renal water, sodium and potassium excretion during sleep. *Horm. Res.*, 7:11–15.
176. del Pozo, E., Varga, L., Schulz, K. D., Künzig, H. J., Marbach, P., López del Campo, G., and Eppenberger, U. (1975): Pituitary and ovarian response patterns to stimulation in the postpartum and in galactorrhea-amenorrhea. *Obstet. Gynecol.*, 46:539–543.
177. del Pozo, E., Varga, L., Wyss, H., Tolis, G., Friesen, H., Wenner, R., Vetter, L.,

and Uettwiler, A. (1974): Clinical and hormonal response to bromocriptine (CB 154) in the galactorrhea syndromes. *J. Clin. Endocrinol. Metab.,* 39:18–26.

178. del Pozo, E., Wyss, H., Lancranjan, I., Obolensky, W., and Varga, L. (1976): Prolactin-induced luteal insufficiency and its treatment with bromocriptine: Preliminary results. In: *Ovulation in the Human,* edited by P. G. Crosignani and D. R. Mishell, pp. 297–299. Academic Press, New York.

179. del Pozo, E., Wyss, H., Tolis, G., Lancranjan, I., Alcañiz, J., and Naftolin, F. (1977): Prolactin and inappropriate luteal function. *Am. J. Obstet. Gynecol. (in press).*

180. Prange-Hansen, A. (1971): The effect of adrenergic receptor blockade on the exercise-induced serum growth hormone rise in normals and juvenile diabetics. *J. Clin. Endocrinol. Metab.,* 33:807–812.

181. Prange-Hansen, A., Lundbeak, K., Mortimer, C. H., Besser, G. M., Hall, R., and Schally, A. V. (1975): Growth hormone release inhibiting hormone: Its action in normals, acromegalics and diabetics. In: *Hypothalamic Hormones,* edited by M. Motta, P. G. Crosignani, and L. Martini, pp. 337–345. Academic Press, New York.

182. Quadri, S. K., and Meites, J. (1973): Effect of ergocornine and CG 603 on blood prolactin and GH in rats bearing a pituitary tumor. *Proc. Soc. Exp. Biol. Med.,* 14:837–841.

183. Quik, M., and Sourkes, T. L. (1977): Central dopaminergic and serotoninergic systems in the regulation of adrenal tyrosine-hydroxylase. *J. Neurochem.,* 28:137–147.

184. Re, R. N., Kourides, I. A., Ridgway, E. C., Weintraub, B. D., and Maloof, F. (1976): The effect of glucocorticoid administration on human pituitary secretion of thyrotropin and prolactin. *J. Clin. Endocrinol. Metab.,* 43:338–346.

185. Reichlin, S. (1973): The physiology of growth hormone regulation pre and post-immunoassay eras. *Metabolism,* 22:987–993.

186. Reichlin, S. (1974): Regulation of somatotrophic hormone secretion. In: *Handbook of Physiology-Endocrinology, Vol. 4,* edited by E. Knobil and W. H. Sawyer, pp. 405–447. Williams & Wilkins, Baltimore.

187. Rivier, C., Vale, W., Ling, N., Brown, M., and Guillemin, R. (1977): Stimulation in vivo of the secretion of prolactin and growth hormone by β-endorphin. *Endocrinology,* 100:238–241.

188. Robyn, C., Vekemans, M., Delvoye, P., Joostens-Defleur, V., Caufriez, A., and L'Hermite, M. (1976): Prolactin and fertility control in women. In: *Growth Hormone and Related Peptides,* edited by A. Pecile and E. E. Müller, pp. 396–406. Excerpta Medica, Amsterdam.

189. Rolland, R., de Jong, F. H., Schellekens, L. A., and Lequin, R. M. (1975): The role of prolactin in the restoration of ovarian function during the early post-partum period in the human female. II. A study during inhibition of lactation by bromoergocryptine. *Clin. Endocrinol.,* 4:27–38.

190. Rolland, R., Schellekens, L. A., and Lequin, R. M. (1974): Successful treatment of galactorrhea and amenorrhea and subsequent restoration of ovarian function by a new ergot alkaloid 2-bromo-α-ergocryptine. *Clin. Endocrinol.,* 3:155–166.

191. Roulier, R., Mattei, A., Reuter, A., and Franchimont, P. (1976): Étude de la prolactine dans les stérilités et les hypogonadismes masculins. *Ann. Endocrinol. (Paris),* 37:285–286.

192. Rubin, A. L., Levin, S. R., Bernstein, R. I., Tyrrell, J. B., Noacco, C., and Forsham, P. H. (1973): Stimulation of growth hormone by luteinizing-hormone releasing-hormone in active acromegaly. *J. Clin. Endocrinol. Metab.,* 37:160–162.

193. Rubin, R. T., Couin, P. R., Lubin, A., Poland, R. E., and Pirke, K. M. (1975): Nocturnal increase of plasma testosterone in men: Relation to gonadotropins and prolactin. *J. Clin. Endocrinol. Metab.,* 40:1027–1033.

194. Ruch, W., Jaton, A. L., Bucher, B., Marbach, P., and Doepfner, W. (1976): Alpha adrenergic control of growth hormone in adult male rats. *Experientia,* 32:529–531.

195. Sachdev, Y., Tunbridge, W. M. G., Weightman, D. R., Gomez-Pan, A., Duns, A., and Hall, R. (1975): Bromocriptine therapy in acromegaly. *Lancet,* 13:1164–1168.

196. Saidi, K., Wenn, R. V., and Sharif, F. (1977): Bromocriptine for male infertility. *Lancet,* 1:250.
197. Schulz, K. D., del Pozo, E., Lose, K. H., Künzig, H. J., and Geiger, W. (1975): Successful treatment of mastodynia with the prolactin inhibitor bromocriptine (CB 154). *Arch. Gynäkol.,* 220:83–87.
198. Schulz, K. D., Geiger, W., del Pozo, E., and Künzig, H. J. (1977): Secretion pattern of sex steroids and gonadotropins under prolactin-inhibition in normally cycling women. *Arch. Gynäkol. (in press).*
199. Schulz, K. D., Geiger, W., del Pozo, E., Lose, K. H., Künzig, H. J., and Lancranjan I. (1976): The influence of the prolactin inhibitor bromocriptine (CB 154) on human luteal function in vivo. *Arch. Gynäkol.,* 221:93–96.
200. Schwinn, G., Schwarck, H., McIntosh, C., Milstrey, H. R., Willms, B., and Köbberling, J. (1976): Effect of the dopamine receptor blocking agent pimozide on the growth hormone response to arginine and exercise and on the spontaneous growth hormone fluctuations. *J. Clin. Endocrinol. Metab.,* 43:1183–1185.
201. Seppälä, M., Hirvonen, E., and Ranta, T. (1976): Hyperprolactinemia and luteal insufficiency. *Lancet,* 1:229–230.
202. Seppälä, M., Ranta, T., and Hirvonen, E. (1976): Bromocriptine therapy of secondary amenorrhea. *Lancet,* 1:1154–1156.
203. Serment, H., and Ruf, H. (1955): Note a propos de l'utilisation thérapeutique de la méthyl-ergobasine "per os." *Sem. Hop. Paris,* 31:2675–2676.
204. Shane, J. M., and Naftolin, F. (1974): Effect of ergonovine maleate on puerperal prolactin. *Am. J. Obstet, Gynecol.,* 120:129–131.
205. Smythe, G. A., Brandstater, J. F., and Lazarus, L. (1975): Serotoninergic control of rat growth hormone secretion. *Neuroendocrinology,* 17:245–257.
206. Smythe, G. A., Compton, P. J., and Lazarus, L. (1976): Serotoninergic control of human growth hormone secretion: The actions of L-dopa and 2-bromo-α-ergocryptine. In: *Growth Hormone and Related Peptides,* edited by A. Pecile and E. E. Müller, pp. 222–235. Excerpta Medica, Amsterdam.
207. Smythe, G. A., and Lazarus, L. (1974): Suppression of human growth hormone secretion by melatonin and cyproheptadine. *J. Clin. Invest.,* 54:116–121.
208. Tashjian, A. H., and Hoyt, R. F. (1972): Transient control of organ specific functions in pituitary cells in culture. In: *Molecular Genetics and Developmental Biology,* edited by M. Sussman, pp. 353–387. Prentice Hall, Englewood Cliffs, N.J.
209. Thorner, M. O., and Besser, G. M. (1977): Hyperprolactinemia and gonadal function: Results of bromocriptine treatment. In: *Prolactin and Human Reproduction,* edited by P. G. Crosignani. Academic Press, New York *(in press).*
210. Thorner, M. O., Chait, A., Aitken, M., Benker, G., Bloom, S. R., Mortimer, C. H., Sanders, P., Stuart Mason, A., and Besser, G. M. (1975): Bromocriptine treatment of acromegaly. *Br. Med. J.,* 1:299–303.
211. Thorner, M. O., NcNeilly, A. S., Hagen, C., and Besser, G. M. (1974): Long-term treatment of galactorrhea and hypogonadism with bromocriptine. *Br. Med. J.,* 2:419–422.
212. Tolis, G., Hickey, J., and Guyda, H. (1975): Effects of morphine on serum growth hormone, cortisol, prolactin and thyroid stimulating hormone in man. *J. Clin. Endocrinol. Metab.,* 41:797–800.
213. Tolis, G., and Naftolin, F. (1976): Induction of menstruation with bromocriptine in patients with euprolactinemic amenorrhea. *Am. J. Obstet. Gynec.,* 126:426–429.
214. Tolis, G., Pinter, E. J., and Friesen, H. G. (1975): The acute effect of 2-Bromo-α-ergocryptine (CB 154) on anterior pituitary hormones and free fatty acids in man. *Int. J. Clin. Pharmacol.,* 12:281–283.
215. Turkington, R. W. (1972): Inhibition of prolactin secretion and successful therapy of the Forbes-Albright syndrome with L-dopa. *J. Clin. Endocrinol. Metab.,* 34:306–311.
216. Turkington, R. W., Underwood, L. E., and van Wyk, J. J. (1971): Elevated serum prolactin levels after pituitary-stalk section in man. *N. Engl. J. Med.,* 285:707–710.
217. Tyson, J. E., Hwang, P., Guyda, H., and Friesen, H. G. (1972): Studies on prolactin secretion in human pregnancy. *Am. J. Obstet. Gynecol.,* 113:14–20.

218. Varga, L., Lutterbeck, P. M., Pryor, J. S., Wenner, R., and Erb, H. (1972): Suppression of puerperal lactation with an ergot alkaloid: A double-blind study. *Br. Med. J.,* 2:743–744.

219. Verde, G., Oppizzi, G., Colussi, G., Cremascoli, G., Botalla, L., Müller, E. E., Silvestrini, F., Chiodini, P. G., and Liuzzi, A. (1976): Effect of dopamine infusion on plasma levels of growth hormone in normal subjects and in acromegalic patients. *Clin. Endocrinol.,* 5:419–423.

220. Weiss, G., Klein, S., Shenkman, L., Kataoka, K., and Hollander, C. (1975): Effect of methylergonovine on puerperal prolactin secretion. *Obstet. Gynecol.,* 46: 209–210.

221. Wenner, R. (1975): Les Antiprolactins. *Act. Gynécol.,* 6:91–93.

222. Wright, A. D., McLachlan, M. S., Doyle, F. H., and Russell Fraser, T. (1969): Serum growth hormone levels and size of pituitary tumor in untreated acromegaly. *Br. Med. J.,* 4:582–584.

223. Yanai, R., and Nagasawa, H. (1974): Effect of 2-Br-α-ergocryptine on pituitary synthesis and release of prolactin and growth hormone in rats. *Horm. Metab. Res.,* 5:1–5.

224. Zacur, H. A., Chapanis, N., Lake, C. R., Ziegler, M., and Tyson, J. E. (1975): Galactorrhea-amenorrhea: Psychological interaction with neuroendocrine function. *Am. J. Obstet. Gynecol.,* 125:859–862.

225. Zárate, A., Canales, E. S., Jacobs, L. S., Maneiro, P. J., Soria, J., and Daughaday, W. H. (1973): Restoration of ovarian function in patients with the amenorrhea-galactorrhea syndrome after long-term therapy with L-dopa. *Fertil. Steril.,* 24:340–344.

226. Zárate, A., Canales, E. S., Soria, J., Garrido, J., Jacobs, L. S., and Schally, A. V. (1974): Pituitary secretory reserve in patients with amenorrhea associated with galactorrhea. *Ann. Endocrinol. (Paris),* 35:535–545.

227. Zippel, H. H., Schulz, K. D., and del Pozo, E. (1977): Morphological studies in human proliferating mammary tissues under treatment with the prolactin inhibitor Bromocriptine (CB 154). *Acta Endocrinol. (Khb.) [Suppl.],* 208:42.

Frontiers in Neuroendocrinology, Vol. 5,
edited by W. F. Ganong and L. Martini.
Raven Press, New York © 1978.

Chapter 9

Neuroendocrine Control of Gonadotropin Secretion in the Female Rhesus Monkey

E. Knobil and T. M. Plant

*Department of Physiology, University of Pittsburgh School of Medicine,
Pittsburgh, Pennsylvania 15261*

The time courses of the circulating gonadotropic hormones (LH and FSH) during the menstrual cycle of the rhesus monkey (Fig. 9–1) may be viewed as being the resultant of tonic secretion interrupted, once every 28 days on the average, by an abrupt discharge of these hypophysial hormones followed by ovulation some 36 hr later (29,43,46). These secretory patterns, which closely resemble those in the human female (39), are controlled by seemingly simple negative and positive feedback loops involving two major components: the ovary and the mediobasal hypothalamico-hypophysial apparatus. The following account represents a brief analysis of this control system.

THE OVARIAN COMPONENT OF THE CONTROL SYSTEM

The role of ovarian steroids in the feedback control of gonadotropin secretion in the rhesus monkey has been reviewed in detail previously (21,22). Ovariectomy leads to an increase in circulating gonadotropin levels which reach "steady-state" concentrations in approximately 3 weeks (3). This state is characterized by striking, pulsatile discharges of FSH and LH with a frequency of approximately one per hour (10,24). Therefore, the term "circhoral" has been used to describe this secretory mode (10). Acute closure of the open negative feedback loop by introduction of small physiologic increments in serum estrogen levels results in a prompt inhibition of pulsatile gonadotropin secretion (44) and a consequent reduction in the circulating levels of these hormones (Fig. 9–2). If plasma estrogen concentrations characteristic of those normally observed in the early follicular phase of the cycle are established chronically in ovariectomized females by subcutaneous implants of estradiol-containing Silastic capsules, mean gonadotropin levels which are also characteristic of this stage of the cycle are achieved (18). The administration of progesterone alone, however, even in enormous quantities, has no significant effect on open loop gonadotropin secretion (44). These

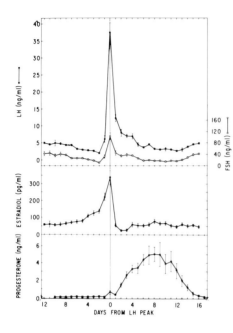

FIG. 9–1. Serum concentrations of LH, FSH, estradiol, and progesterone throughout the menstrual cycle of the rhesus monkey normalized to the day of the preovulatory gonadotropin surge (day 0). Each point represents the mean ± SE of at least 7 observations. From Knobil (21) with permission.

findings have led to the conclusion that estradiol is the principal ovarian component of the negative feedback loop which governs tonic gonadotropin secretion (20,44).

In some experimental circumstances wherein both estradiol and progesterone are administered to ovariectomized monkeys, a synergism between these two steroids in the inhibition of gonadotropin secretion can be demon-

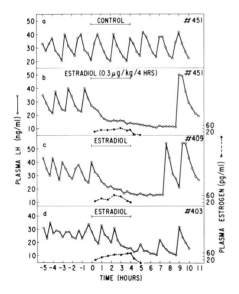

FIG. 9–2. Inhibition of circhoral LH discharges in ovariectomized rhesus monkeys by low physiologic concentrations of plasma estrogen produced with a constant intravenous infusion of estradiol beginning at 0 time. Estrogen concentrations prior to infusion were undetectable. From Yamaji et al. (44) with permission.

strated (20). The physiological significance of this interaction, however, remains obscure because such a synergism between endogenous estrogens and progesterone does not seem to obtain during the luteal phase of the menstrual cycle (11,38; Fig. 9–1). The most likely explanation for the discrepancy between these pharmacological and physiological circumstances is that the ovary normally produces a substance which prevents the negative feedback effect of progesterone.

The preovulatory gonadotropin surge is the consequence of a positive feedback action of estrogen. The effective stimulus is the incremental pattern in serum estradiol concentration which accompanies follicular maturation late in the follicular phase of the menstrual cycle (Fig. 9–1). The administration of estradiol benzoate during the early follicular phase of the cycle, in a manner to mimic this incremental pattern, results in premature gonadotropin discharges indistinguishable from those occurring normally during the menstrual cycle (45). These discharges of LH and FSH can be initiated at any time during the 24-hr day (19,43). The additional observation that estrogen administration alone readily evokes gonadotropin surges in ovariectomized (45) and in adrenalectomized-ovariectomized animals (21) suggests that other steroids are not necessary in this regard (Fig. 9–3). That this stimulatory effect of estrogen on gonadotropin secretion is not a release from negative feedback inhibition can be easily demonstrated by the subcutaneous implantation of estradiol-containing Silastic capsules, which induces characteristic gonadotropin discharges in the presence of continued, elevated serum estrogen concentrations (19). The positive feedback action of estradiol becomes manifest when a physiological increment in serum estradiol is sustained for approximately 36 hr (Fig. 9–4). This rather striking latency can be foreshort-

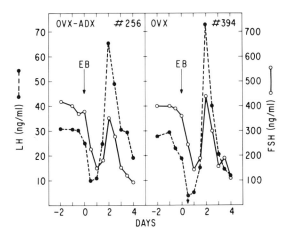

FIG. 9–3. The induction of gonadotropin surges following the subcutaneous injection of estradiol benzoate (EB) (42µg/kg BW) on day 0 in an adrenalectomized-ovariectomized (OVX-ADX) and an ovariectomized (OVX) rhesus monkey. From Knobil (21) with permission.

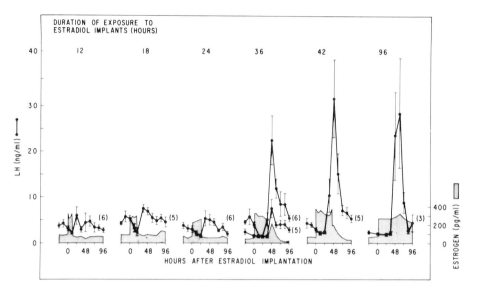

FIG. 9–4. Relationship between the duration of an increment in circulating estrogen and the induction of LH surges in intact rhesus monkeys. The stippled areas designate the mean serum estrogen concentrations before, during, and after the imposition of an estrogen increment by the subcutaneous implantation of estradiol-containing Silastic capsules at 0 time, on day 3 of the menstrual cycle. Each point on the LH curve represents the mean ± SE of the numbers of observations shown in parentheses. Characteristic LH discharges were induced even when the estrogen stimulus was maintained for the entire duration of the surge. From Karsch et al. (19) with permission.

ened somewhat by grossly supraphysiological elevations in serum estradiol (19). These characteristics of the positive feedback action of estradiol have been confirmed in the human female (37,48).

As may be predicted from the foregoing, the time course of gonadotropin secretion observed during the entire menstrual cycle can be replicated experimentally in ovariectomized animals by superimposing increments in serum estradiol concentration, produced by the injection of estradiol benzoate, on the constant levels of the steroid released from Silastic capsules (Fig. 9–5). These observations permit the conclusion that the time courses of LH and FSH secretion throughout the menstrual cycle are controlled by the cyclic pattern of ovarian estrogen secretion during the cycle and that the ovary may be considered as the "Zeitgeber" for the timing of ovulation in the rhesus monkey (18).

THE NEURAL COMPONENT OF THE CONTROL SYSTEM

In the rhesus monkey, as in the rat (41), luteinizing hormone releasing hormone (LRH) plays an essential role in the control of gonadotropin secretion. Placement of large radiofrequency lesions in the mediobasal hypothalamus (MBH) of ovariectomized monkeys, which do not infarct the adenohy-

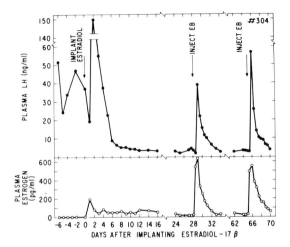

FIG. 9–5. Replication of the secretory pattern of LH, as observed during the menstrual cycle, in an ovariectomized rhesus monkey by superimposing increments in circulating estrogen levels (subcutaneous injections of estradiol benzoate at arrow) upon constant estrogen concentrations achieved by a subcutaneous estradiol-containing Silastic capsule implanted on day 0. From Karsch et al. (18) with permission.

pophysis, results in a profound and permanent inhibition of LH and FSH secretion (35). Passive immunization of ovariectomized animals with specific antisera to LRH (28) produces a similar, albeit transient and less pronounced, inhibition of gonadotropin secretion (Fig. 9–6). Immunoreactive LRH has been demonstrated in the hypothalamus (4,49) and in hypophysial portal blood (9,33) of the rhesus monkey, and, although the macaques seem to be less responsive than other species to single injections of the synthetic decapeptide (2,12,25,27,30), this peculiarity of the genus appears to be of quantitative rather than qualitative significance.

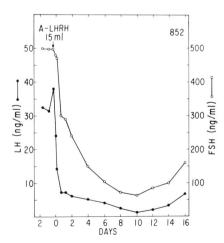

FIG. 9–6. Abrupt suppression of serum LH and FSH concentrations in an ovariectomized rhesus monkey following a single intravenous injection, on day 0, of a specific antiserum to LRH (A-LHRH). From McCormack et al. (28) with permission.

That the release of LRH in the monkey is, at least in part, under the control of catecholaminergic neurons is suggested by the finding that in ovariectomized animals single intravenous injections of α-adrenergic blocking agents, which have been reported not to inhibit pituitary responsiveness to exogenous LRH (42), are followed within minutes by a cessation of pulsatile gonadotropin discharges and a resultant fall in the plasma concentration of these hormones (5). This finding further suggests that the signals which initiate the circhoral pulsatile discharges of gonadotropin originate within the CNS. In this regard, Carmel et al. (9) have reported that the concentration of immunoreactive LRH in pituitary stalk blood from ovariectomized monkeys appears to fluctuate with a frequency not incompatible with that of circhoral LH oscillations in the peripheral circulation (10). On the other hand, the same group of workers has also described a single experiment in which pulsatile LH release was seen following pituitary stalk section, and intercalation of a Silastic barrier, in an ovariectomized animal receiving a constant infusion of LRH (13). The latter observation suggests that the signal for circhoral release of gonadotropin originates within the pituitary itself, but it is difficult to conceive of an integrating mechanism, resident within the hypophysis, which could cause the synchronous discharge of gonadotropins by a vast number of adenohypophysial cells.

In the rhesus monkey, as in the rat (6,15,16), the neural component of the control system which governs tonic gonadotropin secretion is resident in the MBH. Complete surgical disconnection of this structure from the remainder of the brain does not significantly interfere with either the circhoral discharges of LH and FSH or the negative feedback inhibition of their secretion by estradiol (24).

In striking contrast to its effect in the rat (7,15,16,32), however, surgical disconnection of the MBH in the monkey does not appear to interfere with the initiation of estrogen-induced gonadotropin surges nor with spontaneous ovulatory discharges of LH and FSH (24). The MBH "islands" produced in the monkey (Fig. 9–7) were judged to be complete by examination of serial coronal sections of the hypothalamus and were anatomically similar to those described by Halasz and others in the rat (7,15,16). They included the median eminence and arcuate nucleus as well as portions of the ventromedial nucleus, the premamillary region, and the mamillary bodies, but not the suprachiasmatic nucleus and preoptic area. It was concluded from these observations that the neural components of the control system which govern the preovulatory gonadotropin surge in the rhesus monkey are also located within the MBH (24).

This conclusion was difficult to reconcile with the interpretation by Norman et al. (34) of their finding that some lesions in the rostral hypothalamus of the rhesus monkey blocked the positive feedback action of estradiol on gonadotropin release. These lesions caused extensive bilateral damage of the ventromedial preoptic area–anterior hypothalamic area (POA-AHA). Thus,

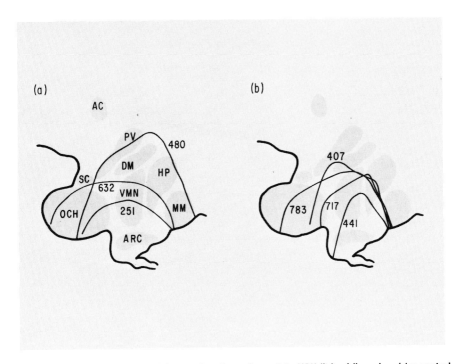

FIG. 9–7. Reconstructions, from serial coronal sections, of complete MBH "islands" produced by surgical disconnection in 7 intact female rhesus monkeys superimposed on diagrammatic parasagittal sections of the hypothalamus, in whom (a) spontaneous and (b) estradiol benzoate-induced gonadotropin surges were observed. The numbers identify individual animals. Hypothalamic nuclei: ARC, arcuate; DM, dorsomedial; VMN, ventromedial; HP, posterior hypothalamic; PV, paraventricular; SC, suprachiasmatic; MM, mamillary body. The optic chiasm and anterior commissure are labeled OCH and AC, respectively. From Krey et al. (24) with permission.

they differed from the complete surgical disconnections described above which left this region of the brain essentially intact. It should be noted, however, that following anterior surgical disconnection of the MBH in female rhesus monkeys extensive areas of necrosis were produced in the POA and AHA without interfering with the positive feedback action of estradiol (24). In addition, corpora lutea or elevated serum progesterone levels were observed in two of the animals studied by Norman et al. (34) several months after placement of bilateral lesions in the POA-AHA. The authors suggested these sequelae of ovulation may be a consequence of "neural reorganization" (34).

The possibility remained, however, that in response to an elevation in estradiol, the ventromedial POA-AHA could produce a neurotransmitter, or LRH itself, which was then transported to the MBH by a non-neural pathway. The recent description of LRH in the organum vasculosum of the lamina terminalis (OVLT) in the rhesus monkey (33,49) provided substance to such speculation. Alternatively, in response to estradiol, the ventromedial POA-

AHA could generate a neural signal that is relayed to the MBH by nerve fibers capable of rapid functional regeneration. If nerve regeneration is the explanation for the continued functioning of the pituitary-ovarian axis in monkeys with MBH "islands," one may wonder why such regeneration should be limited to nerve fibers involved in the control of estrogen-induced gonadotropin discharges since abnormalities in cortisol, thyroxine, and growth hormone secretion as well as unremitting diabetes insipidus, which are also observed in these animals, persist (8,24,26).

These alternative explanations were directly addressed by aspirating all neural tissue dorsal and anterior to the optic chiasm, including the OVLT and the suprachiasmatic nucleus, in a series of ovariectomized female monkeys, and examining the capacity of these preparations to discharge LH and FSH in response to the positive feedback action of estrogen (17). The MBH "peninsulas" that remained following decerebration were continuous with the brainstem and contained the median eminence, arcuate nucleus, mamillary bodies, and varying portions of the ventromedial, dorsomedial, supraoptic, and paraventricular nuclei (Fig. 9–8). The administration of estradiol benzoate, immediately upon completion of the ablation procedure, resulted in massive gonadotropin discharges 18 to 24 hr later (Fig. 9–9). Since there is no reason to believe that the mechanisms underlying estradiol-induced gonadotropin discharges in monkeys with MBH "peninsulas" differ from those in animals with intact nervous systems, it must be concluded that the positive feedback action of this steroid is demonstrable in the absence of any neural or neurohumoral inputs from regions anterior to the MBH.

(a)

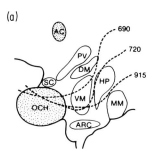

(b)

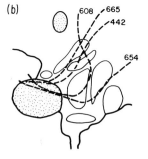

FIG. 9–8. Reconstructions, from serial coronal sections, of the MBH "peninsulas" produced by aspiration in 3 estrogen-treated (a) and 4 control (b) ovariectomized rhesus monkeys superimposed on diagrammatic parasagittal sections of the hypothalamus. The dashed lines demarcate the anterior and dorsal limits of the residual neural tissue. Hypothalamic nuclei as in Fig. 9–7. From Hess et al. (17).

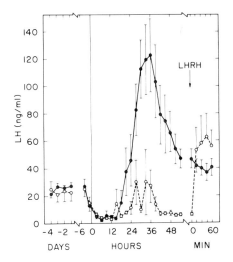

FIG. 9–9. Time courses of serum LH concentrations before and after ablation of all neural tissue rostral to the MBH in 4 estrogen treated (●—●) and 4 control (○—○) monkeys. The completion of the ablation procedure and the simultaneous administration of estradiol benzoate at time 0 are indicated by the vertical line. The severe surgical procedure resulted in a transient inhibition of LH secretion. The intravenous administration of LRH (LHRH), indicated by the arrow, immediately prior to the termination of the experiments induced a release of gonadotropin in the control animals but not in the estrogen-treated group. Each point represents the mean ± SE of 4 observations. FSH responded in like manner. From Hess et al. (17).

We have also attempted to repeat the experiments of Norman et al. (34) by placing radiofrequency lesions in the ventromedial POA-AHA of four intact female monkeys but without the aid of intraventricular radiopaque dyes (36). These lesions extended from the lamina terminalis to the caudal aspect of the optic chiasm and encompassed the suprachiasmatic nucleus and, with one exception, all of the OVLT. Laterally, they extended from midline

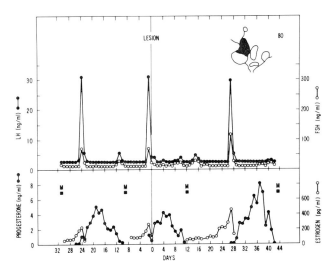

FIG. 9–10. Time courses of serum gonadotropins and ovarian steroid hormones in an intact rhesus monkey before and after placement of a large radiofrequency lesion in the ventromedial POA-AHA on day 0. The reconstruction of the lesion from serial coronal sections of the brain is superimposed on a diagrammatic parasagittal section of the hypothalamus. Note that a spontaneous gonadotropin surge, followed by ovulation, occurred at the appropriate time after the placement of this large lesion. Menstrual periods are indicated by M. For identity of hypothalamic nuclei see Fig. 9–7.

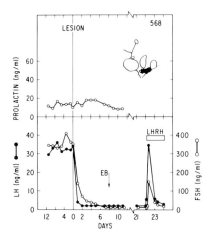

FIG. 9–11. Reduction in serum LH and FSH concentrations and abolition of the positive feedback action of estradiol in an ovariectomized rhesus monkey following placement of a radiofrequency lesion (on day 0) in the arcuate region and the dorsal aspect of the posterior median-eminence. The injection of estradiol benzoate (42 μg/kg BW) on day 8 is indicated by the arrow. The continuous intravenous infusion of LRH (*horizontal bar*) at a dose of 6.8 μg/hr resulted in a transient discharge of gonadotropic hormones. Note that this lesion did not result in a rise in serum prolactin levels.

toward the medial aspects of the supraoptic nuclei. In the dorsoventral plane, the area of destruction reached from the superior surface of the optic chiasm to within approximately 2 mm of the anterior commissure. In one of these animals, a spontaneous ovulatory gonadotropin surge was observed 27 days after placement of the lesion (Fig. 9–10). In two of the other three lesioned animals, characteristic surges of LH and FSH were elicited in response to the injection of estradiol benzoate 1 to 2 months after surgery. Although the remaining animal failed to respond to the positive feedback action of estradiol, so did one of five control animals given repeated injections of estradiol benzoate. We are currently unable to provide a compelling explanation for the discrepancy between our own studies and the observations reported by Normal et al. (34).

That the arcuate nucleus is the primary structure within the MBH responsible for the hypothalamic control of both tonic and surge gonadotropin secretion in the rhesus monkey is suggested by the findings (35) that placement of relatively discrete radiofrequency lesions in the arcuate region of ovariectomized animals caused a rapid fall in serum LH and FSH to undetectable levels and abolished the positive feedback action of estradiol (Fig. 9–11). Placement of larger lesions, which only partially destroyed the arcuate region (10 to 60%), had lesser effects (Fig. 9–12). When the arcuate region was spared entirely by the lesions, LH and FSH secretion did not differ from control (35). The striking deficits in gonadotropin secretion that follow the placement of lesions in the arcuate region cannot be attributed to a generalized reduction in hypophysiotropic stimulation because basal adrenocortical and thyroid function did not appear to be grossly influenced, growth hormone discharge in response to insulin hypoglycemia was not abolished, and elevations in prolactin secretion were not observed (35). The finding that relatively discrete lesions of the arcuate region, which abolish gonadotropin secretion in the rhesus monkey, do not influence basal serum prolactin levels

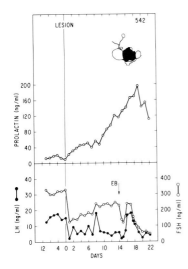

FIG. 9–12. Time courses of serum LH, FSH, and prolactin concentrations in an ovariectomized rhesus monkey before and after placement of a large radiofrequency lesion in the MBH that spared the ventral aspects of the arcuate region. An injection of estradiol benzoate (42 μg/kg BW) on day 14 is indicated by the arrow. Note that gonadotropin secretion was only partially suppressed while circulating prolactin levels increased.

suggests that the areas of the MBH involved in the regulation of gonadotropin release and those which control prolactin secretion are anatomically distinct in this species. It seems reasonable to conclude that the seemingly specific abolition of gonadotropin secretion following arcuate lesions is the consequence of damage to neurons that either secrete LRH or control the secretion of this releasing factor. Whether the majority of the perikarya of these neurons reside primarily within the region of the arcuate nucleus or whether their axons course through this region to the median eminence cannot be definitively answered at present. Although perikarya containing immunoreactive LRH have been identified in the arcuate nucleus of the rhesus monkey, such cell bodies are also diffusely distributed throughout the hypothalamus of this species (4,49).

SITES OF THE FEEDBACK ACTIONS OF ESTRADIOL

The feedback actions of estradiol on gonadotropin secretion may occur at the level of the MBH, there controlling LRH release, or at the level of the adenohypophysis, there modulating the response of the gonadotrophs to hypophysiotropic stimulation, or at both of these levels.

Ferin et al. (14) observed that the pulsatile LH secretion in ovariectomized monkeys was inhibited by the microinjection of estradiol at various sites in the hypothalamus. These same workers, however, later reported that acute intravenous injections of estradiol did not suppress immunoreactive LRH levels in pituitary portal blood (9). Similarly, Neill and his colleagues (33) were unable to detect significant differences between the concentrations of LRH in portal blood collected from ovariectomized animals and from females in the early follicular phase of the cycle. Elevated levels of LRH were observed, however, in animals undergoing estrogen-induced gonadotropin surges, which led Neill et al. (33) to suggest that the positive action of estradiol is exerted primarily at the neural level. On the other hand, less direct evidence based on the augmentation of the gonadotropin response to LRH administration in women (47,48) has suggested that the principal site of the positive action of estrogen may be at the level of the pituitary (48).

This problem has recently been reexamined in ovariectomized rhesus monkeys bearing hypothalamic lesions, which abolish gonadotropin secretion, but in whom essentially normal production of LH and FSH was reestablished by the chronic administration of synthetic LRH (31). Initial attempts to restore gonadotropin secretion in such animals by the continuous intravenous infusion of LRH were markedly unsuccessful. This replacement regimen, while causing an immediate discharge of LH and FSH for 24 to 36 hr, did not result in a sustained elevation of these hormones despite the continued administration of the decapeptide. Unaccountably, the pituitary seemed to become refractory to the sustained hypophysiotropic stimulus with a resultant fall in serum gonadotropins to undetectable levels (Fig. 9–11). When the LRH was administered in a pulsatile mode, however, using constant infusion pumps programmed to deliver a 6-min pulse once per hour, serum LH and FSH concentrations gradually rose from undetectable levels to approximately those observed during the prelesion control period. The administration of estradiol

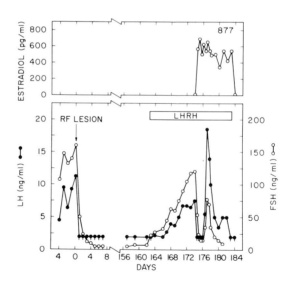

FIG. 9–13. Cessation of tonic gonadotropin secretion in an ovariectomized rhesus monkey by placement of a radiofrequency lesion in the arcuate region on day 0, and its subsequent restoration by a chronic intermittent intravenous infusion of synthetic LRH (horizontal bar) initiated on day 162 (1 μg/min for 6 min every hour). The subcutaneous implantation of estradiol-containing Silastic capsules 12 days later (day 174) resulted in an abrupt decline of LH and FSH levels followed by a discharge of these hormones. The time course of this biphasic gonadotropin response to estrogen administration was similar to that observed in an ovariectomized animal with an intact central nervous system (see Fig. 9–3).

to such animals, while continuing the LRH replacement, resulted in a profound decline in circulating gonadotropin levels followed by an unambiguous discharge of LH and FSH (Fig. 9–13). The time course of this biphasic pattern of gonadotropin secretion is remarkably similar to that observed in response to the negative and positive feedback actions of estradiol in otherwise intact ovariectomized animals (Fig. 9–3). Since endogenous LRH production is abolished in this experimental preparation, the results demonstrate that, in the rhesus monkey, estradiol can exert both its negative and positive feedback actions on LH and FSH secretion at the level of the pituitary gland. However, the experiments do not exclude feedback actions of the steroid at the neural level in the context of a more physiological setting.

These findings are in harmony with our earlier observations that passive immunization with antisera to LRH (28) and administration of a variety of neuroactive drugs (21), both of which inhibit tonic gonadotropin secretion (see above) and block ovulation in the rat (1,23,40), do not interfere with estradiol-induced gonadotropin surges in the rhesus monkey.

CONCLUSION

In the rhesus monkey both the tonic and surge modes of gonadotropin secretion are primarily controlled by the negative and positive feedback actions of estradiol on the mediobasal hypothalamico-hypophysial unit. The neural component of this control system is expressed by the secretion of LRH, a function which appears to require the structural integrity of the arcuate nucleus. The feedback actions of estrogen, which result in both inhibition and discharge of the gonadotropins can, however, be exerted solely at the level of the pituitary gland.

ACKNOWLEDGMENTS

The work conducted in this laboratory has been generously supported by grants from the National Institutes of Health and the Ford Foundation. Dr. Plant is a Postdoctoral Research Fellow of the National Institute of Child Health and Human Development.

REFERENCES

1. Arimura, A., Debeljuk, L., and Schally, A. V. (1974): Blockade of the preovulatory surge of LH and FSH and of ovulation by anti-LH-RH serum in rats. *Endocrinology,* 95:323–325.
2. Arimura, A., Spies, H. G., and Schally, A. V. (1973): Relative insensitivity of rhesus monkeys to the LH-releasing hormone (LH-RH). *J. Clin. Endocrinol. Metab.,* 36:372–374.
3. Atkinson, L. E., Bhattacharya, A. N., Monroe, S. E., Dierschke, D. J., and Knobil, E. (1970): Effects of gonadectomy on plasma LH concentrations in the rhesus monkey. *Endocrinology,* 87:847–849.

4. Barry, J., Giiud, C., and Dubois, M. P. (1975): Topographie des neurones elaborateurs de LRF chez les primates. *Bull Assoc. Anat.,* 59:103–110.
5. Bhattacharya, A. N., Dierschke, D. J., Yamaji, T., and Knobil, E. (1972): The pharmacologic blockade of the circhoral mode of LH secretion in the ovariectomized rhesus monkey. *Endocrinology,* 90:778–786.
6. Blake, C. A., and Sawyer, C. H. (1974): Effects of hypothalamic deafferentation on the pulsatile rhythm in plasma concentrations of luteinizing hormone in ovariectomized rats. *Endocrinology,* 94:730–736.
7. Blake, C. A., Weiner, R. I., Gorski, R. A., and Sawyer, C. H. (1972): Secretion of pituitary luteinizing hormone and follicle stimulating hormone in female rats made persistently estrous or diestrous by hypothalamic deafferentation. *Endocrinology,* 90:855–861.
8. Butler, W. R., Krey, L. C., Espinosa-Campos, J., and Knobil, E. (1975): Surgical disconnection of the medial basal hypothalamus and pituitary function in the rhesus monkey. III. Thyroxine secretion. *Endocrinology,* 96:1094–1098.
9. Carmel, P. W., Araki, S., and Ferin, M. (1976): Pituitary stalk portal blood collection in rhesus monkeys: Evidence for pulsatile release of gonadotropin-releasing hormone (GnRH). *Endocrinology,* 99:243–248.
10. Dierschke, D. J., Bhattacharya, A. N., Atkinson, L. E., and Knobil, E. (1970): Circhoral oscillations of plasma LH levels in the ovariectomized rhesus monkey. *Endocrinology,* 87:850–853.
11. Dierschke, D. J., Yamaji, T., Karsch, F. J., Weick, R. F., Weiss, G., and Knobil, E. (1973): Blockade by progesterone of estrogen-induced LH and FSH release in the rhesus monkey. *Endocrinology,* 92:1496–1501.
12. Ehara, Y., Ryan, K. J., and Yen, S. S. C. (1972): Insensitivity of synthetic LRF in LH-release of rhesus monkeys. *Contraception,* 6:465–478.
13. Ferin, M., Carmel, P. W., and Vande Wiele, R. L. (1974): The neuroendocrine regulation of LH secretion by estrogens in rhesus monkeys. *Adv. Biosci.,* 15:223–234.
14. Ferin, M., Carmel, P. W., Zimmerman, E. A., Warren, M., Perez, R., and Vande Wiele, R. L. (1974): Location of intrahypothalamic estrogen-responsive sites influencing LH secretion in the female rhesus monkey. *Endocrinology,* 95:1059–1068.
15. Halasz, B., and Gorski, R. A. (1967): Gonadotrophic hormone secretion in female rats after partial or total interruption of neural afferents to the medial basal hypothalamus. *Endocrinology,* 80:608–622.
16. Halasz, B., and Pupp, L. (1965): Hormone secretion of the anterior pituitary gland after physical interruption of all nervous pathways to the hypophysiotrophic area. *Endocrinology,* 77:553–562.
17. Hess, D. L., Wilkins, R. H., Moossy, J., Chang, J. L., Plant, T. M., McCormack, J. T., Nakai, Y., and Knobil, E. (1977): Estrogen-induced gonadotropin surges in decerebrated female rhesus monkeys with medial basal hypothalamic peninsulae. *Endocrinology* (in press).
18. Karsch, F. J., Dierschke, D. J., Weick, R. F., Yamaji, T., Hotchkiss, J., and Knobil, E. (1973): Positive and negative feedback control by estrogen of luteinizing hormone secretion in the rhesus monkey. *Endocrinology,* 92:799–804.
19. Karsch, F. J., Weick, R. F., Butler, W. R., Dierschke, D. J., Krey, L. C., Weiss, G., Hotchkiss, J., Yamaji, T., and Knobil, E. (1973): Induced LH surges in the rhesus monkey: Strength-duration characteristics of the estrogen stimulus. *Endocrinology,* 92:1740–1747.
20. Karsch, F. J., Weick, R. F., Hotchkiss, J., Dierschke, D. J., and Knobil, E. (1973): An analysis of the negative feedback control of gonadotropin secretion utilizing chronic implantation of ovarian steroids in ovariectomized rhesus monkeys. *Endocrinology,* 93:478–486.
21. Knobil, E. (1974): On the control of gonadotropin secretion in the rhesus monkey. *Recent Prog. Horm. Res.,* 30:1–36.
22. Knobil, E., Dierschke, D. J., Yamaji, T., Karsch, F. J., Hotchkiss, J., and Weick, R. F. (1972): Role of estrogen in the positive and negative control of LH secretion during the menstrual cycle of the rhesus monkey. In: *Gonadotropins,* edited by

B. B. Saxena, G. G. Belling, and H. M. Gandy, pp. 72–86. John Wiley & Sons, New York.

23. Koch, Y., Chobsieng, P., Zor, U., Fridkin, M., and Lindner, H. R. (1973): Suppression of gonadotropin secretion and prevention of ovulation in the rat by antiserum to synthetic gonadotropin releasing hormone. *Biochem. Biophys. Res. Commun.*, 55:623–629.

24. Krey, L. C., Butler, W. R., and Knobil, E. (1975): Surgical disconnection of the medial basal hypothalamus and pituitary function in the rhesus monkey. I. Gonadotropin secretion. *Endocrinology*, 96:1073–1087.

25. Krey, L. C., Butler, W. R., Weiss, G., Weick, R. F., Dierschke, D. J., and Knobil, E. (1973): Influences of endogenous and exogenous gonadal steroids on the actions of synthetic LRF in the rhesus monkey. In: *Hypothalamic Hypophysiotropic Hormones*, edited by C. Gual and E. Rosemberg, pp. 39–47. Excerpta Medica, Amsterdam.

26. Krey, L. C., Lu, K.-H., Butler, W. R., Hotchkiss, J., Piva, F., and Knobil, E. (1975): Surgical disconnection of the medial basal hypothalamus and pituitary function in the rhesus monkey. II. GH and cortisol secretion. *Endocrinology*, 96:1088–1093.

27. Levitan, D., Beitins, I. Z., Milton, G., Barnes, A., and McArthur, J. W. (1977): Insensitivity of bonnet monkeys to (D-Ala^6, Des-Gly^{10}) LHRH ethylamide, a potent new luteinizing hormone releasing hormone analogue in rats and mice. *Endocrinology*, 100:918–922.

28. McCormack, J. T., Plant, T. M., Hess, D. L., and Knobil, E. (1977): The effect of luteinizing hormone releasing hormone (LHRH) antiserum administration on gonadotropin secretion in the rhesus monkey. *Endocrinology*, 100:663–667.

29. Monroe, S. E., Atkinson, L. E., and Knobil, E. (1970): Patterns of circulating luteinizing hormone and their relation to plasma progesterone levels during the menstrual cycle of the rhesus monkey. *Endocrinology*, 87:453–455.

30. Mori, J., and Hafez, E. S. E. (1973): Release of LH by synthetic LH-RH in the monkey, *Macaca fascicularis*. *J. Reprod. Fertil.*, 34:155–157.

31. Nakai, Y., Plant, T. M., Hess, D. L., Keogh, E. J., and Knobil, E. (1977): On the sites of the negative and positive feedback actions of estradiol in the control of gonadotropin secretion in the rhesus monkey. Presented at 59th Annual Meeting of the Endocrine Society. Abstract #298.

32. Neill, J. D. (1972): Sexual differences in the hypothalamic regulation of prolactin secretion. *Endocrinology*, 90:1154–1159.

33. Neill, J. D., Patton, J. M., Dailey, R. A., Tsou, R. C., and Tindall, G. T. (1977): Luteinizing hormone releasing hormone (LHRH) in pituitary stalk blood of rhesus monkeys: relationship to level of LH release. *Endocrinology*, 101:430–434.

34. Norman, R. L., Resko, J. A., and Spies, H. G. (1976): The anterior hypothalamus: How it affects gonadotropin secretion in the rhesus monkey. *Endocrinology*, 99:59–71.

35. Plant, T. M., Krey, L. C., Moossy, J., McCormack, J. T., Hess, D. L., and Knobil, E. (1978): The arcuate nucleus and the control of gonadotropin and prolactin secretion in the female rhesus monkey (*Macaca mulatta*). *Endocrinology (in press)*.

36. Plant, T. M., Moossy, J., Hess, D. L., Nakai, Y., McCormack, J. T., and Knobil, E. (1977): The rostral hypothalamus and gonadotropin secretion in the rhesus monkey. Proceedings of the Annual Meeting of the Society for Study of Reproduction, Austin, Texas.

37. Reiter, E. V., Kulin, H. E., and Hamwood, S. M. (1974): The absence of positive feedback between estrogen and luteinizing hormone in sexually immature girls. *Pediatr. Res.*, 8:740–745.

38. Resko, J. A., Norman, R. L., Niswender, G. D., and Spies, H. G. (1974): The relationship between progestins and gonadotropins during the late luteal phase of the menstrual cycle in rhesus monkeys. *Endocrinology*, 94:128–135.

39. Ross, G. T., Cargille, C. M., Lipsett, M. B., Rayford, P. L., Marshall, J. R., Strott, C. A., and Rodbad, D. (1970): Pituitary and gonadal hormones in women during spontaneous and induced ovulatory cycles. *Recent Prog. Horm. Res.*, 26:1–48.

40. Sawyer, C. A. (1969): Regulatory mechanisms of secretion of gonadotrophic hor-

mones. In: *The Hypothalamus,* edited by W. Haymaker, E. Anderson, and W. J. H. Nauta, pp. 389–430. Charles C. Thomas, Springfield, Ill.

41. Sawyer, C. H. (1975): Some recent developments in brain-pituitary-ovarian physiology. *Neuroendocrinology,* 17:97–124.
42. Spies, H. G., and Norman, R. L. (1975): Interaction of estradiol and LHRH on LH release in rhesus females: Evidence for a neural site of action. *Endocrinology,* 97:685–692.
43. Weick, R. F., Dierschke, D. J., Karsch, F. J., Butler, W. R., Hotchkiss, J., and Knobil, E. (1973): Periovulatory time courses of circulating gonadotropic and ovarian hormones in the rhesus monkey. *Endocrinology,* 93:1140–1147.
44. Yamaji, T., Dierschke, D. J., Bhattacharya, A. N., and Knobil, E. (1972): The negative feedback control by estradiol and progesterone of LH secretion in the ovariectomized rhesus monkey. *Endocrinology,* 90:771–777.
45. Yamaji, T., Dierschke, D. J., Hotchkiss, J., Bhattacharya, A. N., Surve, A. H., and Knobil, E. (1971): Estrogen induction of LH release in the rhesus monkey. *Endocrinology,* 89:1034–1041.
46. Yamaji, T., Peckham, W. D., Atkinson, L. E., Dierschke, D. J., and Knobil, E. (1973): Radioimmunoassay of rhesus monkey follicle-stimulating hormone (RhFSH). *Endocrinology,* 92:1652–1659.
47. Yen, S. S. C., Lasley, B. L., Wang, C. F., Leblanc, H., and Siler, T. M. (1975): The operating characteristics of the hypothalamic-pituitary system during the menstrual cycle and observations of biological action of somatostatin. *Recent Prog. Horm. Res.,* 31:321–357.
48. Young, J. R., and Jaffe, R. B. (1976): Strength-duration characteristics of estrogen effects on gonadotropin response to gonadotropin releasing hormone in women. II. Effects of varying concentrations of estradiol. *J. Clin. Endocrinol. Metab.,* 42:432–442.
49. Zimmerman, E. A., and Antunes, J. L. (1976): Organization of the hypothalamic-pituitary system: Current concepts from immunohistochemical studies. *J. Histochem. Cytochem.,* 24:807–815.

Frontiers in Neuroendocrinology, Vol. 5,
edited by W. F. Ganong and L. Martini.
Raven Press, New York © 1978.

Chapter 10

The Role of the Autonomic Nervous System and Somatostatin in the Control of Insulin and Glucagon Secretion

*John E. Gerich and Mara Lorenzi

*Metabolic Research Unit, University of California,
San Francisco, California 94143*

Modulation of glucose homeostasis during perturbations of the internal and external environment is an important function of the autonomic nervous system (29,54,89,129). Innervation of the liver (160) and of glucose-consuming tissues such as muscle (10) as well as neurally mediated changes in blood flow (102) are no doubt involved in this process. Additionally, there is mounting evidence (149,162,186) that both the sympathetic and the parasympathetic nervous system may affect glucose homeostasis by directly altering pancreatic A and B cell secretion of glucagon and insulin—major glucoregulatory hormones (172). The secretion of somatostatin, a peptide originally isolated from the hypothalamus (174) and now recognized to be a normal secretory product of pancreatic D cells (68), also appears to be under autonomic control (8,157). The facts that this peptide inhibits the release of insulin and glucagon under a variety of conditions when administered exogenously (68), that it has a half-life less than 1 min, and that it has not been detected in the general circulation suggest that it may function as a local regulator of insulin and glucagon secretion. Although data on pancreatic D cell function are still limited, this review will attempt to summarize the actions of the autonomic nervous system on the secretion of insulin, glucagon, and somatostatin keeping in mind the possibility that islet somatostatin may modify or mediate some of the actions of the autonomic nervous system on insulin and glucagon release.

FUNCTIONAL ORGANIZATION OF PANCREATIC ISLETS

Numerous cell types are found within pancreatic islets (50); in most mammalian species, however, A cells containing glucagon, B cells containing insulin, and D cells containing somatostatin account for more than 95% of the cells present. Immunohistochemical studies in rat and man (136) indicate these cells normally constitute about 20, 70, and 10% of the islet cell mass,

---

* Present address: Diabetes and Metabolism Research Laboratory, Mayo Medical School and Mayo Clinic, Rochester, Minnesota 55901.

respectively, and are not distributed randomly in islets (Fig. 10–1, *left*): A cells occur at the periphery closely associated with D cells and occasional B cells; the center of the islet is occupied by B cells with only rare A and D cells. This organization has prompted the suggestion (137) that islets may contain two functionally distinct regions—a heterocellular "cortex" containing A, B, and D cells where vascular and neural elements are prominent and a homocellular "medulla" containing mainly B cells. The heterocellular component could be a dynamic region where inhibition of glucagon release by insulin (74) and of insulin release by insulin (98) may be mediated by D cells. The most conspicuous disruption of this organization of islet cells occurs in diabetic animals and man (136,143) (Fig. 10–1, *right*): B cells and insulin release are diminished; there is an increase in A and D cells. Release of glucagon is excessive (173), but the secretory profile of the increased D cell population is not as yet known. Indeed, the accumulation of somatostatin in diabetic islets may indicate impaired somatostatin release which might contribute to the overabundant glucagon secretion in diabetes.

NORMAL   DIABETIC

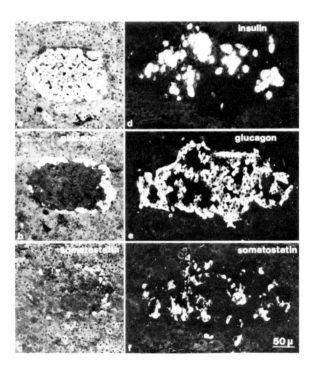

FIG. 10–1. Distribution of A, B, and D cells in pancreases from normal rats (a, b, c) and rats made diabetic with streptozotocin (d, e, f). Fluorescein-labeled antiserum. Magnification in (d, e, f) greater than in (a, b, c.) Courtesy of L. Orci (136).

Most studies (68) have failed to find a clear difference in sensitivity of A and B cells to inhibitory effects of somatostatin. Nevertheless, the asymmetric distribution of D cells in close proximity to A cells (136) suggests that somatostatin may exert a more dominant influence on glucagon release. The recent finding (144) that glucagon but not insulin augments somatostatin release from canine pancreases perfused *in vitro* supports the notion that somatostatin may function as part of a negative feedback of glucagon on glucagon release. Furthermore, this peptide may mediate the suppressive action of glucose on glucagon release (70) since glucose stimulates somatostatin secretion (158). The most convincing evidence to date that endogenous somatostatin functions as a local regulator of pancreatic islet hormone secretion is the demonstration that antisomatostatin serum when incubated with cultured rat islets causes a 10-fold increase in glucagon release; under the same conditions insulin release is not enhanced (9). This provides support for a more important role of somatostatin in governing A cell function than B cell function. However, A and B cells differ in their sensitivity to somatostatin depending on the intensity of their stimulation (76), the particular secretogogues employed (44,69), and the prevailing neural input to these cells.

The mechanism by which somatostatin inhibits insulin and glucagon release is not yet known. Release of each hormone to all known secretogogues is at least partially if not totally blocked by somatostatin both *in vivo* and *in vitro* (68). Like other polypeptide hormones, somatostatin presumably binds initially to cell membrane receptors. However, as yet, no such receptors have been demonstrated. Indeed, the presence of gap junctions between islet cells (134) and the recent report of a cytosol protein which binds somatostatin (133) suggest that the peptide may act intracellularly after transmission through gap junctions from adjacent cells without first binding cell surface receptors.

Originally it was thought that somatostatin might inhibit pancreatic hormone release by diminishing islet cAMP levels since the characteristic increase of islet cAMP accompanying glucose-induced insulin release was not observed in presence of somatostatin (43). Subsequent work has cast doubt on this mechanism since islet hormone responses to cAMP itself are prevented by somatostatin (166), and glucagon-stimulated insulin release is inhibited by somatostatin without its altering glucagon activation of adenylate cyclase (159). Presently it seems more likely that somatostatin inhibits insulin and glucagon release by interfering with some aspect of islet calcium metabolism. Release of both these hormones is calcium dependent (71). During hormone secretion, calcium efflux from islets transiently decreases (117) and calcium uptake by islets increases (23). This is thought to result in an increase in the intraislet free calcium concentration which triggers or at least modulates islet hormone release (86). Somatostatin diminishes islet calcium uptake (14, 135); elevation of extracellular calcium concentration (14,39,59) or addition of the divalent cation ionophore A23187 (60) has been reported to at least partially restore the inhibition of insulin and glucagon secretion due to somatostatin. However, not all intraislet calcium compartments are involved in hormone secretion (87), and alterations in islet calcium uptake have not been determined during reversal of somatostatin inhibition by the divalent cation ionophore and by augmentation of extracellular calcium. Moreover, since somatostatin diminishes the electrical activity of pancreatic islets which usually accompanies insulin release (139), this action could represent its prime mechanism for inhibiting hormone secretion.

INNERVATION OF PANCREATIC ISLETS

Islet innervation has been recently reviewed (162,186). Nerves to the pancreas contain preganglionic parasympathetic fibers from the dorsal trunk of

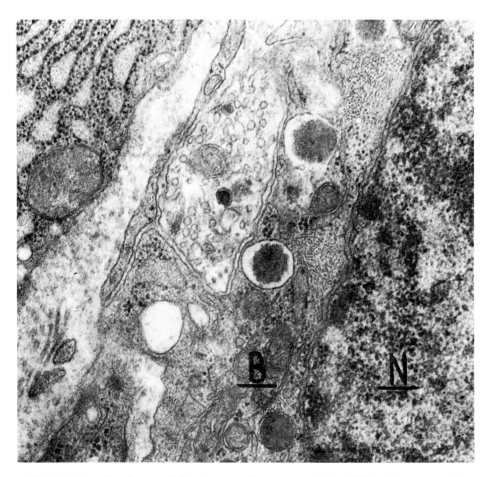

FIG. 10–2. Nerve fiber (*upper center*) in close opposition to pancreatic B cell (B) in rabbit pancreas. N, nucleus of B cell. Courtesy of T. Ban (7).

the vagus nerve and postganglionic sympathetic fibers from the greater and middle splanchnic nerves which originate in the celiac and superior mesenteric plexuses (20,107). Afferent fibers arising within the pancreas may reach the spinal cord and higher centers along these same pathways, but little information is available on this subject. Although nerve terminals have been observed at the periphery of islets, it is generally thought that most fibers enter the islets accompanying blood vessels (37). Both myelinated and nonmyelinated fibers are found, but the latter type usually predominates (11). The presence of both cholinergic and adrenergic nerve fibers within islets has been established by fluorescence microscopy (30,49), autoradiography (47,48), and enzymatic histochemistry (37,48). Thus certain nerve terminals have been shown to contain cholinesterase (37,48), whereas others contain catecholamines (30,49) or take up injected catecholamine precursors (47,48). Ultrastructural studies have identified three types of nerve terminals (162): cholinergic with 30 to 50 nm agranular vesicles; adrenergic with 30 to 50 nm dense-cored structures; and a third distinct but as yet uncharacterized type with 60 to 200 nm dense-cored vesicles. Ratios of cholinergic and adrenergic endings vary with species, but these data must be viewed as only semiquantitative. No selective association of nerve terminals with a particular cell type has been found; sometimes more than one type of nerve ending is seen associated with the same cell (48,109).

Figure 10–2 illustrates a typical synapse between an autonomic nerve fiber and a B cell. Gap junctions have been observed between nerve endings and islet cells (138). Since such areas have low electrical resistance and allow passage of low molecular weight substances, conceivably electrical as well as chemical signals may affect islet cell secretion. Moreover, since gap junctions exist between islet cells themselves (134), these cells could behave as a syncitium whereby discrete electrical signals could be multiplied and transmitted rapidly throughout the whole islet. Some nerve terminals end "en distance" (109) without any islet cell nearby. Release of neurotransmitters from these endings into the islet intercellular space could conceivably affect a number of islet cells.

EFFECTS OF NEUROTRANSMITTERS ON PANCREATIC ISLET CELL FUNCTION

Norepinephrine and acetylcholine, the neurohormones of the sympathetic and parasympathetic nervous system, and epinephrine, the principal catecholamine of the adrenal medulla, have been shown to alter insulin and glucagon secretion under a variety of conditions. Recent preliminary studies indicate that these neurohormones may also affect somatostatin secretion (157). Other neurotransmitters such as dopamine and serotonin alter A and B cell secretion (114,151), and dopamine has been found in the circulation at concentrations similar to those of norepinephrine (35). However, since neither dopamine nor serotonin occurs in endings within pancreatic islets and since they appear to function as intracellular modulators rather than as neuro-transmitters in this tissue, they are not discussed further.

Catecholamines

Effects of Epinephrine and Norepinephrine

Coore and Randle (36) first demonstrated that epinephrine inhibited glu-cose-induced insulin release from slices of rabbit pancreas; this and a similar action of norepinephrine have been repeatedly confirmed in other *in vitro* systems (27,28,97,157,178). Both these catecholamines inhibit insulin re-lease *in vivo* when infused into man or other species (31,62,72,94,146,153). Leclercq-Meyer and co-workers (111) first reported that epinephrine in-creased glucagon release from isolated rat pancreatic islets. Shortly thereafter, Gerich and his colleagues (72) (Fig. 10–3) demonstrated that infusion of epinephrine simultaneously stimulated glucagon release and inhibited insulin secretion in man. These results have been confirmed in the dog (97) and rat (168,177). Data concerning the effects of catecholamines on somatostatin se-cretion are limited; in one study (158) epinephrine was reported to inhibit somatostatin release from isolated rat islets during stimulation by glucose.

Although the concentration of norepinephrine released at nerve terminals is unknown, most of the above studies have employed amounts of norepi-nephrine and epinephrine which are likely to exceed the circulating levels of these catecholamines found even in the most stressful situations (33,38). In one study (31), however, epinephrine infused at a rate of 3 ng/kg/min caused a 50% reduction of insulin responses to infused glucose. This dose might produce plasma levels similar to the ones observed in man under certain

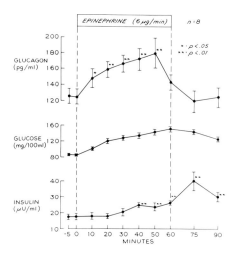

FIG. 10–3. Stimulation of glucagon secretion and inhibition of insulin response to concurrent hyper-glycemia during infusion of epinephrine in man. From Gerich et al. (72).

conditions. No similar data are available for epinephrine-induced glucagon secretion. At present the relative importance of circulating catecholamines of
adrenal origin versus neurogenous norepinephrine acting locally on islet hormone secretion remains to be clarified.

Synthetic Adrenergic Receptor Agonists and Antagonists

There are two general categories of catecholamine receptors whose activation usually causes effects in a given tissue—alpha- and beta-adrenergic receptors (2). The latter have recently been subdivided into beta$_1$ and beta$_2$
types (99). The availability of synthetic adrenergic agonists and antagonists
with varying specificities for the different receptors has provided a means of
evaluating the receptor mechanism by which catecholamines alter islet hormone release. Alpha-adrenergic blocking agents such as phentolamine reverse
inhibition of insulin release by epinephrine (62,94,97,119,146,153) and
norepinephrine (97,119), whereas alpha-adrenergic agonists such as methoxamine inhibit insulin release (73,146). Isoproterenol, a relatively pure beta-
adrenergic agonist, stimulates insulin (73,94,97,108,115) and glucagon release (72,97,108). The stimulation is reversed by propranolol (73), a highly
specific beta receptor blocker, and is unaffected by phentolamine. Epinephrine
stimulation of glucagon release in the dog (97) and man (75) is also blocked
by propranolol.

Isoproterenol has recently been reported to stimulate somatostatin release
from perfused dog pancreases (157); this action was prevented by simultaneous infusion of propranolol, and thus a beta-adrenergic mechanism seems
likely. However, since insulin (158) and glucagon (144) have been reported
to stimulate somatostatin release, it is unclear whether these results indicate a
direct action of isoproterenol on D cells or an indirect effect mediated by
enhanced release of insulin and glucagon. Somatostatin itself inhibits insulin
and glucagon responses to isoproterenol (76) and to epinephrine (75,178).

Whether glucagon release is affected by alpha-adrenergic mechanisms is
controversial at the present time. In the duck (170) activation of these receptors was reported to stimulate glucagon release. In the dog no evidence
was found for the presence of alpha receptors on A cells (97). In man (73),
however, phentolamine blocked suppression of circulating glucagon levels
due to infusion of methoxamine and itself caused a rise in plasma glucagon.
These results suggest that in man A and B cells behave similarly with respect
to alpha- and beta-adrenergic receptors.

Studies employing adrenergic antagonist have provided evidence that
endogenous catecholamines modulate insulin and glucagon secretion in man.
Infusion of phentolamine increases circulating insulin and glucagon in man
fasted overnight, whereas infusion of propranolol has the opposite effect
(73,153). These data suggest that alpha-adrenergic tone down-modulates release of these hormones while beta-adrenergic tone simultaneously up-regu-

lates secretion. It should be pointed out, however, that infusions of alpha- or beta-adrenergic blockers have been reported not to affect circulating insulin and glucagon levels in humans fasted for 60 hr (176), and no differences in insulin responses to glucose have been found in adrenalectomized or sympathectomized individuals (24). Furthermore, adrenergic receptor antagonists are not totally specific in their actions (61,99).

Mechanism of Action

Stimulation of beta-adrenergic receptors elevates pancreatic islet cAMP levels through activation of adenylate cyclase, whereas stimulation of alpha-adrenergic receptors lowers islet cAMP levels (6,110,118,130,169). It is generally accepted that augmentation of islet hormone release owing to beta receptor activation is due to elevation of islet cAMP levels (70), but doubt has arisen about the mechanism whereby alpha-adrenergic receptor activation inhibits islet hormone release (148). Simultaneous inhibitory and stimulatory effects of mixed adrenergic agents are difficult to explain solely on the basis of alterations in cAMP levels, and there are quantitative inconsistencies between the effects of epinephrine on islet hormone release and its diminution of islet cAMP levels (130). Exogenous cAMP does not reverse inhibition of insulin release by epinephrine (118). Islets previously exposed to epinephrine exhibit increased insulin responses to subsequent stimulation by acetylcholine (28). Since this increase is dependent on the prevailing extracellular calcium concentration during exposure to epinephrine (27) and since epinephrine has been reported to increase calcium efflux (22) and to decrease calcium uptake by pancreatic islets (120), alpha-adrenergic inhibition of insulin release may primarily involve alteration of islet calcium metabolism rather than diminution of intracellular cAMP levels. This is supported by the fact that a calcium ionophore (183) can reverse epinephrine inhibition of insulin release *in vitro*. It must be emphasized, however, that the respective roles of calcium and cAMP in insulin release are poorly understood (76), as are the interactions of adrenergic agents and calcium (163).

Acetylcholine and Parasympathomimetic Agents

Acetylcholine augments insulin (27,28,96,97,119,170) and glucagon (96,97,170) release *in vitro* through activation of muscarinic receptors, since these hormonal responses are blocked by atropine. At low glucose concentrations, acetylcholine evokes little insulin release. However, it is an effective stimulant of glucagon secretion over a wide range of glucose levels, its effect being more pronounced at low glucose levels (96). Metacholine, a synthetic analogue of acetylcholine, increases fasting insulin levels in the dog (105) and man (103). Atropine, although not affecting basal insulin levels (147), has been reported to diminish insulin responses to oral but not intravenous glucose (88). In various species basal glucagon levels (20,107) and glucagon responses to intravenous arginine (20) and to insulin-induced hypoglycemia (19,20) are diminished by atropine. In one study (157), acetylcholine diminished somatostatin release from perfused dog pancreases. This observation raises the possibility that acetylcholine augments insulin and glucagon secretion partially through deinhibition (i.e., decreasing the influence of adjacent D cells). The molecular events mediating cholinergic effects on islet hormone release are not known; but, as in other tissues (66,78,93), elevation of islet cGMP may be involved.

PERIPHERAL NERVE STIMULATION AND DENERVATION

There is now substantial evidence that direct as well as indirect manipulation of neural input to the pancreas results in alterations of immunoreactive insulin and glucagon secretion (for review see 186); no similar data are presently available for somatostatin release. The effect of alterations in systemic glucose levels on efferent discharges of vagal fibers innervating the pancreas and of splanchnic nerve fibers innervating the adrenal has been studied by Niijima (131,132). Both intracarotid and intravenous infusions of glucose (but not mannose) decrease adrenal nerve discharges and increase vagal discharges; opposite effects are seen during hypoglycemia (insulin administration) and intracellular glucopenia (2-deoxyglucose infusion). Transsection of the spinal cord at the level of T_5 and bilateral transsection of the cervical vagi abolishes these changes in adrenal nerves and pancreatic vagal branches, respectively. These results provide further evidence for glucose-sensitive areas within the central nervous system (4,5,141,161,165) and for efferent pathways modulating adrenal (79) and pancreatic hormone secretion.

Electrical stimulation of pancreatic nerves containing both sympathetic and parasympathetic fibers augments insulin and glucagon secretion in the dog (122,147). Atropinization inhibits these insulin responses but has no effect on glucagon responses which are nevertheless suppressible by hyperglycemia. These observations suggest that the augmentation of insulin release following pancreatic nerve stimulation is almost exclusively parasympathetic and that the augmentation of glucagon release involves a sympathetic mechanism. A parasympathetic influence on glucagon release is not necessarily excluded, since such an effect might not be apparent due to simultaneous sympathetic stimulation.

Electrical stimulation of the vagus—either branch in the neck and the dorsal trunk in the abdomen—increases circulating insulin levels in the dog (12,58,106,107) and baboon (41). This response is prevented by atropine. Similar effects have been observed following vagal stimulation of a perfused rabbit pancreas (52), indicating that insulin secretion is affected directly at the pancreatic level. Circulating glucagon levels are augmented during electrical stimulation of the thoracic vagus (105) and dorsal trunk of the sub-diaphragmatic vagus (107). Unfortunately, no comparable studies of soma-tostatin release have been performed.

Section of the vagus nerve has yielded variable results. After acute va-gotomy, a transient decrease in fasting serum insulin levels unaccompanied by impairment of insulin responses to intravenous glucose has been observed in the dog (58); nevertheless, in various species chronically vagotomized, fasting insulin (20,81,155) and glucagon (20,155) levels are normal. In rats vagotomy decreases insulin responses to oral but not intravenous glucose (81); in man diminished insulin responses to oral glucose in patients with truncal vagotomy compared to those with selective vagotomy have been re-ported (155). Additionally, impaired insulin release during stress hyper-glycemia (125) and elimination of conditioned insulin release (184) have been reported in vagotomized animals suggesting that parasympathetic modu-lation of insulin secretion is not limited to meal-related phenomena. Gluca-gon responses to insulin-induced hypoglycemia are diminished by vagotomy in the calf (19), and in patients with truncal vagotomy compared to those with selective vagotomy (20).

Electrical stimulation of splanchnic nerves carrying sympathetic fibers to pancreatic islets increases both insulin and glucagon release in intact dogs (104) and in adrenalectomized calves (18) independent of changes in pan-creatic blood flow. Presumably glucagon released under these conditions pro-vides an explanation for the glycogenolysis found in adrenalectomized calves after splanchnic nerve stimulation (42). Pretreatment with atropine does not alter hormonal responses to splanchnic nerve stimulation, but pretreatment with propranolol diminishes insulin release (184). In these same studies glucagon responses to splanchnic nerve stimulation were reported as being uninfluenced by either alpha- or beta-adrenergic receptor blockade. However, the marked changes in arterial glucose levels make these results difficult to interpret in view of the extreme sensitivity of the pancreatic A cell to altera-tions in glucose levels (70). Chemical stimulation of sympathetic nerve terminals with scorpion toxin (101) causes release of norepinephrine from perfused rat pancreases associated with augmentation of glucagon secretion. The latter is blocked by somatostatin and phentolamine as well as by pro-pranolol. Thus, local catecholamine release as observed in perfused dog pan-creases following abrupt diminution of the perfusate glucose concentration to hypoglycemic levels (34) may provide a partial explanation for the charac-teristic release of glucagon during hypoglycemia (77). However, only minor diminution in glucagon responses to hypoglycemia was found after section of splanchnic nerves in adrenalectomized calves (19). Moreover, normal glu-cagon responses to hypoglycemia have been reported in adrenalectomized man (46) and in traumatically sympathectomized patients with complete cervical cord transsection (140). These observations need not exclude a role of the sympathetic system in mediating A cell responses to hypoglycemia since there is evidence that low spinal sympathetic reflexes may be involved (79,124). Nevertheless, in one study (176) neither alpha- nor beta-adrenergic blockade altered glucagon responses to hypoglycemia. Thus, the sympathetic nervous system may play some role in mediating glucagon responses to hypoglycemia, but clearly it is not an essential one.

In contrast to this, section of splanchnic nerves has provided clear evidence for a role of the sympathetic nervous system in inhibiting insulin release during hypoglycemia (126). When pancreases of dogs made hypoglycemic by functional hepatectomy were cross-perfused with blood having elevated glucose concentrations, markedly diminished insulin responses were found. Section of splanchnic nerves of hepatectomized animals restored normal insulin responses.

ROLE OF THE CENTRAL NERVOUS SYSTEM

The hypothalamus is often regarded as the integrative center for autonomic homeostatic responses (8,129). Descending sympathetic pathways originating in the medial preoptic area and medial hypothalamus are believed to reach the spinal medulla via the dorsal longitudinal fasciculus (7). Synapses in the intermediolateral column of the spinal cord between segments T_1 and L_2 give rise to preganglionic nerve fibers which end either in ganglia of the sympathetic chain or in peripheral ganglia lying within the abdominal cavity (112). Descending parasympathetic pathways may originate either in the parasympathetic area A (septal region, preoptic stratum, and hypothalamic periventricular stratum) or in the parasympathetic area C (septal region, lateral preoptic area, and lateral hypothalamic area) (7). The stria medullaris and medial forebrain bundle, which connects the lateral preoptic area and lateral hypothalamus with the rhinencephalon, midbrain, and pontine tegmentum, are believed to participate in the parasympathetic function of the hypothalamus. Preganglionic parasympathetic fibers which synapse in ganglia within the pancreas arise in the dorsal nucleus of the vagus in the floor of the fourth ventricle (128) and are carried to the pancreas in the vagus nerve.

Little information is available regarding afferent autonomic pathways to the hypothalamus. However, there is evidence for the presence of "glucoreceptors" (4,5,132,141,161) and also of insulin-sensitive areas (32,141,165, 187) within the hypothalamus so that direct chemical or humoral influences on hypothalamic autonomic centers may result in efferent signals to the endocrine pancreas. For example, hyperglycemia caused by intravenous glucose infusion increases the frequency of neuronal electrical activity in the medial hypothalamus and decreases neuronal electrical activity in the lateral hypothalamus. Insulin-induced hypoglycemia causes the opposite alterations of neuronal electrical activity in these areas (4). Whether such changes occur in hypothalamic autonomic neurons has not been established, but it seems likely in view of concomitant changes in the electrical discharges of splanchnic nerves and the vagus under similar conditions (132).

More than 100 years ago Claude Bernard demonstrated that puncture of the floor of the fourth ventricle resulted in hyperglycemia and glycosuria in dogs (13). Although these studies may be considered the first evidence for participation of central nervous system in glucose homeostasis, they could not identify intervening hormonal mechanisms. More recently electrical stimulation of discrete areas of the central nervous system (40,56,57) has been shown to alter insulin and glucagon secretion. In a series of elegant studies, Frohman and Bernardis (56) found that electrical stimulation of the rat ventromedial hypothalamus (VMH) results in hyperglycemia, increased plasma glucagon levels, and suppression of insulin release. Prior adrenalectomy did not affect the immediate hyperglycemic and glucagon responses but did prevent the inhibition of insulin release, suggesting that sympathetic discharge of adrenomedullary catecholamines had suppressed pancreatic B cell function and that direct neural action on pancreatic A cells had caused release of glucagon. Nevertheless, neither central administration of 6-hydroxydopamine nor intraperitoneal injection of alpha- and beta-adrenergic blocking agents altered glucose and pancreatic hormonal responses to VMH stimulation (57). The reasons for this failure to confirm sympathetic mediation of metabolic-hormonal responses to VMH stimulation are unclear but may involve differences in the accessibility of postjunctional receptors to locally discharged neurotransmitters and exogenously administered antagonists. Few data are available on the hormonal effects of electrical stimulation of the ventrolateral hypothalamus (VLH). Immediate fasting insulin levels appear unaffected (56,164), but later, in conjunction with induction of compulsive food intake, hyperglycemia and excessive insulin responses occur (164). There is morphologic evidence for alterations of pancreatic D cell function following stimulation of VMH and VLH in the rat (8). As shown in Fig. 10–4, VMH stimulation results in margination of somatostatin-containing granules along the D cell plasma membrane and diminution of the total number of cytoplasmic granules—changes usually associated with increased hormone secretion. VLH stimulation causes accumulation of granules suggesting suppressed secretory activity. These alterations are consistent with the recent studies of Samols and colleagues (157) indicating sympathetic stimulatory and parasympathetic inhibitory influences on somatostatin release from canine pancreases perfused *in vitro*.

Specific structures in the ventromedial hypothalamus probably function as a "satiety center," which may oppose the activity of the "feeding center" located in the ventrolateral hypothalamus (3,8). Lateral hypothalamic lesions are generally followed by aphagia and loss of body weight (3,167). Destruction of ventromedial hypothalamic nuclei in adult rats is accompanied by obesity, hyperphagia, and increased glucose and insulin levels (3,53,82–

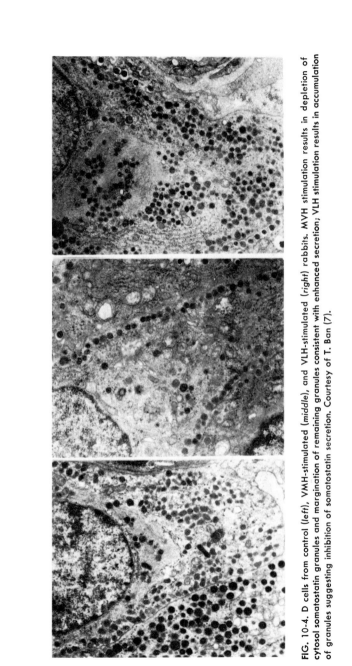

FIG. 10-4. D cells from control (*left*), VMH-stimulated (*middle*), and VLH-stimulated (*right*) rabbits. MVH stimulation results in depletion of cytosol somatostatin granules and margination of remaining granules consistent with enhanced secretion; VLH stimulation results in accumulation of granules suggesting inhibition of somatostatin secretion. Courtesy of T. Ban (7).

84,123). Insulin responses to such maneuvers have been difficult to interpret due to the different feeding patterns observed; for example, it is unclear whether the hyperinsulinism that accompanies VMH destruction has an etiologic role in the development of the characteristic obesity or whether it represents a mere consequence of the hyperphagia and tissue resistance due to weight gain (95). Recent evidence (55,92,150) attributes a causative role to neurally induced changes in insulin secretion in the development of the syndrome, especially since obesity and hyperinsulinism do not develop after subdiaphragmatic vagotomy (150). This observation suggests an important role for the VMH in regulation of insulin secretion: the destruction of the VMH may "disinhibit" lateral hypothalamic activity with consequent activation of parasympathetic pathways leading to augmented release of insulin. No data exist concerning the effects of destructive lesions of the VMH and VLH on glucagon and somatostatin secretion.

POTENTIAL AUTONOMIC INFLUENCE ON PANCREATIC A, B, AND D CELL FUNCTION IN CERTAIN PATHOPHYSIOLOGIC SITUATIONS

Intake of Nutrients

Hunger (80), anticipation of a meal (142), and sham-feeding (90) induce insulin secretion. This probably occurs via a vagal (parasympathetic) pathway since similar conditioned insulin responses are blocked by vagotomy or atropinization (184,185) and may be physiologically important in the disposal of meals. Ingestion of glucose elicits a greater and more sustained insulin response than comparable hyperglycemia caused by intravenous glucose administration (45). The "potentiating" factors are probably insulinotropic enterohormones (70) released by a local reflex effect of glucose involving a vagal mechanism; atropine (88) and nonselective vagotomy (81,155) diminish insulin responses to oral glucose but not to intravenous glucose. Part of this vagally mediated enhancement of insulin release could be due to diminution of inhibitory pancreatic D cell influence since acetylcholine has been reported to block somatostatin release *in vitro* (157). Excessive vagal stimulation might contribute to the syndrome of reactive hypoglycemia; anticholinergic drugs depress insulin secretion and normalize the glycemic response to oral glucose in these patients (145,175). The role of the sympathetic nervous system in hormonal responses to nutrient intake is unclear. Chronic adrenergic insufficiency due to either bilateral adrenalectomy or cervical sympathectomy is not associated with abnormalities in glucose-induced insulin release in man (24), whereas in rats functional sympathectomy of pancreatic islets with 6-hydroxydopamine results in glucose intolerance, diminished insulin responses to oral glucose, and impaired insulin release from pancreatic islets *in vitro* despite normal islet insulin content (26).

Postabsorptive State and Starvation

Mobilization of substrates from endogenous stores during fasting involves diminution of insulin release and augmented glucagon secretion (1,121). The role of the sympathetic nervous system in these hormonal responses is controversial (25,176). Augmented sympathetic activity, inferred from increased urinary excretion of catecholamines during starvation (33), could conceivably impair insulin release while sensitizing pancreatic A cells to small decrements in glucose levels (73,153). The failure of adrenergic blockers to modify plasma glucagon and insulin levels during 72 hr of starvation (176) and the unaffected substrate responses in fasted sympathectomized man (25) argue against this hypothesis. However, alpha-adrenergic blockade has been reported to increase basal insulin levels in overnight fasted man (153) and to reverse diminished insulin responses to glucose observed after prolonged fasting (127). A possible parasympathetic contribution to the maintenance of basal glucagon levels in fasted man has been suggested (20), but its role is unclear since there is no evidence that vagotomy diminishes tolerance to fasting. Furthermore, basal insulin levels are not affected after this procedure (20,81,155). The interplay of autonomic-induced changes in endogenous somatostatin release with the other pancreatic hormones in a concerted adjustment to caloric deprivation awaits investigation.

Stress

Stress states, whether psychological or physical, are associated with activation of the sympathetic and parasympathetic systems. Characteristic changes in A cell (15) and B cell function (15,70,148) occur which foster the mobilization of endogenous substrates. Thus in various species and under both experimental or spontaneous conditions, exercise (21,51,63,64,85,116), trauma (113), surgery (11,156), burns (182), infection (67,152,154), myocardial infarction (180), anoxia (100,148), hypoglycemia (65,77,91, 176), uncontrolled diabetes mellitus (171), pain (16), and anxiety (17) have all been reported to induce a state of relative or absolute insulin deficiency and glucagon excess. The involvement of the autonomic nervous system in mediating these hormonal responses seems likely, but in very few instances is firm evidence available. However, an adrenergic contribution to exercise-induced hyperglucagonemia (64,85,116) and suppression of insulin release in hypoglycemia (179) and trauma (181) have been established. So has a parasympathetic contribution to glucagon stimulation by hypoglycemia (20). No data are available concerning alterations in pancreatic D cell function in these conditions.

SUMMARY AND CONCLUSIONS

Autonomic innervation to A, B, and D cells of pancreatic islets and the ability of exogenous and endogenous autonomic neurotransmitters to affect insulin and glucagon release are firmly established. Data on the influence of the autonomic nervous system on somatostatin secretion are presently limited and its possible local mediation of sympathetic and parasympathetic effects on insulin and glucagon release is intriguing but still speculative. There is evidence that alterations in glucose availability can initiate neural signals from the central nervous system to the pancreas which subsequently modify islet hormone secretion. However, autonomic influences in conditions other than those associated primarily with changes in glucose availability are not firmly established, and the pathophysiologic significance to the organism as a whole of such regulation remains to be critically evaluated.

ACKNOWLEDGMENTS

This study was supported in part by funds provided by the Bureau of Medicine and Surgery, Navy Department, for CI 6–48–859; and in part by grants from the Susan Greenwall Foundation of New York City; the Levi J. and Mary Skaggs Foundation, Oakland, California; the Ellis L. Phillips Foundation of Jericho, New York; and by USPHS grant AM 1276(05).

REFERENCES

1. Aguilar-Parada, E., Eisentraut, A., and Unger, R. (1969): Effects of starvation on plasma pancreatic glucagon in normal man. *Diabetes,* 18:717–723.
2. Ahlquist, R. (1948): A study of adrenotropic receptors. *Am. J. Physiol.,* 153:586–600.
3. Anand, B., and Brobeck, J. (1951): Hypothalamic control of food intake in rats and cats. *Yale J. Biol. Med.,* 24:123–140.
4. Anand, B., Chhina, G., Sharma, K., Dua, S., and Singh, B. (1964): Activity of single neurons in the hypothalamic feeding centers: Effect of glucose. *Am. J. Physiol.,* 207:1146–1154.
5. Anand, B., Dua, S., and Singh, B. (1961): Electrical activity of the hypothalamic feeding centers under the effect of changes in blood chemistry. *Electroencephalogr. Clin. Neurophysiol.,* 13:54–59.
6. Atkins, T., and Matty, A. (1971): Adenyl cyclase and phosphodiesterase activity in the isolated islets of Langerhans of obese mice and their lean litter mates: The effect of glucose, adrenaline and drugs on adenyl cyclase activity. *J. Endocrinol.,* 51:67–78.
7. Ban, T. (1966): The septo-preoptico-hypothalamic system and its autonomic function. *Prog. Brain Res.,* 21:1–43.
8. Ban, T. (1975): Fiber connections in the hypothalamus and some autonomic functions. *Pharmacol. Biochem. Behav.,* 3 (Suppl. 1):3–13.
9. Barden, N., Lavoie, M., Alvarado-Urbina, G., Cote, J., and Dupont, A. (1977): A physiologic role of somatostatin in the control of insulin and glucagon secretion. *Fed. Proc.,* 36:298.
10. Bass, A., and Hudlicka, O. (1960): Utilization of oxygen, glucose, unesterified fatty acids, carbon dioxide, and lactic acid in normal and denervated muscle in situ. *Physiol. Bohemoslov.,* 9:401–407.
11. Benscome, S. (1959): Studies on the terminal autonomic nervous system with special reference to the pancreatic islets. *Lab. Invest.,* 8:629–646.
12. Bergman, R., and Miller, R. (1973): Direct enhancement of insulin secretion by vagal stimulation of the isolated pancreas. *Am. J. Physiol.,* 225:481–486.

13. Bernard, C. (1849): Chiens rendus diabetiques. *C. R. Soc. Biol. (Paris)*, 1:60–78.
14. Bhathena, S., Perrino, P., Voyles, N., Smith, S., Wilkins, S., Coy, D., Schally, A., and Recant, L. (1976): Reversal of somatostatin inhibition of insulin and glucagon secretion. *Diabetes*, 25:1031–1040.
15. Bloom, S. (1973): Glucagon, a stress hormone. *Postgrad. Med. J.*, 49 (Suppl. 1): 607–611.
16. Bloom, S., Daniel, P., Johnston, D., Ogawa, O., and Pratt, O. (1972): Changes in glucagon level associated with anxiety or stress. *Psychol. Med.*, 2:426–427.
17. Bloom, S., Daniel, P., Johnston, D., Ogawa, O., and Pratt, O. (1973): Release of glucagon, induced by stress. *Q. J. Exp. Physiol.*, 58:99–108.
18. Bloom, S., Edwards, A., and Vaughan, N. (1973): The role of the sympathetic innervation in the control of plasma glucagon concentration in the calf. *J. Physiol. (Lond.)*, 233:457–466.
19. Bloom, S., Edwards, A., and Vaughan, N. (1974): The role of the autonomic innervation in the control of glucagon release during hypoglycemia in the calf. *J. Physiol. (Lond.)*, 236:611–623.
20. Bloom, S., Vaughan, N., and Russell, R. (1974): Vagal control of glucagon release in man. *Lancet*, 2:546–549.
21. Böttger, I., Schlein, E., Faloona, G., Knochel, J., and Unger, R. (1972): The effect of exercise on glucagon secretion. *J. Clin. Endocrinol. Metab.*, 35:117–125.
22. Brisson, G., and Malaisse, W. (1973): The stimulus-secretion coupling of glucose-induced insulin release. XI. Effects of theophylline and epinephrine on ^{45}Ca efflux from perfused islets. *Metabolism*, 22:455–465.
23. Brisson, G., Malaisse-Lagae, F., and Malaisse, W. (1972): The stimulus-secretion coupling of glucose-induced insulin release. VII. A proposed site of action for adenosine-3′,5′-cyclic monophosphate. *J. Clin. Invest.*, 51:232–241.
24. Brodows, R., Pi-Sunyer, F., and Campbell, R. (1974): Insulin secretion in adrenergic insufficiency in man. *J. Clin. Endocrinol. Metab.*, 38:1103–1108.
25. Brodows, R., Campbell, R., Al-Aziz, A., and Pi-Sunyer, F. (1976): Lack of central autonomic regulation of substrate during early fasting in man. *Metabolism*, 25:803–807.
26. Burr, I., Jackson, A., Culbert, S., Sharp, P., Felts, P., and Olson, W. (1974): Glucose intolerance and impaired insulin release following 6-hydroxydopamine administration in intact rats. *Endocrinology*, 94:1072–1076.
27. Burr, I., Slonim, A., Burke, V., and Fletcher, T. (1976): Extracellular calcium and adrenergic and cholinergic effects on islet beta cell function. *Am. J. Physiol.*, 231:1246–1249.
28. Burr, I., Slonim, A., and Sharp, R. (1976): Interactions of acetylcholine and epinephrine on the dynamics of insulin release in vitro. *J. Clin. Invest.*, 58:230–239.
29. Cannon, W., Newton, H., Bright, E., Menkin, V., and Moore, R. (1929): Some aspects of the physiology of animals surviving complete exclusion of sympathetic nerve impulses. *Am. J. Physiol.*, 89:84–107.
30. Cegrell, L. (1968): Adrenergic nerves and monoamine containing cells in the mammalian endocrine pancreas. *Acta Physiol. Scand. [Suppl.]*, 314:17–23.
31. Cerasi, E., Luft, R., and Efendic, S. (1971): Antagonism between glucose and epinephrine regarding insulin secretion: A dose-response study in man. *Acta Med. Scand.*, 190:411–417.
32. Chen, M., Woods, S., and Porte, D. (1975): Effect of cerebral intraventricular insulin on pancreatic insulin secretion in the dog. *Diabetes*, 24:910–914.
33. Christensen, N. (1974): Plasma norepinephrine and epinephrine in untreated diabetics, during fasting and after insulin administration. *Diabetes*, 23:1–8.
34. Christensen, N., and Iversen, J. (1973): Release of large amounts of noradrenaline from the isolated perfused canine pancreas during glucose deprivation. *Diabetologia*, 9:396–399.
35. Christensen, N., Mathias, C., and Frankel, H. (1976): Plasma and urinary dopamine: Studies during fasting and exercise and in tetraplegic man. *Eur. J. Clin. Invest*, 6:403–409.
36. Coore, H., and Randle, P. (1964): Regulation of insulin secretion studied with pieces of rabbit pancreas incubated in vitro. *Biochem. J.*, 93:66–78.

37. Coupland, R. (1958): The innervation of the pancreas of the rat, cat, and rabbit as revealed by the cholinesterase technique. *J. Anat.*, 92:143–149.
38. Cryer, P. (1976): Isotope-derivative measurements of plasma norepinephrine and epinephrine in man. *Diabetes*, 25:1071–1082.
39. Curry, D., and Bennett, L. (1974): Reversal of somatostatin inhibition of insulin secretion by calcium. *Biochem. Biophys. Res. Commun.*, 60:1015–1019.
40. Curry, D., and Joy, R. (1974): Direct CNS modulation of insulin secretion. *Endocrinol. Res. Commun.*, 1:229–237.
41. Daniel, P., and Henderson, J. (1967): The effect of vagal stimulation on plasma insulin and glucose levels in the baboon. *J. Physiol. (Lond.)*, 192:317–327.
42. Edwards, A., and Silver, M. (1970): Glycogenolytic response to stimulation of the splanchnic nerves in adrenalectomized calves. *J. Physiol. (Lond.)*, 211:109–124.
43. Efendic, S., Grill, V., and Luft, R. (1975): Inhibition by somatostatin of glucose induced 3':5'-monophosphate (cyclic AMP) accumulation and insulin release in isolated pancreatic islets of the rat. *FEBS Lett.*, 55:131–133.
44. Efendic, S., and Luft, R. (1975): Studies on the inhibitory effect of somatostatin on glucose induced insulin release in the isolated perfused rat pancreas. *Acta Endocrinol. (Kbh.)*, 78:510–516.
45. Elrick, H., Stimmler, L., Hlad, C., Jr., and Arai, Y. (1964): Plasma insulin response to oral and intravenous glucose administration. *J. Clin. Endocrinol.*, 24:1076–1082.
46. Ensinck, J., Walter, R., Palmer, J., Brodows, R., and Campbell, R. (1976): Glucagon responses to hypoglycemia in adrenalectomized man. *Metabolism*, 25:227–232.
47. Ericson, L. (1971): Uptake of H^3-5-hydroxytryptophan by noradrenergic nerves in the mouse pancreas studied with electron microscopic autoradiography. *Z. Zellforsch. Mikrosk. Anat.*, 113:441–449.
48. Esterhuizen, A., Spriggs, T., and Lever, J. (1968): Nature of islet cell innervation in the cat pancreas. *Diabetes*, 17:33–36.
49. Falck, B., and Hellman, B. (1963): Evidence for the presence of biogenic amines in pancreatic islets. *Experientia*, 19:139–140.
50. Falkmer, S., and Patent, G. (1972): Comparative and embryological aspects of the pancreatic islets. In: *Handbook of Physiology, Section 7, Endocrinology, Vol. I*, pp. 1–24. American Physiological Society, Washington, D.C.
51. Felig, P., Wahren, J., Hendler, R., and Ahlborg, G. (1972): Plasma glucagon levels in exercising man. *N. Engl. J. Med.*, 287:184–185.
52. Findlay, J., Gill, J., Lever, J., Randle, P., and Spriggs, T. (1969): Increased insulin output following stimulation of the vagal supply to the perfused rabbit pancreas. *J. Anat.*, 104:580–584.
53. Friedman, M. (1972): Effects of alloxan diabetes on hypothalamic hyperphagia and obesity. *Am. J. Physiol.*, 222:174–178.
54. Frohman, L. (1971): The hypothalamus and metabolic control. *Pathobiol. Annu.*, 1:353–372.
55. Frohman, L., and Bernardis, L. (1968): Growth hormone and insulin levels in weanling rats with ventromedial hypothalamic lesions. *Endocrinology*, 82:1125–1132.
56. Frohman, L., and Bernardis, L. (1971): Effect of hypothalamic stimulation on plasma glucose, insulin and glucagon levels. *Am. J. Physiol.*, 221:1596–1603.
57. Frohman, L., Bernardis, L., and Stachura, M. (1974): Factors modifying plasma insulin and glucose responses to ventromedial hypothalamic stimulation. *Metabolism*, 23:1047–1056.
58. Frohman, L., Ezdink, E., and Javid, R. (1967): Effect of vagotomy and vagal stimulation on insulin secretion. *Diabetes*, 16:443–448.
59. Fujimoto, W. (1975): Somatostatin inhibition of glucose-, tolbutamide-, theophylline, cytochalasin B-, and calcium-stimulated insulin release in monolayer cultures of rat endocrine pancreas. *Endocrinology*, 97:1494–1500.
60. Fujimoto, W., and Ensinck, J. (1976): Somatostatin inhibition of insulin and glucagon secretion in rat islet culture: Reversal by ionophore A23187. *Endocrinology*, 98:259–262.
61. Furman, B., and Tayo, F. (1974): Effect of some B-adrenoreceptor blocking drugs on insulin secretion in the rat. *J. Pharm. Pharmacol.*, 26:512–517.

62. Gagliardo, J., Bellone, C., Doria, I., Sanchez, J., and Pereyra, V. (1970): Adrenergic regulation of basal serum glucose, NEFA, and insulin levels. *Horm. Metab. Res.*, 2:318–322.
63. Galbo, H., Holst, J., and Christensen, N. (1975): Glucagon and plasma catecholamine responses to graded and prolonged exercise in man. *J. Appl. Physiol.*, 38:70–76.
64. Galbo, H., Holst, J., Christensen, N., and Hilsted, J. (1976): Glucagon and plasma catecholamines during beta-receptor blockade in exercising man. *J. Appl. Physiol.*, 40:855–863.
65. Garber, A., Cryer, P., Santiago, J., Haymond, W., Pagliara, A., and Kipnis, D. (1976): The role of adrenergic mechanisms in the substrate and hormonal response to insulin-induced hypoglycemia in man. *J. Clin. Invest.*, 58:7–15.
66. George, W., Polson, J., O'Toole, A., and Goldberg, N. (1970): Elevation of guanosine 3′,5′ cyclic phosphate in rat heart after perfusion with acetyl choline. *Proc. Natl. Acad. Sci. U.S.A.*, 66:398–403.
67. George, D., Rayfield, E., and Wannemacher, R. (1974): Altered glucoregulatory hormones during acute pneumococcal sepsis in the rhesus monkey. *Diabetes*, 23:544–549.
68. Gerich, J. (1976): Somatostatin and the endocrine pancreas. In: *Current Topics in Molecular Endocrinology, Vol. III: Hypothalamus and Endocrine Function*, edited by F. Labrie, J. Meites, and G. Pellitier, pp. 127–143. Plenum Press, New York.
69. Gerich, J., Charles, M., and Grodsky, G. (1974): Characterization of the effects of arginine and glucose on glucagon and insulin release from the perfused rat pancreas. *J. Clin. Invest.*, 54:833–841.
70. Gerich, J., Charles, M., and Grodsky, G. (1976): Regulation of pancreatic insulin and glucagon secretion. *Annu. Rev. Physiol.*, 38:353–388.
71. Gerich, J., Frankel, B., Fanska, R., West, L., Forsham, P., and Grodsky, G. (1974): Calcium dependency of glucagon secretion from the in vitro perfused rat pancreas. *Endocrinology*, 94:1381–1385.
72. Gerich, J., Karam, J., and Farsham, P. (1973): Stimulation of glucagon secretion by epinephrine in man. *J. Clin. Endocrinol. Metab.*, 37:479–481.
73. Gerich, J., Langlois, M., Noacco, C., Schneider, V., and Forsham, P. (1974): Adrenergic modulation of pancreatic glucagon secretion in man. *J. Clin. Invest.*, 53:1441–1446.
74. Gerich, J., Lorenzi, M., Tsalikian, E., Bohannon, N., Schneider, V., Karom, J., and Forsham, P. (1976): Effects of acute insulin withdrawal and administration on plasma glucagon responses to intravenous arginine in insulin-dependent diabetic subjects. *Diabetes*, 25:955–960.
75. Gerich, J., Lorenzi, M., Tsalikian, E., and Karam, J. (1976): Studies on the mechanism of epinephrine-induced hyperglycemia in man: Evidence for participation of pancreatic glucagon secretion. *Diabetes*, 25:65–71.
76. Gerich, J., Lovinger, R., and Grodsky, G. (1975): Inhibition by somatostatin of glucagon and insulin release from the perfused rat pancreas in response to arginine, isoproterenol, and theophylline: Evidence for a preferential effect on glucagon secretion. *Endocrinology*, 96:749–754.
77. Gerich, J., Schneider, V., Dippe, S., Langlois, M., Noacco, C., Karam, J., and Forsham, P. (1974): Characterization of the glucagon response to hypoglycemia in man. *J. Clin. Endocrinol. Metab.*, 38:77–82.
78. Goldberg, N., Haddox, M., Estensen, R., White, J., Lopez, C., and Hadden, J. (1974): Evidence for a dualism between cyclic GMP and cyclic AMP in the regulation of cell proliferation and other cellular processes. In: *Cyclic AMP, Cell Growth and the Immune Response*, edited by W. Brown, L. Lichtenstein, and C. Parker, pp. 247–262. Springer-Verlag, New York.
79. Goldfien, A. (1966): Effects of glucose deprivation on the sympathetic outflow to the adrenal medulla and adipose tissue. *Physiol. Rev.*, 18:303–311.
80. Goldfine, I., Abraira, C., Gruenewald, D., and Goldstein, M. (1970): Plasma insulin levels during imaginary food ingestion under hypnosis. *Proc. Soc. Exp. Biol. Med.*, 133:274–276.
81. Hakanson, R., Liedberg, G., and Lundquist, I. (1971): Effect of vagal denervation on insulin release after oral and intravenous glucose. *Experientia*, 27:460–461.

82. Hales, C., and Kennedy, G. (1964): Plasma glucose, non-esterified fatty acid and insulin concentrations in hypothalamic-hyperphagic rats. *Biochem. J.,* 90:620–624.
83. Han, P., and Frohman, L. (1970): Hyperinsulinemia in tube fed hypophysectomized rats bearing hypothalamic lesions. *Am. J. Physiol.,* 219:1632–1636.
84. Han, P., Yu, Y., and Chow, S. (1970): Enlarged pancreatic islets of tube-fed hypophysectomized rats bearing hypothalamic lesions. *Am. J. Physiol.,* 218:769–771.
85. Harvey, W., Faloona, G., and Unger, R. (1974): The effects of adrenergic blockade on exercise-induced hyperglucagonemia. *Endocrinology,* 94:1254–1258.
86. Hellman, B., Sehlin, J., and Taljedal, I. (1971): Calcium uptake by pancreatic beta cells as measured with the aid of ^{45}Ca and mannitol-^{3}H. *Am. J. Physiol.,* 221:1795–1801.
87. Hellman, B., Sehlin, J., and Taljedal, I. (1976): Calcium and secretion: Distinction between two pools of glucose-sensitive calcium in pancreatic islets. *Science,* 194:1421–1423.
88. Henderson, J., Jefferys, D., Jones, R., and Stanley, D. (1976): The effect of atropine on the insulin release caused by oral and intravenous glucose in human subjects. *Acta Endocrinol. (Kbh.),* 83:772–780.
89. Himms-Hagen, J. (1967): Sympathetic regulation of metabolism. *Pharmacol. Rev.,* 19:368–461.
90. Hommel, H., Fischer, V., Retzlaff, K., and Knäfler, H. (1972): The mechanism of insulin secretion after oral glucose administration. *Diabetologia,* 8:111–116.
91. Horwitz, D., Rubinstein, A., Reynolds, C., Molnar, G., and Vanaihara, N. (1975): Prolonged suppression of insulin release by insulin-induced hypoglycemia: Demonstration by C-peptide assay. *Horm. Metab. Res.,* 7:449–452.
92. Hustvedt, B., and Lovo, A. (1972): Correlation between hyperinsulinemia and hyperphagia in rats with ventromedial hypothalamic lesions. *Acta Physiol. Scand.,* 84:29–33.
93. Illiano, G., Tell, P., Siegel, M., and Cuatrecasas, P. (1973): Guanosine 3'-5'-cyclic monophosphate and the action of insulin and acetyl choline. *Proc. Natl. Acad. Sci. USA,* 70:2443–2447.
94. Imura, H., Kato, Y., Ikeda, M., Moumoto, M., and Yawata, M. (1971): Effects of adrenergic-blocking or stimulating agents on plasma growth hormone, immunoreactive insulin and blood free fatty acid and levels in man. *J. Clin. Invest.,* 50:1069–1079.
95. Inoue, S., Mullen, Y., and Bray, G. (1977): Pancreatic beta cell transplantation prevents the development of hypothalamic obesity. *Clin. Res.,* 25:160A.
96. Iversen, J. (1973): Effect of acetyl choline on the secretion of glucagon and insulin from the isolated, perfused canine pancreas. *Diabetes,* 22:381–387.
97. Iversen, J. (1973): Adrenergic receptors and the secretion of glucagon and insulin from the isolated perfused canine pancreas. *J. Clin. Invest.,* 52:2102–2116.
98. Iversen, J., and Miler, D. (1971): Evidence for a feedback inhibition of insulin on insulin secretion in the isolated perfused canine pancreas. *Diabetes,* 20:1–9.
99. Jenkinson, D. (1974): Classification and properties of peripheral adrenergic receptors. *Br. Med. Bull.,* 29:142–147.
100. Johnston, D., and Bloom, S. (1973): Plasma glucagon levels in the term human infant and effect of hypoxia. *Arch. Dis. Child.,* 48:451–454.
101. Johnson, D., and Ensinck, J. (1976): Stimulation of glucagon secretion by scorpion toxin in the perfused rat pancreas. *Diabetes,* 25:645–649.
102. Jorfeldt, I., and Wahren, J. (1971): Leg blood flow during exercise in man. *Clin. Sci. (Lond.),* 41:459–473.
103. Kajinuma, H., Kaneto, A., Kuzuya, T., and Nakao, K. (1968): Effects of methacholine on insulin secretion in man. *J. Clin. Endocrinol.,* 28:1384–1388.
104. Kaneto, A., Kajinuma, H., and Kosaka, K. (1975): Effect of splanchnic nerve stimulation on glucagon and insulin output in the dog. *Endocrinology,* 96:143–150.
105. Kaneto, A., Kajinuma, H., Kosaka, K., and Nakao, K. (1968): Stimulation of insulin secretion by parasympathomimetic agents. *Endocrinology,* 83:651–658.
106. Kaneto, A., Kosaka, K., and Nakao, K. (1967): Effects of stimulation of the vagus nerve on insulin secretion. *Endocrinology,* 80:530–536.

107. Kaneto, A., Miki, E., and Kosaka, K. (1974): Effects of vagal stimulation on glucagon and insulin secretion. *Endocrinology,* 95:1005–1010.
108. Kaneto, A., Miki, E., and Kosaka, K. (1975): Effect of beta and beta₂ adrenoreceptor stimulants infused intrapancreatically on glucagon and insulin secretion. *Endocrinology,* 97:1166–1173.
109. Kobayashi, S., and Fujita, T. (1969): Fine structure of mammalian and avian pancreatic islets with special reference to D cells and nervous elements. *Z. Zellforsch.,* 100:340–363.
110. Kuo, W., Hodgins, D., and Kuo, J. (1973): Adenylate cyclase in islets of Langerhans: Isolation of islets and regulation of adenylate cyclase activity by various hormones and drugs. *J. Biol. Chem.,* 248:2705–2711.
111. Leclercq-Meyer, V., Brisson, G., and Malaisse, W. (1971): Effect of adrenaline and glucose on release of glucagon and insulin *in vitro. Nature [New Biol.],* 231:248–249.
112. Lenman, J. (1975): *Clinical Neurophysiology,* pp. 226–244. Blackwell Scientific Publications, Oxford.
113. Lindsey, A., Santeusanio, F., Braaten, J., Faloona, G., and Unger, R. (1974): Pancreatic alpha-cell function in trauma. *J.A.M.A.,* 227:757–761.
114. Lorenzi, M., Tsalikian, E., Bohannon, N., Schmitt, J., Gerich, J., and Karam, J. (1977): Dopamine during alpha- and beta-adrenergic blockade in man: Effect of plasma glucagon, insulin, prolactin and growth hormone. *Endocrinology,* 100:135 (abstract).
115. Loubatieres, A., Mariani, M., Sorel, G., and Savi, L. (1971): The action of beta adrenergic blocking and stimulating agents on insulin secretion: Characterization of the type of beta receptor. *Diabetologia,* 7:127–132.
116. Luyckx, A., and Lefebvre, P. (1973): Exercise-induced glucagon secretion. *Postgrad. Med. J.,* 49:620–623.
117. Malaisse, W. (1973): Insulin secretion: Multifactorial regulation for a single process of release. *Diabetologia,* 9:167–173.
118. Malaisse, W., Brisson, G., and Malaisse-Lagae, F. (1976): The stimulus-secretion coupling of glucose-induced insulin release. *J. Lab. Clin. Med.,* 76:895–902.
119. Malaisse, W., Malaisse-Lagae, F., Wright, P., and Ashmore, L. (1967): Effects of adrenergic and cholinergic agents upon insulin secretion in vitro. *Endocrinology,* 80:975–978.
120. Malaisse-Lagae, F., and Malaisse, W. (1971): Stimulus-secretion coupling of islets of Langerhans. *Endocrinology,* 88:72–80.
121. Marliss, E., Aoki, T., Unger, R., Soeldner, J., and Cahill, G., Jr. (1970): Glucagon levels and metabolic effects in fasting man. *J. Clin. Invest.,* 49:2256–2270.
122. Marliss, E., Girardier, L., Seydoux, J., Wollheim, C., Kanazawa, Y., Orci, L., Renold, A., and Porte, D. (1973): Glucagon release induced by pancreatic nerve stimulation in the dog. *J. Clin. Invest.,* 52:1246–1259.
123. Martin, J., Konijnendijk, W., and Bouman, P. (1974): Insulin and growth hormone secretion in rats with ventromedial hypothalamic lesions maintained on restricted food intake. *Diabetes,* 23:203–208.
124. Mathias, C., Christensen, N., Corbett, J., Frankel, H., and Spalding, J. (1976): Plasma catecholamines during paroxysmal neurogenic hypertension in quadraplegic man. *Circ. Res.,* 39:204–208.
125. Miller, R. (1970): Effects of vagotomy and splanchnicotomy on blood insulin and sugar concentrations in the conscious monkey. *Endocrinology,* 86:642–651.
126. Miller, R., Ward, T., and Joyce, M. (1976): Direct neural inhibition of insulin secretion in response to systemic hypoglycemia. *Am. J. Physiol.,* 230:1090–1094.
127. Misbin, R., Edgar, P., and Lockwood, D. (1970): Adrenergic regulation of insulin secretion during fasting in normal subjects. *Diabetes,* 19:688–693.
128. Mitchell, G. (1953): *Anatomy of the Autonomic Nervous System.* Livingston, London.
129. Monnier, M. (1968): *Functions of the Nervous System, Vol. 1: General Physiology, Autonomic Functions,* pp. 410–417. Elsevier Publishing Company, Amsterdam.
130. Montague, W., and Cook, J. (1971): The role of adenosine 3'5' cyclic monophos-

phate in the regulation of insulin release by isolated islets of Langerhans. *Biochem., J.,* 122:115–120.
131. Niijima, A. (1975): The effect of 2-deoxy-D-glucose and D-glucose on the efferent discharge rate of sympathetic nerves. *J. Physiol. (Lond.),* 251:231–243.
132. Niijima, A. (1975): Studies on the nervous regulatory mechanism of blood sugar levels. *Pharmacol. Biochem. Behav.,* 3 (Suppl. 1):139–143.
133. Ogawa, N., Thompson, T., and Friesen, H. (1976): Soluble somatostatin binding protein. *Clin. Res.,* 24:661A.
134. Orci, L. (1974): A portrait of the pancreatic B-cell. *Diabetologia,* 10:163–187.
135. Oliver, J. (1976): Inhibition of calcium uptake by somatostatin in isolated rat islets of Langerhans. *Endocrinology,* 99:910–913.
136. Orci, L., Baetens, D., Rufener, C., Amherdt, M., Ravazzola, M., Studer, P., Malaisse-Lagae, F., and Unger, R. (1976): Hypertrophy and hyperplasia of somatostatin-containing D-cells in diabetes. *Proc. Natl. Acad. Sci. USA,* 73:1338–1342.
137. Orci, L., and Unger, R. (1975): Functional subdivision of islets of Langerhans and possible role of D cells. *Lancet,* 2:1243–1244.
138. Orci, L., Unger, R., and Renold, A. (1973): Structural coupling between pancreatic islet cells. *Experientia,* 29:1015–1018.
139. Pace, C., Conant, S., and Murphy, M. (1976): Somatostatin inhibition of electrical activity in cultured rat islet cells. *Diabetes,* 25 (Suppl. 1):390.
140. Palmer, J., Henry, D., Bensen, J., Johnson, D., and Ensinck, J. (1976): Glucagon response to hypoglycemia in sympathectomized man. *J. Clin. Invest.,* 57:522–525.
141. Pansepp, J. (1974): Hypothalamic regulation of energy balance and feeding behavior. *Fed. Proc.,* 33:1150–1165.
142. Parra-Covarrubias, A., Rivera-Rodriquez, I., and Almaraz-Ugalde, A. (1971): Cephalic phase of insulin secretion in obese adolescents. *Diabetes,* 20:800–802.
143. Patel, Y., and Weir, G. (1976): Increased somatostatin content of islets from streptozotocin-diabetic rats. *Clin. Endocrinol.,* 5:191–194.
144. Patton, G., Dobbs, R., Orci, L., Vale, W., and Unger, R. (1976): Stimulation of pancreatic immunoreactive somatostatin release by glucagon. *Metabolism,* 25 (Suppl. 1):1499–1500.
145. Permutt, M., Keller, D., and Santiago, J. (1977): Cholinergic blockade in reactive hypoglycemia. *Diabetes,* 26:121–127.
146. Porte, D. (1967): A receptor mechanism for the inhibition of insulin release by epinephrine in man. *J. Clin. Invest.,* 46:86–94.
147. Porte, D., Girardier, L., Seydoux, J., Kanazawa, Y., and Posternak, H. (1973): Neural regulation of insulin secretion in the dog. *J. Clin. Invest.,* 52:210–214.
148. Porte, D., and Robertson, R. (1973): Control of insulin secretion by catecholamines, stress and the sympathetic nervous system. *Fed. Proc.,* 23:1792–1796.
149. Porte, D., Woods, S., Mei, C., Smith, P., and Ensinck, J. (1975): Central factors in the control of insulin and glucagon secretion. *Pharmacol. Biochem. Behav.,* 3 (Suppl. 1):127–133.
150. Powley, T., and Opsahl, C. (1974): Ventromedial hypothalamic obesity abolished by subdiaphragmatic vagotomy. *Am. J. Physiol.,* 226:25–33.
151. Quickel, K., Feldman, J., and Lebovitz, H. (1971): Inhibition of insulin secretion by serotonin and dopamine: Species variation. *Endocrinology,* 89:1295–1302.
152. Rayfield, E., Curnow, R., George, D., and Beisel, W. (1973): Impaired carbohydrate metabolism during a mild viral illness. *N. Engl. J. Med.,* 289:618–621.
153. Robertson, R., and Porte, D. (1973): Adrenergic modulation of basal insulin secretion in man. *Diabetes,* 22:1–8.
154. Rocha, D., Santeusanio, F., Faloona, G., and Unger, R. (1973): Abnormal pancreatic alpha-cell function in bacterial infections. *N. Engl. J. Med.,* 288:700–703.
155. Russell, R., Thomson, J., and Bloom, S. (1974): The effect of truncal and selective vagotomy on the release of pancreatic glucagon, insulin and enteroglucagon. *Br. J. Surg.,* 61:821–824.
156. Russell, R., Walker, C., and Bloom, S. (1975): Hyperglucagonemia in the surgical patient. *Br. Med. J.,* 1:10–12.
157. Samols, E., Weir, G., Patel, Y., Loo, S., and Gabbay, K. (1977): Autonomic

control of somatostatin and pancreatic polypeptide secretion by the isolated perfused canine pancreas. *Clin. Res. (in press)*.

158. Schauder, P., McIntosh, C., Arends, J., Arnold, R., Frerichs, H., and Creutzfeldt, W. (1976): Somatostatin and insulin release from isolated rat pancreatic islets stimulated by glucose. *FEBS Lett.*, 68:225–227.

159. Shapiro, S., Sumkya, E., Fleischer, N., and Baum, S. (1975): Regulation of in vitro insulin release from a transplantable Syrian hamster insulinoma. *Endocrinology*, 97:442–447.

160. Shimazu, T., and Amakawa, A. (1968): Regulation of glucogen metabolism in liver by the autonomic nervous system. *Biochem. Biophys. Acta*, 165:335–341.

161. Shimazu, T., Fukuda, A., and Ban, T. (1966): Reciprocal influences of the ventromedial and lateral hypothalamic nuclei on blood glucose level and liver glycogen content. *Nature*, 210:1178–1179.

162. Smith, P., and Porte, D. (1976): Neuropharmacology of the pancreatic islets. *Annu. Rev. Pharmacol. Toxicol.*, 16:269–285.

163. Steer, M., Atlas, D., and Levitzki, A. (1975): Inter-relationships between beta-adrenergic receptors, adenylate cyclase and calcium. *N. Engl. J. Med.*, 292:401–414.

164. Steffens, A., Mogenson, G., and Stevenson, J. (1972): Blood glucose, insulin, and free fatty acids after stimulation and lesions of the hypothalamus. *Am. J. Physiol.*, 222:1446–1452.

165. Szabo, O., and Szabo, A. (1975): Neuropharmacologic characterization of insulin sensitive CNS glucoreceptor. *Am. J. Physiol.*, 229:663–668.

166. Taminato, T., Seino, Y., Goto, Y., and Imura, H. (1975): Interaction of somatostatin and calcium in regulating insulin release from isolated pancreatic islets of rats. *Biochem. Biophys. Res. Commun.*, 66:928–934.

167. Teitelbaum, P., and Epstein, A. (1962): The lateral hypothalamic syndrome: Recovery of feeding and drinking after lateral hypothalamic lesions. *Psychol. Rev.*, 69:74–80.

168. Toyota, T., Sato, S., Kudo, M., Abe, K., and Goto, Y. (1975): Secretory regulation of endocrine pancreas: Cyclic AMP and glucagon secretion. *J. Clin. Endocrinol. Metab.*, 41:81–89.

169. Turtle, J., and Kipnis, D. (1967): An adrenergic receptor mechanism for the control of cyclic 3'5' adenosine monophosphate synthesis in tissues. *Biochem. Biophys. Res. Commun.*, 28:797–802.

170. Tyler, J., and Kajinuma, H. (1972): Influence of adrenergic and cholinergic agents in vivo on pancreatic glucagon and insulin secretion. *Diabetes*, 21 (Suppl. 1):332.

171. Unger, R. (1971): Glucagon and the insulin:glucagon molar ratio in diabetes and other catabolic illnesses. *Diabetes*, 20:834–838.

172. Unger, R. (1974): Alpha and beta cell interrelationships in health and disease. *Metabolism*, 23:581–593.

173. Unger, R. (1976): Diabetes and the alpha cell. *Diabetes*, 25:136–151.

174. Vale, W., Brazeau, P., Rivier, C., Brown, M., Boss, B., Rivier, J., Burgus, R., Ling, N., and Guillimen, R. (1975): Somatostatin. *Recent Prog. Horm. Res.*, 34:365–397.

175. Veverbrants, E., Olsen, W., and Arky, R. (1969): Role of gastrointestinal factors in reactive hypoglycemia. *Metabolism*, 18:6–12.

176. Walter, R., Dudl, R., Palmer, J., and Ensinck, J. (1974): The effect of adrenergic blockade on the glucagon responses to starvation and hypoglycemia in man. *J. Clin. Invest.*, 54:1214–1220.

177. Weir, G., Knowlton, S., and Martin, D. (1974): Glucagon secretion from the perfused rat pancreas: Studies with glucose and catecholamines. *J. Clin. Invest.*, 54:1403–1412.

178. Weir, G., Knowlton, S., and Martin, D. (1974): Somatostatin inhibition of epinephrine-induced glucagon secretion. *Endocrinology*, 95:1744–1746.

179. Widström, A., and Cerasi, E. (1973): On the action of tolbutamide in normal man. 1. Role of adrenergic mechanisms in tolbutamide-induced insulin release

during normoglycaemia and induced hypoglycaemia. *Acta Endocrinol. (Khb.)*, 72:506–518.

180. Willerson, J., Hutcheson, D., Leshin, S., Faloona, G., and Unger, R. (1974): Serum glucagon and insulin levels and their relationship to blood glucose values in patients with acute myocardial infarction and acute coronary insufficiency. *Am. J. Med.*, 57:747–753.

181. Wilmore, D., Long, J., Mason, A., and Pruitt, B. (1976): Stress in surgical patients as a neurophysiologic reflex response. *Surg. Gynecol. Obstet.*, 142:257–269.

182. Wilmore, D., Moylan, J., Pruitt, B., Lindsey, C., Faloona, G., and Unger, R. (1974): Hyperglucagonemia after burns. *Lancet*, 1:73–75.

183. Wollheim, C., Blondel, B., Trueheart, P., Renold, A., and Sharp, P. (1975): Calcium induced insulin release in monolayer culture of the endocrine pancreas. *J. Biol. Chem.*, 250:1354–1360.

184. Woods, S. (1972): Conditioned hypoglycemia: Effect of vagotomy and pharmacologic blockade. *Am. J. Physiol.*, 223:1424–1427.

185. Woods, S., Hutton, R., and Makous, W. (1970): Conditioned insulin secretion in the albino rat. *Proc. Soc. Exp. Biol. Med.*, 133:964–968.

186. Woods, S., and Porte, D. (1974): Neural control of the endocrine pancreas. *Physiol. Rev.*, 54:596–619.

187. Woods, S., and Porte, D. (1975): Effect of intracisternal insulin on plasma glucose and insulin in the dog. *Diabetes*, 24:905–909.

Frontiers in Neuroendocrinology, Vol. 5,
edited by W. F. Ganong and L. Martini.
Raven Press, New York © 1978.

Chapter 11

Opioid Peptides and the Opiate Receptor

George R. Uhl,
Steven R. Childers,
and
Solomon H. Snyder

*Departments of Pharmacology and Experimental Therapeutics
and Psychiatry and Behavioral Sciences,
Johns Hopkins University School of Medicine,
Baltimore, Maryland 21205*

The identification of several hypothalamic releasing factors as peptides highlights the relevance of brain peptides for neuroendocrinology. The recognition that some of these peptides exist in substantial levels in numerous extrahypothalamic areas in specific neuronal systems suggests that they may have synaptic roles in general brain function, possibly as neurotransmitters. Recently, peptides with opiate-like activity have been isolated and characterized in brain and pituitary. These opioid peptides were detected on the basis of their interactions with the opiate receptor in the tissues. This review describes properties of replicators and of opioid peptides.

Several striking pharmacological properties of opiates suggested that they must interact with specific receptor sites in the brain. Some opiates are extremely potent. For instance, etorphine (Fig. 11–1) is 5,000 to 10,000 times more potent than morphine in eliciting analgesia, possessing milligram potency comparable to D-lysergic acid diethylamide (LSD). Actions at such low doses imply that pharmacological effects are mediated through specific receptors for which the drug has very high affinity. Similarly, the stereospecificity of the effects of most opiates suggests actions at specific receptor sites; the $(-)$-isomers of most opiates are thousands of times more potent than $(+)$-isomers.

The properties of opiate antagonists also favor the receptor concept for opiate actions. Pure antagonists such as naloxone (Fig. 11–1) elicit no analgesic or euphoric actions themselves but block those of opiate agonists such as morphine. Most known opiate antagonists, such as nalorphine or levallorphan, seem "contaminated" with some agonist effects since they also elicit analgesia. Mixed agonist-antagonists such as pentazocine elicit analgesia, yet are markedly less addicting than pure agonists. Apparently their antagonist properties block the addicting features which might arise from their agonist propensities. Identification of such safer analgesics is a major goal in

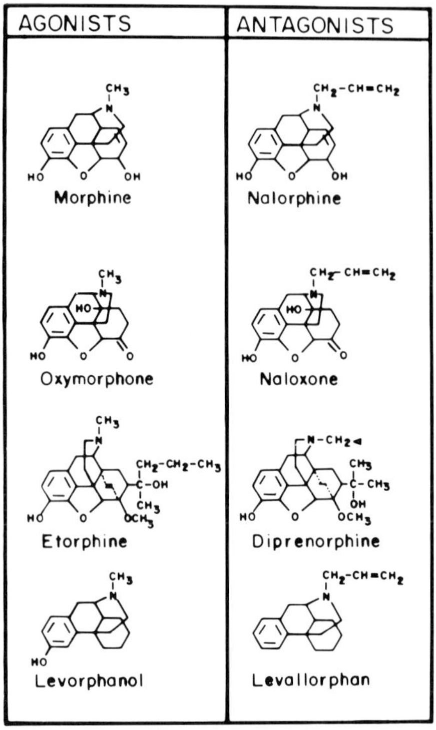

FIG. 11–1. Structures of representative opiate agonists and antagonists.

new opiate drug development which may be facilitated by studies of the opiate receptor.

If specific opiate receptors exist, biochemical receptor labeling techniques might be able to demonstrate their existence and their properties. Goldstein et al. (42) suggested that the known specificity of opiates' pharmacological activities could be used to identify hypothesized receptor sites. He detected binding of ^{3}H-levorphanol to mouse brain homogenates, a small fraction of which was stereospecific (42). After purification, however, it became apparent that this stereospecific binding involved cerebrosides, not proteins, and was distinct from the pharmacologically relevant opiate receptor. Subsequent use of ^{3}H-opiates of higher specific activity and assay conditions allowing the washing away of nonspecifically bound ligand permitted identification of pharmacologically relevant opiate receptor binding (101,129,133,134). This binding exhibited not only stereospecificity and other parallels with known pharmacology, but also high affinity, saturability, and reversibility. These are all criteria for the identification of receptors by binding studies (26).

The identification and characterization of specific receptors for opiates raised questions regarding their normal physiological role. The idea that opiates were in fact mimicking the action of some naturally occurring endogenous substance at these receptors was explored through attempts to extract, isolate, and characterize such a substance. Hughes (47), Pasternak and associates (83,84), and Terenius and Wahlstrom (135) found material in brain extracts that exhibited opiate agonist properties. These substances were purified and characterized as a mixture of two pentapeptides, H-Tyr-Gly-Gly-Phe-Met-OH (methionine-enkephalin) and H-Tyr-Gly-Gly-Phe-Leu-OH (leucine-enkephalin) by Hughes et al. using pig brain (48). Their findings were confirmed in calf brain by Simantov and Snyder (125). Other investigators have found larger peptides with opiate agonist properties. Goldstein and collaborators found larger opioid peptides in pituitary extracts (137). The observation that the sequence of met-enkephalin was contained in the 91-amino acid sequence of the pituitary peptide β-lipotropin aided in the isolation of several endorphins. These peptides with opioid activities, consisting of various lengths of the β-lipotropin sequence and including met-enkephalin's sequence, were isolated from the pituitary (68,70).

This review concentrates on topics that have been of particular interest in our laboratory: the identification and characterization of opiate receptors and opioid peptides, their brain and pituitary distributions, and their possible roles in normal and drug-altered brain and pituitary functions.

NOMENCLATURE

The terms met-enkephalin, leu-enkephalin, α-endorphin, β-endorphin (or C-fragment), and γ-endorphin refer to sequenced peptides (Table 11–1). The term enkephalin, originally used to describe the substance with opioid activity contained in crude brain extracts (47), is now used in reference to the two specific pentapeptides. Ambiguity has surrounded the use of the term "endorphin," however, since it has been used in three ways. First, it is used as a generic term for the sequenced opioid peptides including the enkephalin pentapeptides, α-, β-, and γ-endorphins (41). Secondly, "endorphin" has been applied as a descriptive term designating substances with morphine-like activity but unspecified structure in pituitary extracts (110). Finally, it has been employed in reference to the specific sequenced peptides, α-, β-, and γ-endorphin (127). For the purposes of this review, we have designated the two pentapeptides "enkephalin" (Table 11–1), the larger sequenced peptides as "endorphins," and any peptide with opioid activity as an "opioid peptide."

IDENTIFICATION OF OPIATE RECEPTOR BINDING

The introduction of radiolabeled opiates of high specific radioactivity and of rapid, thorough techniques for separating bound from unbound opiates has permitted the demonstration of substantial opiate receptor binding. This procedure, as developed in our laboratory, uses a crude total particulate membrane fraction prepared from rat brain. Incubation of this preparation at

TABLE 11–1. *Amino acid sequence of β-lipotropin and its biologically active constituent peptides*

	1
β-Lipotropin:	NH$_2$Glu-Leu-Ala-Gly-Ala-Pro-Pro-Glu-Pro-Ala-Arg-Asp-Pro-Glu-Ala-Pro-Ala-Glu-
	20
	Gly-Ala-Ala-Ala-Arg-Ala

		37
β-Lipotropin: (continued)	Glu-Leu-Glu-His-Gly-Leu-Val-Ala-Glu-Ala-Gln-Ala-Ala-Glu-Lys-Lys-Asp-Glu-Gly-Pro-Tyr-Lys	
β-MSH		Ala-Glu-Lys-Lys-Asp-Glu-Gly-Pro-Tyr-Arg-

	47	61
β-Lipotropin: (continued)	Met-Glu-His-Phe-Arg-Try-Gly-Ser-Pro-Pro-Lys-Asp-Lys-Arg-Tyr-Gly-Gly-Phe-Met-Thr- Ser-Glu-Lys-Ser-	
β-MSH: (continued)	Met-Glu-His-Phe-Arg-Try-Gly-Ser-Pro-Pro-Lys-Asp	
ACTH$_{4-10}$:	Met-Glu-His-Phe-Arg-Try-Gly	
α-Endorphin:		Tyr-Gly-Gly-Phe-Met-Thr-Ser-Glu-Lys-Ser
β-Endorphin:		Tyr-Gly-Gly-Phe-Met-Thr-Ser-Glu-Lys-Ser
Methionine-enkephalin:		Tyr-Gly-Gly-Phe-Met

	76	91
β-Lipotropin: (continued)	Gln-Thr-Pro-Leu-Val-Thr-Leu-Phe-Lys-Asn-Ala-Ile-Val-Lys-Asn-Ala-His-Lys-Lys-Gly-Gln- OH	
α-Endorphin: (continued)	Gln-Thr-Pro-Leu-Val-Thr	
β-Endorphin: (continued)	Gln-Thr-Pro-Leu-Val-Thr-Leu-Phe-Lys-Asn-Ala-Ile-Val-Lys-Asn-Ala-His-Lys-Lys-Gly-Gln- OH	

37° C before binding studies are begun increases the binding of labeled opiates, presumably by allowing release and degradation of endogenous opioid substances (88). Labeled and unlabeled drugs are incubated with the membranes for 40 min at 25° C. Membrane-bound ligand is then separated from unbound ligand by trapping the membranes on glass fiber filters, or by centrifuging them into a pellet. Thorough washing of the membranes is followed by assay of the associated radioactivity by liquid scintillation spectrometry. Specific binding is the difference between radiolabeled ligand associated with membranes in the presence of unlabeled pharmacologically inactive dextrorphan and membrane-associated ligand in the presence of its active isomer, levorphanol.

In addition to stereospecificity, however, binding must fulfill a number of other criteria to be considered to be related to physiologically relevant opiate receptors. Binding should have high affinity; ^{3}H-naloxone binding has a dissociation constant of about 0.4 nm (86). Binding is selective, since addition of high concentrations of numerous nonopiate drugs to incubation media does not displace ^{3}H-naloxone binding to brain membranes. Finally, binding affinities of a series of opiates should parallel their relative pharmacological activities. Two kinds of evidence support the pharmacological parallels. First, potencies of numerous opiates in reducing ^{3}H-naloxone binding to brain membranes correlate closely with their relative potencies in producing analgesia. In cases where discrepancy exists between receptor affinity and pharmacological potency, the lack of correlation may be explained by *in vivo* transformations of the drugs into compounds of different activity, or by the variable abilities of different drugs to cross the blood-brain barrier. For example, codeine is about one-fifth as potent as morphine as an analgesic, but displays less than 1/3,000 of morphine's receptor affinity. However, this finding is consistent with the fact that codeine has no analgesic activity itself, but acts only after an O-demethylation reaction that converts it to morphine (143). The 5,000 to 10,000-fold greater potency of etorphine than of morphine is related to its 20-fold affinity for the opiate receptor (102) and its 300-fold greater ability to penetrate the blood-brain barrier (45).

A second approach to establishing parallels between binding and pharmacological potencies of drugs involves the use of simpler, smooth muscle systems, such as the guinea pig ileum and mouse vas deferens. Pharmacologically, these tissues seem to possess opiate receptors, since morphine and other

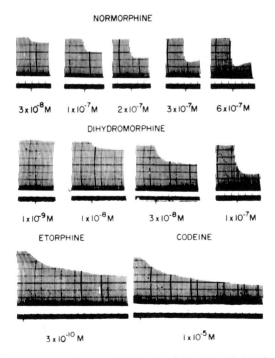

FIG. 11–2. Inhibition of the electrically induced contractions of the guinea pig intestine longitudinal muscle and myenteric plexus preparation by normorphine, dihydromorphine, etorphine, and codeine. The upper trace in each case represents the degree of contraction of the muscle which was supramaximally stimulated every 10 sec for 1.5 msec. The lower trace is a time scale with the upward deflections representing 1-min intervals. The downward deflection indicates the addition of the drug under study. A separate muscle strip was used for each of the drugs. From Creese and Snyder (25).

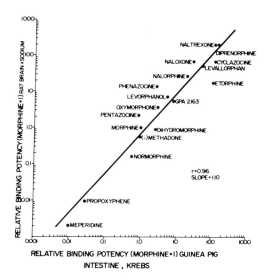

FIG. 11–3. Correlation between the relative potencies of opiates to inhibit ^{3}H-naloxone binding in guinea pig intestine and rat brain homogenates. The relative potencies of opiates were calculated from ED_{50} determinations for each drug to inhibit stereospecific ^{3}H-naloxone binding in either homogenates of the guinea pig intestine longitudinal and myenteric plexus preparation (assayed in Krebs-Tris, 37°C, pH 7.4) or homogenates of rat brain (assayed in 0.05 M Tris + 100 mM NaCl, 25°C, pH 7.7). The ED_{50} for morphine was taken as the standard in each system and given the value of 1. The ED_{50} values for the intestine are the means of two separate determinations. From Creese and Snyder (25).

opiate agonists inhibit their electrically induced contraction (89) (Fig. 11–2). Opiate antagonists block the agonist-induced inhibition. Kosterlitz and Waterfield (60) showed that the potencies of various opiates in producing this effect parallel their analgesic potencies. Creese and Snyder (25) demonstrated close correlation between the affinity of opiates for guinea pig ileal binding sites and their effects on electrically induced contractions (25). Binding to brain also parallels binding to intestine (Fig. 11–3).

These parallels between the binding and pharmacological potencies of opiate drugs convincingly support the notion that the sites which mediate pharmacological effects of opiates are labeled in binding studies.

AGONIST AND ANTAGONIST FORMS
OF THE OPIATE RECEPTOR

Stereospecific receptor binding has been demonstrated for opiate agonists and antagonists in two ways. The binding of a number of tritiated opiates has been studied directly; agents examined include ^{3}H-naloxone, ^{3}H-etorphine, ^{3}H-dihydromorphine, ^{3}H-nalorphine, ^{3}H-levallorphan, ^{3}H-levorphanol, ^{3}H-oxymorphone, and ^{3}H-morphine (103,129,148). Since it is not practical to obtain all opiates in tritiated form, however, the potencies of unlabeled opiates in displacing the specific binding of a standard ^{3}H-agonist, such as ^{3}H-dihydromorphine, or a standard antagonist, such as ^{3}H-naloxone, are routinely used to assess agonist and antagonist properties of a novel drug.

Certain manipulations of binding assay conditions differentially affect the binding of agonists and antagonists. These manipulations, involving selected ions, temperature changes, and protein-modifying reagents, have both theoretical and practical importance. They offer a practical *in vitro* method for identifying novel drugs as opiate agonists, antagonists, or mixed agents, and perhaps provide some insight into the molecular mechanism for differentiation between agonist and antagonist drug activities.

Incubation in media containing sodium reduces the binding of a number of ^{3}H-agonists (57,97,102,130). Binding of ^{3}H-antagonists, on the other hand, is enhanced in the presence of sodium (Fig. 11–4) (103). The effect of sodium is highly specific; only lithium, whose atomic radius and biological activities are similar to those of sodium, can mimic the actions of sodium, whereas other monovalent cations are essentially ineffective. As the presence of an endogenous ligand for the opiate receptor became apparent, some of sodium's effectiveness in enhancing the binding of exogenous ^{3}H-antagonists was explicable on the basis of its enhancement of the removal of enkephalin from the receptor. The sodium-induced reduction in agonist potency, however, cannot be attributed to such a phenomenon.

The divalent cation manganese selectively increases binding of ^{3}H-agonists, having no effect on ^{3}H-antagonist binding, even in thoroughly prewashed

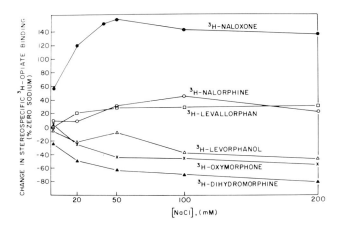

FIG. 11–4. Effect of sodium chloride on stereospecific binding of three ^{3}H-opiate agonists and three ^{3}H-opiate antagonists. Each ^{3}H-opiate was incubated in the presence of levallorphan (100 nM) and dextrallorphan (100 nM) with varied concentrations of sodium chloride and standard rat brain homogenate which had been washed twice. ^{3}H-naloxone (1 nM), ^{3}H-nalorphine (4 nM), ^{3}H-levallorphan (8.6 nM), ^{3}H-levorphanol (6 nM), ^{3}H-oxymorphone (40 nM), and ^{3}H-dihydromorphine (1 nM), when incubated at 25°C for 30 min in the standard binding assay, gave the following stereospecific control (zero sodium) values, respectively: 1,292 ± 115 cpm, 355 ± 30 cpm, 2,170 ± 195 cpm, 1,023 ± 95 cpm, 694 ± 51 cpm, and 2,570 ± 141 cpm.

membrane preparations from which dissociation of native opioid peptides is less of a concern (85). Manganese may act physiologically to lower the sensitivity of the opiate receptor to sodium, since manganese reduces the potency of sodium in inhibiting ^{3}H-agonist binding fivefold.

Ion effects *in vitro* can be used to predict pharmacological properties of novel drugs. A pure antagonist, for example, has the same potency in inhibiting ^{3}H-naloxone binding with or without sodium. A pure agonist, on the other hand, is 12- to 60-fold less potent in the presence of sodium. A drug with mixed agonist-antagonist properties is affected to an intermediate degree.

Temperature of incubation also differentially affects the binding of agonists and antagonists. Increasing temperatures from 0° to 30° C reduces ^{3}H-antagonist binding while tripling ^{3}H-agonist binding (24,122).

Protein-modifying reagents and enzymatic treatments also differentially alter agonist and antagonist binding. Pretreatment of membrane preparations with sulfhydryl reagents, including iodoacetamide, *N*-ethylmaleimide, and mercuriacetate (88), reduces ^{3}H-agonist binding, while not affecting ^{3}H-antagonist binding. Simon and Groth (128) showed that *N*-ethylmaleimide inactivation of receptor binding could be prevented by the presence of an agonist or antagonist, suggesting proximity of an SH group to the binding site. The enzymes trypsin, chymotrypsin, and phospholipase A reduce binding of agonists more than that of antagonists (87). Phospholipase C and D and neuraminidase have negligible effects on the binding of either agonists or antagonists.

The effects of ions and protein-modifying reagents, as well as the close structural similarities between opiate agonists and antagonists, have suggested a hypothetical working model for the opiate receptor (86). In this model, the opiate receptor macromolecule is envisioned as existing in two interconvertible forms, one of which has higher affinity for agonists, the other of which has higher affinity for antagonists. Sodium might shift the equilibrium between these two receptor states in favor of increasing proportions of "antagonist state" receptors, whereas protein-modifying reagents and enzymes might interfere with the interconversion. This model has been useful heuristically; however, its relationship to the actual molecular mechanisms of the opiate receptor has not been definitely established or disproved.

ENKEPHALIN

The discovery of receptors in the brain that specifically recognize opiates raises important questions concerning these receptors' physiological role, since most animals do not come into contact with opiates. One answer to these questions is that the opiate receptor is normally associated with a neurotransmitter system or systems with which exogenous opiates interact.

Depletion of opiate receptor binding following transmitter-specific lesions would help to associate the opiate receptor with a known neurotransmitter system. To study this possibility, lesions of known cholinergic, noradrenergic, serotoninergic, and dopaminergic pathways were followed by examination of residual opiate receptor binding (61,132). Lesions of the septal area destroyed cholinergic projections to the hippocampus but failed to reduce hippocampal opiate receptor binding. Destruction of the locus ceruleus interrupted ascending norepinephrine-containing projections to the ipsilateral cerebral cortex, with no associated changes in opiate receptor binding. Raphé lesions depleted serotonin in the forebrain, although opiate receptor binding remained unaffected. Finally, lesions of the nigrostriatal dopamine pathway with 6-hydroxydopamine did not alter striatal opiate receptor binding. This lack of exclusive association of the opiate receptor with presynaptic elements of any of these transmitter systems suggests that the opiate receptor might be associated with previously unidentified neurotransmitter systems.

Such a novel transmitter system would perhaps involve an endogenous opiate receptor ligand, that should therefore presumably display opioid properties. Hughes (47) showed that brain extracts mimicked the ability of morphine and other opiate agonists to inhibit electrically induced contractions of the guinea pig ileum and mouse vas deferens. Furthermore, these actions of brain extracts were blocked by naloxone and other opiate agonists. In our laboratory, Pasternak et al. (88) observed that preincubation of membrane preparations at 37° C enhanced subsequent ³H-naloxone binding. This finding suggested that an endogenous ligand that was released and/or metabolized was present in these preparations. Later studies (83,135) showed that the brain extracts, like morphine, could displace ³H-opiate binding to brain membranes.

Characterization of the "morphine-like factor" in brain was first accomplished by Hughes and his colleagues (47). These studies demonstrated that the morphine-like factor was a low molecular weight substance ($< 1,000$) sensitive to proteolytic enzymes such as carboxypeptidase and leucine aminopeptidase, but not to trypsin. A similar low molecular weight substance was detected in brain (135) and in human cerebrospinal fluid (136) by displacement of ³H-dihydromorphine binding. Pasternak et al. (83,84) also assayed the factor by receptor binding and showed that it possessed opiate agonist properties and a regional brain distribution parallel to that of the opiate receptor. Isolation of the morphine-like factor was first accomplished by Hughes et al. (49) who named the isolated factor "enkephalin." Purified enkephalin is a low molecular weight peptide that was purified from porcine brain by a procedure which included extraction with 0.1 M HCl, adsorption chromatography on Amberlite XAD-2, and gel filtration on Sephadex G-15 (131). The resulting preparation revealed only one ninhydrin-positive spot by high-voltage electrophoresis at pH 2, 3.5, and 6.5. Bioassay of purified enkephalin in the mouse vas deferens assay revealed that enkephalin mimics morphine in a dose-dependent manner which is completely blocked by low concentrations of naloxone. Later, Hughes et al. (48) reported that enkephalin is a mixture of two pentapeptides, H-Tyr-Gly-Gly-Phe-Met-OH (methionine-enkephalin; met-enkephalin) and H-Tyr-Gly-Gly-Phe-Leu-OH (leucine-enkephalin; leu-enkephalin). Sequences were determined by sequential degradation by the dansyl-Edman procedure and mass spectrometric analysis. Mass spectra of a mixture of the two synthetic peptides were identical to that of natural enkephalin, thus indicating that enkephalin from pig brain consists of a mixture of leu- and met-enkephalin. The ratio of met- to leu-enkephalin in pig brain is approximately 4 to 1. In addition, there is close agreement between the pharmacological activities of the natural and synthetic peptides, as assayed on the mouse vas deferens and guinea pig ileum. These findings were confirmed using bovine brain (125), except that the ratio of met- to leu-enkephalin is reversed as compared to pig brain (i.e., met- to leu-enkephalin ratio was 1 to 4).

Detailed studies have evaluated the interactions of enkephalins with the opiate receptor. In bioassays, met-enkephalin is 20 times more potent than normorphine in the vas deferens and equipotent with normorphine in guinea pig ileum (48). Leu-enkephalin has half the potency of met-enkephalin in the vas deferens but only one-fifth the potency of met-enkephalin in the guinea pig ileum (48). Naloxone, at a concentration of 900 nM, completely blocks these effects. Studies of enkephalin binding to brain opiate receptors (125,126) show that both enkephalins compete for opiate receptor binding with affinities resembling that of morphine (Fig. 11–5). Met-enkephalin is twice as potent as leu-enkephalin in reducing binding of ^{3}H-naloxone, whereas both peptides are equipotent in reducing binding of the agonist ^{3}H-dihydromorphine.

In measuring enkephalin binding in brain, one must be careful to avoid the rapid degradation of enkephalin by brain membrane preparations which occurs at 25° and 37° C. At 25° C, as little as 40 min of incubation results in 80% destruction of enkephalin. At 37° C, 85% destruction occurs after 20 min of incubation. However, no significant destruction occurs at 0°. Degradation of enkephalin at the higher temperatures can be prevented by the antibiotic bacitracin (50 μg/ml) (126). At this concentration, bacitracin itself does not affect ^{3}H-naloxone binding, but it does protect enkephalin for 40 min at 25° C and 20 min at 37° C. Further studies of enkephalin degradation (44) show that rapid destruction occurs in human plasma as well as rat brain homogenates. The half-life of enkephalin in plasma is about 2 min; in brain homogenates, enkephalin is completely destroyed within 1 min at 37° C at a brain protein concentration of 3 mg/ml. Examination of degradation products by thin-layer chromatography showed that deactivation occurs by cleavage of the Try-Gly amide bond. Pert et al. (94) attempted to stabilize this bond by the substitution of Gly^2 by a D-amino acid which would presumably block the accessibility of this crucial bond to proteolytic enzymes. The introduction of D-Ala into position 2, thus creating $D-Ala^2$-met-enkephalin, produces an analogue with a potency equivalent to that of met-enkephalin

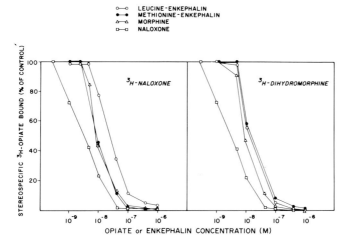

FIG. 11–5. Concentration dependence for inhibition of ³H-naloxone and ³H-dihydromorphine binding by enkephalins and other opiates. Incubations were performed at 0° for 2 hr in the standard binding assay containing 1.4 nM ³H-dihydromorphine. From Simantov and Snyder (126).

in receptor binding, but which is not rapidly degraded. Therefore, D-Ala²-met-enkephalin can be studied under conditions that completely destroy enkephalins.

Following these studies of unlabeled enkephalins, ³H-enkephalin became available for direct binding studies. In our laboratory, studies (123) show that ³H-enkephalin binding to rat brain membranes is saturable, with half-maximal binding at a concentration of 1 nM. Scatchard analysis reveals two distinct linear components with a high-affinity dissociation constant of 0.64 nM and a low-affinity dissociation constant of 2.6 nM. Binding of ³H-met-enkephalin is also stereospecific, with levorphanol displaying a 10,000-fold greater potency in displacing ³H-met-enkephalin than dextrorphan (82). In general, the drug specificity of ³H-met-enkephalin binding is similar to that obtained with ³H-opiates, although some discrepancies have been noted (123).

Sodium and manganese effects on enkephalin binding have been used to infer the relative agonist or antagonist properties of these peptides. Sodium reduces the potencies of met- and leu-enkephalin as inhibitors of ³H-naloxone binding by 12- and 20-fold, respectively (126). In the presence of manganese, the ability of both enkephalins to inhibit ³H-naloxone binding is increased approximately twofold. The findings are consistent with an agonist role for the enkephalins. Direct studies of ³H-naloxone binding to brain membranes (123) support this conclusion by demonstrating that in the presence of sodium, ³H-met-enkephalin binding is reduced 90 to 95%, with an almost total loss of high-affinity binding sites.

Although this competition for the same receptor site suggests an under-

lying structural similarity between opiate alkaloids and enkephalin pentapeptides, such similarities between these two classes of apparent opiate receptor
agonists may not be apparent at first glance. Enkephalin does possess two
aromatic rings that could conceivably arrange themselves in a conformation
that would resemble the conformation of opiates. Evidence for such a conformation has been obtained using nuclear magnetic resonance spectroscopy
(51,112). In $^2H_6$-DMSO solution, met-enkephalin has a β_1- turn involving
its gly-gly-phe-met portion. This allows a hydrogen bond between the $-NH$
of the met_5 and the $-CO$ of the gly_2 residues. This conformation would allow
the distance between enkephalin's tyrosine $-OH$ and the N-terminal amino
group to be the same as the phenol-ammonium distance in morphine (112).
The spatial orientation of ammonium groups in both compounds is also
similar (112). The similarity in receptor activity between opiates and enkephalins could be based on key structural correspondences such as these.

Based on biochemical studies, then, the pentapeptides met- and leu-
enkephalin seem to be physiological agonist ligands for brain receptors with
which opiates interact.

ENDORPHINS

The identification of enkephalin pentapeptides as likely endogenous ligands
of the opiate receptor does not preclude the possibility that other peptides
might perform the same functions. Studies of the pituitary have been particularly important in the identification of peptides which, although larger
than enkephalin, seem to also have activity in opiate membrane binding and
opiate-sensitive smooth muscle preparations.

Preliminary evidence for such peptides came from the work of Goldstein
and his colleagues (137), who demonstrated that pituitary extracts contained
peptides with morphine-like activities in the guinea pig ileum preparation.
Gel filtration showed that these pituitary peptides were over five times larger
than enkephalin, with molecular weights between 3,000 and 3,500. A clue to
the structure of the pituitary peptides was given by Hughes et al. (48), who
observed that the sequence of met-enkephalin was identical to that of residues
61 to 65 in the 91-amino acid pituitary peptide β-lipotropin (β-LPH) (Table
11–1). This peptide, isolated by Li (67) in 1964, has lipolytic activity in
several systems and contains the amino acid sequence of β-melanocyte
stimulating hormone (β-MSH). The discovery that β-LPH also contains the
sequence of met-enkephalin led to the suggestion that other β-LPH fragments
might exist in the pituitary and also possess opioid activity. This suggestion
was confirmed by Li and Chung (68), who isolated a peptide with opioid
activity from camel pituitaries and identified it as the 61 to 91 COOH-
terminal amino acid residues of β-LPH. This peptide, termed C-fragment or
β-endorphin, contains the sequence of met-enkephalin as its NH_2-terminal
amino acids and is 3.4 times more potent than normorphine in opiate re-

ceptor binding assays. Independently, Bradbury et al. (10) isolated β-endorphin from pituitary. These workers found that β-endorphin is 10 times more potent than morphine and 30 times more potent than met-enkephalin in displacing ^{3}H-naloxone from opiate receptor preparations (12). However, much of this apparent affinity difference between β-endorphin and the enkephalins is related to the more rapid degradation of enkephalin than of β-endorphin by brain membrane preparations. The different binding properties of β-endorphin and enkephalin suggest that β-endorphin is not degraded to enkephalin but instead possesses opioid activity of its own. Goldstein's group (22) studied the properties of synthetic peptides and found that although β-endorphin is more potent than met-enkephalin in displacing ^{3}H-etorphine binding, the two peptides are equipotent in the guinea pig ileum assay. Furthermore, neither β-LPH nor β-MSH has any appreciable opioid effects in these two systems. Other opioid fragments of β-LPH have been identified by Guillemin and associates (70,71). α-Endorphin, consisting of β-LPH residues 61 to 76, has 0.36 times the receptor binding potency of met-enkephalin; γ-endorphin, β-LPH residues 61 to 77, has 0.23 times the binding potency of met-enkephalin. Therefore, β-endorphin is the most potent of the known naturally occurring opioid peptides. In addition, the effects of β-endorphin are of longer duration than those of the other fragments of β-LPH, presumably because of decreased degradation rates.

The finding that all sequenced opioid peptides (see also 65,140) have sequences contained in the structure of β-LPH indicates that this 91-amino acid peptide could serve as a precursor, or prohormone, for opioid peptides. No direct confirmation for this hypothesis has as yet been obtained. Preliminary studies on the synthesis of opioid peptides from β-LPH have taken advantage of the fact that β-LPH itself has no opioid activity. Thus Lazarus et al. (66) has shown that incubation of β-LPH with rat brain extracts generates opioid activity, presumably by breaking β-LPH into opioid peptides. This activity disappears after 2-hr incubation as the peptides are degraded. These findings were extended by Bradbury et al. (11) who demonstrated that pig pituitary contains a trypsin-like enzyme which rapidly cleaves the bond between Arg and Tyr. Such a cleavage would result in the formation of β-endorphin. Therefore, it seems likely that β-endorphin could be formed in the pituitary from β-LPH. The manner in which met-enkephalin might be formed from β-endorphin or β-LPH, or the possible origins of leu-enkephalin, are problems that have not yet been solved.

Although the higher molecular weight opioid peptides are present primarily in pituitary, recent evidence indicates that they are present in brain as well. Goldstein and co-workers (111) identified two peptides in brain that could be distinguished from enkephalin by molecular weight (1,200 to 1,600 and 3,000 to 5,000) and by sensitivity to trypsin. Such findings raise the question of which opioid peptides are most predominant in brain. This question can best be answered by the development of assay procedures which specifically

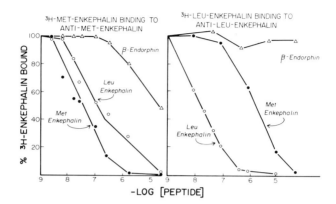

FIG. 11–6. ³H-enkephalin binding to antienkephalin sera. Sera from enkephalin-immunized or -nonimmunized guinea pigs were incubated with 4.6 nM ³H-met-enkephalin or 2.2 nM ³H-leu-enkephalin. Specific binding was determined as the difference between the total binding in the absence of unlabeled enkephalin or in the presence of 4×10^{-5} enkephalin. From Simantov et al. (116).

distinguish between enkephalins and other opioid peptides. The traditional assay procedures (i.e., radioreceptor binding and guinea pig ileum bioassays) detect all opioid peptides and cannot distinguish between individual peptides. The recent development of radioimmunoassays for enkephalins (116,123, 145; R. J. Miller, K.-J. Chang, B. Cooper, and P. Cuatrecasas, *personal communication*) provides an opportunity for this distinction. The enkephalin radioimmunoassay not only distinguishes between met- and leu-enkephalin but also distinguishes enkephalins from higher molecular weight opioid peptides. For example, in our laboratory, antiserum directed against either met- or leu-enkephalin cross-reacts with β-endorphin only at a 1,000-fold molar excess of the latter peptide (Fig. 11–6). When the radioimmunoassay is combined with the radioreceptor assay, estimates can be made concerning levels of different opioid peptides. In pituitary, large amounts of opioid activity are detected by radioreceptor assay (210,000 β-endorphin equivalents per gram tissue), whereas no significant amount of enkephalin is detected by radioimmunoassay (< 2 pmole enkephalin per gram tissue). Therefore, in pituitary the larger opioid peptides, presumably endorphins, predominate. In brain, however, there are not large differences between enkephalin levels measured by radioimmunoassay and total opioid levels measured by radioreceptor assay, indicating only low levels of larger peptides in brain (116).

Studies of brain opioid peptide content before and after pituitary ablation further indicate that brain opioid peptides are not derived from pituitary precursors (17). Thus enkephalins appear to represent the major brain opioid peptides while endorphins predominate in the pituitary.

OTHER OPIOID PEPTIDES

Still other opioid peptides may be present in peripheral tissues. Pert et al. (98) recently reported isolation of a small opioid peptide (MW 600) from human plasma on the basis of competition for receptor binding. This peptide, termed anodynin, was distinguishable from enkephalin by its stability in the presence of proteolytic enzymes and by different mobility in thin-layer chromatography. Studies of guinea pig kidney (115), which possesses opiate receptor binding of an anomalous nature, reveal the presence of a substance which inhibits kidney opiate binding more than that of brain. Until these substances are better characterized and their relationship to sequenced opioid peptides is established, however, their significances are difficult to evaluate.

OPIATE RECEPTOR "SECOND MESSENGERS"

In several biochemically characterized systems, "second messenger" substances appear to transmit information about events taking place at the cell membrane to the rest of the cell. The binding of opiates or opioid peptides to their specific membrane receptors could also be signaled to the rest of opiate-sensitive cells by modulation of second messengers, such as cyclic nucleotides. If this is the case, then opiates should indeed affect these cyclic nucleotide systems. This modulation should also show parallels with receptor pharmacology; effects of opiate agonists on cyclic nucleotide levels should be stereospecific, and the relative effects of a series of opioid drugs should correlate well with their relative receptor affinities and pharmacological potencies.

Collier and Roy (20) have shown that morphine inhibits prostaglandin (PGE_1)-stimulated adenylate cyclase in rat brain homogenates. The inhibition is mimicked by other agonists whose effects roughly correspond to their *in vivo* potencies, is stereospecific, and is blocked by naloxone. In addition, several reports (see 146) have shown a decrease of dopamine-stimulated adenylate cyclase with morphine in brain, an effect which was reversed by naloxone. However, studies in rat brain (15) have not reproduced these effects. Research with a neuroblastoma × glioma cell line that contains opiate receptors pharmacologically similar to those of brain (54) has demonstrated that morphine inhibits both basal and PGE_1-stimulated adenylate cyclase (114,138). All these effects on neuroblastoma × glioma cells are stereospecific and blocked by naloxone. Long-term exposure of these cells to morphine (i.e., "addicted cells") causes adenylate cyclase activity to return to normal; when addicted cells are withdrawn by brief exposure to naloxone, adenylate cyclase activity dramatically increases (56). These findings led to the suggestion that addicted cells adapt to morphine by an increase in adenylate cyclase. Thus, in tolerant cells cyclic AMP levels are normal. When the opiate is withdrawn, cyclic AMP levels rise above normal, thus indicating dependence.

The discovery that morphine inhibits adenylate cyclase suggests that endogenous opiate peptides might act in the same way. In slices of rat neostriatum, both leu- and met-enkephalin mimic the effect of morphine in decreasing cyclic AMP and increasing cyclic GMP levels, as long as degradation is inhibited by bacitracin (81). These effects are blocked by naloxone. Klee and Nirenberg (55) demonstrated that both enkephalins inhibit basal and PGE$_1$-stimulated adenylate cyclase in neuroblastoma × glioma cells. Although leu-enkephalin is less active as an inhibitor than met-enkephalin, both peptides are significantly more potent than morphine.

Modulation of cyclic nucleotide systems thus does seem to be a pharmacologically relevant sequel to opiate or opioid-peptide binding to opiate receptors. Interactions with prostaglandin-stimulated adenylate cyclase, for example, suggest that opiates may also indirectly modify other cyclase-coupled events through their effects on the adenylate cyclase.

ADDICTION AND ANALGESIA

Continuing goals in the study of the brain systems with which opiates interact have been the hopes that such studies might help to elucidate mechanisms of addiction, and that these inquiries might possibly lead to the development of less-addictive analgesics.

Both enkephalin and β-endorphin produce analgesia when administered intracerebroventricularly or into the periaqueductal gray (5,14,16,79). The relatively higher potency of D-Ala-met-enkephalin (91), which is more slowly metabolized than enkephalin, suggests that the low potency and transient nature of met-enkephalin's effects might be due to degradation. However, leu-enkephalin is also a consistently less potent analgesic than met-enkephalin in these studies. Both enkephalin and β-endorphin effects are naloxone-reversible, suggesting that they are due to interactions with opiate receptors.

These opioid peptides produce analgesia; unfortunately, on repeated administration, they also seem to lead to the addictive phenomena of tolerance and physical dependence. Repeated administration of enkephalin (16,142) and of endorphin (141) have resulted in the development of tolerance to the effects of these peptides. Moreover, cross-tolerance between enkephalin and morphine is demonstrable by successive treatments with both compounds. Physical dependence to enkephalin and endorphin is seen by noting withdrawal symptoms when naloxone is injected into animals after courses of administration of these opioid peptides (72,91,144).

Enkephalin has apparent reinforcing properties when injected intracerebroventricularly. Rats will sustain lever-pressing behavior in order to self-administer enkephalin into the lateral ventricle (7). This may suggest an association of these peptides with reward and drive-reduction systems in the brain (6) as postulated for the noradrenergic brain systems with which other classes of addictive drugs interact.

Apparently, then, the isolation of opioid peptides has not yet allowed a dissociation between the analgesic and the addictive properties of opiate receptor agonists.

Clues as to the mechanism of addiction might be provided by the elucidation of opiate receptor and opioid peptide mechanisms. One approach, as seen above, has been to hypothesize a relationship between addiction and changes in cyclic nucleotides. Decreased cyclic AMP levels seen in cell lines after acute opiate exposure are thought to return to normal with the development of tolerance, and to overshoot normal levels as opiates are withdrawn. Another potential mechanism for addiction is found in the regulatory processes that presumably regulate opioid peptide release. In this model, prolonged brain exposure to opiates might lead to diminution of presynaptic opiate peptide release, by feedback regulation. As the release of endogenous opioid peptide slowed, tolerance would occur when receptors, previously exposed to exogenous opiates and endogenous opioid peptides, were exposed only to opiates. Withdrawal could take place in the period when opiate drugs had been removed, but opioid peptide release had not yet been resumed.

Preliminary experiments in our laboratory (124) indicated that morphine addiction causes an increase in opioid peptides levels in rat brain, as assayed by competition for receptor binding. However, radioimmunoassay and an improved radioreceptor assay for enkephalin fail to reveal a change in levels with chronic morphine administration (18,34).

DISTRIBUTION OF THE OPIATE RECEPTOR AND OPIOID PEPTIDES

Studies of the distribution of opiate receptors and opioid peptides in various bodily organs, in different subcellular fractions, in different species, at several development stages, and in different brain and pituitary regions have been of interest, sometimes suggesting sites of action for opioid drugs.

Subcellular Distribution

Selective centrifugation techniques allow separation from brain homogenates of populations of subcellular particles rich in synaptosomes, the pinched-off nerve endings in which various neurotransmitter candidates are concentrated. If opioid peptides and opiate receptor binding are enriched at synapses, then they should be concentrated in synaptosomal fractions.

Opiate receptor binding is indeed concentrated in the synaptosome-containing crude mitochondrial (P_2) fraction, in a more purified synaptosome preparation derived from sucrose gradient subfractionation of unlysed P_2 fractions, and in bands enriched in synaptosomal ghosts and damaged synaptosomes obtained from sucrose gradient subfractionation of lysed P_2 fractions (100).

Enkephalin, measured by radioreceptor assay of brain homogenate extracts, is also enriched in the crude mitochondrial pellet and in discontinuous gradient P_2 subfractions with more purified synaptosomes (121). When lysed P_2 fractions are applied to sucrose gradients, however, enkephalin activity is associated with the lysate and with several membrane-containing fractions (121). Subcellular fractionation of the pituitary shows that opioid peptide activity, presumably endorphins, is associated with "secretory granules" (104).

The localization of both the opiate receptor and enkephalin in synaptosomal subcellular fractions is therefore consistent with a synaptic role for this receptor and its apparent physiological ligand.

Tissue Distribution

Substantial ^{3}H-opiate binding and enkephalin activities are found in brain, but not in many other organs. ^{3}H-naloxone binding to guinea pig heart, stomach, and pancreas, for example, is less than one-sixth of binding to whole brain (132). Binding to the guinea pig intestine, as seen above, has properties similar to those of binding to brain membranes (25). Binding with properties different from that seen in the brain has been observed in kidney and liver membranes (115).

Enkephalin activity is similarly concentrated in brain but not in other tissues such as the lung, liver, kidney, or heart (47,131). Immunohistofluorescence studies do show enkephalin immunoreactivity in the walls of the intestine (31). The fact that both enkephalin and the opiate receptor are preferentially localized to the brain and intestine suggests that enkephalin may fit into the emerging paradigm of peptides with brain and gut localizations (90).

Phylogenetic Distribution

The phylogenetic distributions of both the opiate receptor and of the enkephalins reveal a striking discontinuity. In invertebrates, virtually no enkephalin activity or receptor binding can be detected (93,117). The nervous systems of even the most primitive vertebrates, such as the hagfish, display substantial levels of opiate receptor binding and enkephalin, as measured by radioreceptor assay (93,117). There is no clear trend toward either increasing or decreasing amounts of enkephalin activity and opiate receptor density from more primitive to more advanced vertebrates. Nevertheless, the presence of enkephalinergic systems seems to clearly distinguish vertebrates from invertebrates.

Ontogenetic Distribution

Opiate receptor binding (19,35) and enkephalin as measured by radioreceptor assay (35) seem to develop in parallel in the fetal and neonatal rat. At 2 weeks gestational age, enkephalin activity precedes the initial development of receptor binding. The receptor binding and enkephalin activities develop at a rapid rate until birth, level off for the first postnatal week, and then climb to adult levels in strikingly parallel fashion. This parallelism is similar to that observed with several other transmitter-synthetic enzymes and their receptors (23,32).

Brain/Pituitary Regional Distribution

The anatomic circuitry underlying physiological processes affected by opiates is fairly well understood only in a few instances. It might be hypothesized, however, that enkephalinergic synapses should be found somewhere in the brain pathways involved with each opiate-modulated physiological process. Hints of conceivable sites of opiates' interactions with these ongoing physiological processes have made the study of the brain and pituitary regional distributions of the opiate receptor, enkephalin, and endorphins a subject of intense interest.

Regional distribution studies of receptor binding and of enkephalin levels have each been carried out both in test-tube studies of macroscopically dissected tissue samples from various brain regions and in histological studies on brain sections. Endogenous opioid peptide activity extracted from dissected brain regions has been measured by competition for opiate receptor binding (83) or by activity on smooth muscle preparations (47). More recently, radioimmunoassays specific for each of the enkephalins have allowed regional measurement of these peptides; enkephalin seems to constitute the majority of endogenous opioid activity, or the pituitary (116). Histologic autoradiographic localization of the opiate receptor is based on observations by Pert et al. (95) After intravenous injections of the potent opiate antagonist ^{3}H-diprenorphine, most of the drug found in the brain is unmetabolized, and is specifically bound to opiate receptors. Brains taken from rats 1 hr after ^{3}H-diprenorphine injection can be frozen, sectioned, and processed for autoradiography. Opiate receptor densities in a given brain area are then proportional to the density of exposed silver grains seen over the region when viewed in a light microscope. If grains represent true receptor binding, pharmacologically active unlabeled opiates should compete for binding, reducing grain number, while inactive isomers should not have this effect. When the active opiate levorphanol is injected along with the ^{3}H-diprenorphine, the number of grains seen overlying areas with high receptor density drops dramatically; this effect is not seen when the inactive isomer dextrallorphan is coinjected with the ^{3}H-diprenorphine (96).

Enkephalins and other endorphins are seen in tissue sections by the technique of indirect immunohistofluorescence (21). Enkephalin distribution has been studied by Elde et al. (31) and in this laboratory (119). In our laboratory, antisera characterized in radioimmunoassay as having high titer, selectivity, and affinity for enkephalin are incubated with formalin-fixed, cryostat-cut brain sections. After washing, a fluorescein-conjugated anti-IgG is applied, depositing fluorescent material wherever the primary antibody is bound. Following further washes, specimens are viewed in a fluorescence microscope. Criteria for specificity include the absence of fluorescence in adjacent control sections stained with preimmune serum or with serum adsorbed with enkephalin (Fig. 11–7A,B).

Much of the central nervous system has been mapped using dissection techniques for the opiate receptor and for enkephalin. Histologic autoradiographic studies of opiate receptor distribution and initial immunohistofluorescence studies of brain enkephalin distribution have been completed as well. α- and β-Endorphin fluorescence has been seen in the pituitary and in certain other brain regions (8). The level of anatomic resolution of macrodissection techniques is not very high, whereas that of light microscopic ³H-autoradiography of reversible ligands is somewhat greater. Immunohistochemical methods have a potential for the elucidation of a considerable degree of cellular structural detail about enkephalin- and endorphin-containing neuronal systems. This degree of detail is now being sought with, for example, the use of axoplasmic transport inhibitors to increase cell body peptide concentrations (R. Elde, *personal communication*). As this is written, extensive description is available only of the regional densities of axons and nerve terminals. However, the density of neuronal cell bodies seems to parallel the density of axons and terminals in several regions examined (139; R. Elde, *personal communication;* G. Uhl, R. Goodman, M. Kuhar, and S. Snyder, *submitted*).

Spinal Cord

Opiate receptor binding and enkephalin are present in the spinal cord gray matter. High densities of both are found in laminae I and II (107), a region implicated in nociception (52) and in responsiveness to morphine (53).

Dissection studies (64) of receptor binding show binding in monkey spinal cord to be greatly enriched in laminae I to III, intermediate in the remainder of spinal gray matter, and very low in white matter (Table 11–2). Further, section of the dorsal roots leads to substantial reduction in receptor binding in laminae I to III; binding elsewhere in the cord is unchanged.

Receptor autoradiography confirms this picture, showing dense grains overlying laminae I and II of rat spinal cord, fewer grains over the remaining gray matter, and even fewer grains over white matter (1,96) (Fig. 11–8).

Some enkephalin activity is detectable by radioreceptor assay on dissected fragments of both dorsal and ventral spinal cord (118) (Table 11–2). Enkephalin immunohistofluorescence is seen in much of the spinal gray matter as well as in the white matter adjacent to the lateral aspect of laminae I and

$\longrightarrow$

FIG. 11–7. Enkephalin immunohistofluorescence. (A): Globus pallidus (GP) and striatum (cp). (B): Area similar to A stained with enkephalin-absorbed antiserum. (C): Ventral horn (VH) of spinal cord. (D): Dorsal horn of spinal cord. LT, Lissauer's tract; sg, substantia gelatinosa. Bars = 25 μm (119).

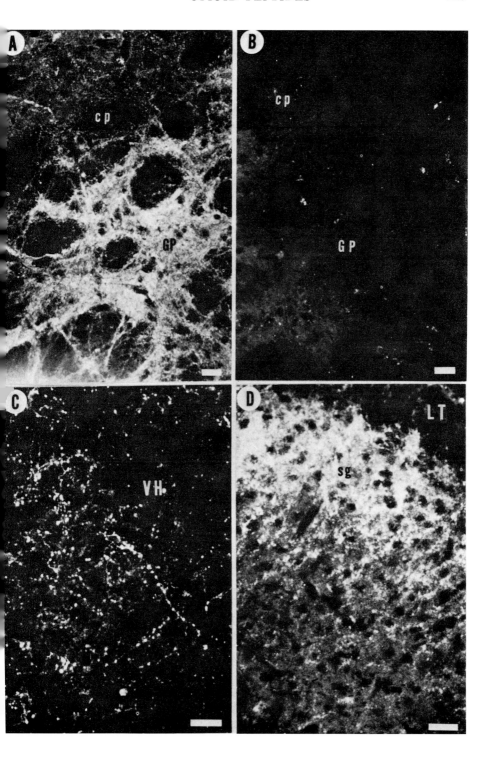

II (31,119). In the gray matter, fluorescence is most concentrated in laminae I and II (Figs. 11–7,11–8) and in the area around the central canal. Long enkephalin-fluorescent fibers are evident in the ventral horn (Fig. 11–7C). At high cervical levels, the "substantia gelatinosa" of the nucleus caudalis

TABLE 11–2. *Distribution of enkephalin activity and opiate receptor binding in monkey brain regions*

Region	Enkephalin concentration (units/mg protein)	Opiate receptor density[a] (fmole stereospecific [3H] dihydromorphine bound/mg protein)
Cerebral cortex		
Superior temporal gyrus	0.88 ± 0.11	10.8
Inferior temporal gyrus	0.53 ± 0.07	6.0
Postcentral gyrus	0.46 ± 0.05	2.8
Precentral gyrus	0.41 ± 0.07	3.4
Temporal pole	0.36 ± 0.07	
Frontal pole	0.35 ± 0.04	11.9
Occipital pole	0.24 ± 0.04	2.3
White matter areas		
Corpus callosum posterior	0.56 ± 0.05	< 2 (Whole)
Corpus callosum anterior	0.53 ± 0.05	
Optic chiasma	0.40 ± 0.06	< 2
Corona radiata	0.34 ± 0.02	< 2
Limbic cortex		
Amygdala	1.68 ± 0.16	65.1 (Anterior) 34.1 (Posterior)
Hippocampus	0.52 ± 0.07	12.5
Hypothalamus		
Anterior hypothalamus	4.20 ± 0.47	24.3
Posterior hypothalamus	1.35 ± 0.11	24.7
Thalamus		
Medial thalamus	0.57 ± 0.04	24.6
Lateral thalamus	0.25 ± 0.02	7.8
Pulvinar	0.19 ± 0.02	
Extrapyramidal areas		
Head of caudate nucleus	5.28 ± 0.40	19.4
Globus pallidus interior	4.96 ± 0.41	7.7 (Whole globus pallidus)
Globus pallidus exterior	4.92 ± 0.34	
Body of caudate nucleus	3.04 ± 0.37	9.0
Tail of caudate nucleus	1.72 ± 0.20	8.9
Putamen	0.96 ± 0.07	11.7
Midbrain		
Periaqueductal gray	1.48 ± 0.16	31.1
Raphe area	1.08 ± 0.06	8.2
Superior colliculi	0.72 ± 0.05	10.6
Inferior colliculi	0.46 ± 0.03	6.7
Cerebellum-lower brainstem		
Floor of fourth ventricle	1.14 ± 0.08	6.3
Lower medulla oblongata	0.44 ± 0.04	5.8
Deep nucleus	0.17 ± 0.02	
Cerebellar cortex	0.16 ± 0.02	< 2
Spinal cord (cervical)		
Dorsal cord (white and grey)	0.72	3.1 (White)
Ventral cord (white and grey)	0.72	3.3 (White)

[a] Derived from 61 and 118.

of nerve V is also densely fluorescent. Interestingly, preliminary studies appear to indicate that the spinal cord lacks appreciable α- and β-endorphin fluorescence (F. Bloom, *personal communication*).

Enkephalin in laminae I and II seems well positioned to interact with the dense receptor population seen there. Rhizotomy experiments suggest that a substantial portion of the opiate receptors in these laminae are found on afferent axons; indeed, the region of laminae II to III seems to contain a relatively large number of axoaxonic synapses (105,106). Opiates applied locally to the spinal cord have been shown to cause analgesia (149). The synapses on afferent neurons could be the anatomic substrate for this opiate-induced attenuation of nociceptive input. Enkephalinergic modulation of information throughout the spinal gray could also take place via gelatinosa synapses on dendritic processes of cells with perikarya located in deeper laminae or by way of the enkephalin fibers seen in other dorsal and ventral horn regions. Communications between different spinal segments might occur via the enkephalin fibers noted to run in the dorsal horn fasciculus proprius lateral to laminae I and II.

An extensive literature suggests that brainstem modulation of nociceptive input (see below) may, at least in part, involve pathways descending to the spinal cord, perhaps from the nucleus raphé magnus (reviewed in 78). If these pathways used enkephalin as a transmitter, enkephalin fluorescence

Enkephalin   Opiate Receptor

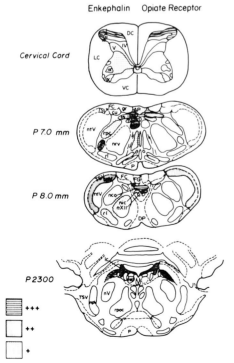

FIG. 11–8. Distributions of enkephalin (*left*) and opiate receptors (*right*) at different levels of the spinal cord and medulla. Abbreviations are as follows: amb, nucleus ambiguus; AP, area postrema; cu, nucleus cuneatus; DC, dorsal column; DP, decussatio pyramidis; FC, fasciculus cuneatus; FG, fasciculus gracilis; gr, nucleus gracilis; io, nucleus olivaris inferior; LC, lateral column; lc, locus ceruleus; nco, nucleus commissuralis; nic, nucleus intercalatus; npV, nucleus principis nerve trigemenii; nrv, nucleus reticularis medullae oblongata pars ventralis; ntd, nucleus tegmenti dorsalis Gudden; nts, nucleus tractus solitarius; ntV, nucleus tractus spinalis nervi trigemini; nV, nucleus origini nerve trigemini; NX, nucleus originis dorsalis vagi; nXII, nucleus originis nervi hypoglossi; P, tractus corticospinalis; rl, nucleus reticularis parvocellularis; rpoc, nucleus reticularis pontis caudalis; sgV, substantia gelatinosa trigemini; ts, tractus solitarius; TSV, tractus spinalis nervi trigemini; VC, ventral column. Derived from (63,64,119).

might be expected to be reduced in spinal segments below cord hemisections. Preliminary evidence from hemisection experiments in the rat (R. Elde, *personal communication*) and in the monkey (R. LaMotte, G. Uhl, M. J. Kuhar, and S. H. Snyder, *unpublished observations*) suggests that substantial enkephalin fluorescence in laminae I and II is not contained in the descending processes of neurons with cell bodies located at supraspinal levels. Since cutting dorsal roots also fails to substantially lower spinal cord enkephalin fluorescence (R. Elde, *personal communication;* R. LaMotte, G. Uhl, M. J. Kuhar, and S. H. Snyder, *unpublished observations*), it would seem that enkephalin is contained in interneurons in laminae I and II of the spinal cord.

Medulla Oblongata/Cerebellum/Pons

Opiate receptor binding and enkephalin activities are particularly evident in certain cranial nerve nuclei and in the floor of the fourth ventricle. The cerebellum and cerebellar deep nuclei, on the other hand, contain low levels of both enkephalin and opiate receptors.

Dissection studies of receptor binding have shown moderate binding to monkey lower medulla and the floor of the fourth ventricle, although only low binding to cerebellar, pontine, and pyramidal tract fragments could be demonstrated (46,61) (Table 11–2).

Receptor autoradiography (1) shows dense grains overlying the "substantia gelatinosa" of the nucleus caudalis of nerve V (Fig. 11–8). The dorsal part of the mesencephalic nucleus of V has moderate grain density, merging into the densely labeled parabrachial nuclei; other fifth nerve nuclear regions show lower densities. Regions associated with the tenth nerve (the nucleus tractus solitarius, nucleus commissuralis, and rostral nucleus ambiguus) show heavy grain densities, whereas moderate densities are seen over the vagal motor nuclei and along fibers of the vagus nerve. The locus ceruleus and periventricular gray matter have high receptor densities, while the area postrema, outermost layer of the dorsal cochlear nucleus, and the pontine tegmentum show moderate grain densities. Areas with receptor grain densities that are low, but nevertheless greater than the very low densities associated with white matter and cerebellar regions, include the reticular formation, olives, dorsal column nuclei, and most motor nuclei (1).

Enkephalin activity in radioreceptor dissection studies is most concentrated in the floor of the fourth ventricle, the periaqueductal gray, and the raphé area (118). The colliculi and caudal medulla have moderate levels, whereas cerebellar activity is very low (Table 11–2). Radioimmunoassay also shows moderate enkephalin levels in rat brainstem and medulla, with less in the cerebellum (123) (R. J. Miller, *personal communication*).

Enkephalin immunofluorescence is dense in the "substantia gelatinosa" of the fifth nerve; the parabrachial nuclei are also densely fluorescent (Fig.

11–8). Vagus nerve-associated structures with moderate to dense flourescence include the nucleus of the tractus solitarius, nucleus commissuralis, and nucleus ambiguus (31,119). Cranial nerve nuclei VII and XII are also densely fluorescent, as is the floor of the fourth ventricle. The area of the locus ceruleus and the pontine central gray show moderate fluorescence; the cerebellum shows relatively little.

The convergence of enkephalin and opiate receptor distributions in certain brainstem areas allows speculation about localization of opiate effects to apparent enkephalinergic synapses in these sites. Depression of respiration by opiates has been thought to involve central respiratory centers, some of which apparently lie in the floor of the fourth ventricle, whereas others are located in the vicinity of the nucleus ambiguus (50,63). Additionally, vagal afferent input is apparently of importance (43); electrical stimulation of the vagus classically causes early termination of inspiration, for example (13). The finding of opiate receptors along the course of the vagus nerve suggests that opiates might act through axoaxonic synapses to modulate vagal afferent input, some of which might be relevant to respiratory control. Thus, the opiate receptor and enkephalin densities in the vagal nucleus, as well as around the nucleus of the solitary tract, and the enkephalin density around the nucleus ambiguus suggest that these medullary centers might also be areas where opiates interact with respiratory control mechanisms. The depressant effects of opiates on cough and vomit reflexes might be mediated by dense enkephalin/opiate receptor systems in nuclei associated with the ninth, tenth, and twelfth cranial nerves which are involved with these reflexes. Nausea might be mediated at the "chemoreceptor trigger zone" lying in the floor of the fourth ventricle (9).

Mesencephalon

The midbrain contains substantial amounts of opiate receptor binding and enkephalin activity. Regions with concentrations of these activities include the periaqueductal gray, interpeduncular nucleus, and accessory optic systems.

Dissection and autoradiographic studies of receptor distribution show moderate to high binding densities in the periaqueductal gray, and in regions of the interpeduncular nucleus (2,46,61; Table 11–2, Fig. 11–9). The lateral part of the fasciculus retroflexus, carrying axons which travel to the interpeduncular nucleus, is overlayed with moderate autoradiographic grain density also. Components of the accessory optic system, the dorsal, lateral, and especially the medial terminal nuclei, are all heavily labeled. Regions of the raphé nuclei, of the superior colliculus, and of the probably optically associated fibers coursing through the substantia nigra are moderately labeled; the substantia nigra pars reticulata and the red nucleus show sparse grains (2).

Moderate enkephalin activity measured by radioreceptor assay is seen in the periaqueductal gray and raphé regions of monkey brain, with somewhat

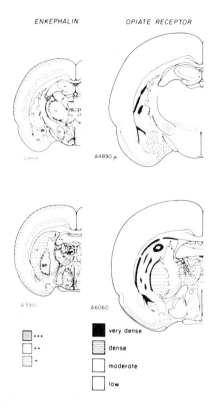

FIG. 11–9. Distribution of enkephalin (*left*) and opiate receptors (*right*) at certain levels of the diencephalon and telencephalon. Abbreviations are as follows: abl, nucleus amygdaloideus basalis, pars lateralis; ac, nucleus amygdaloideus centralis; cp, nucleus caudatus putamen; ha, nucleus anterior (hypothalami); hl, nucleus laterlis (hypothalami); hvma, nucleus ventromedialis (hypothalami), pars anterior; pt, nucleus paratenialis; tmm, nucleus medialis thalami, pars medialis; tr, nucleus reticularis thalami; tv, nucleus ventralis thalami; FH, fimbria hippocampi; GP, globus pallidus; HI, hippocampus; SM, stria medullaris thalami; ZI, zona incerta. Derived from (113,119).

less in the colliculi (118). Immunohistofluorescence studies reveal enkephalin in the periaqueductal gray, extending laterally into other regions of the midbrain tegmentum (Fig. 11–9). Moderate fluorescence is demonstrable in the dorsal portion of the inferior colliculus and overlying the raphé nuclei (31,119).

Preliminary studies of β-endorphin fluorescence show apparent fluorescent cell bodies and processes in the periaqueductal gray (F. Bloom, *personal communication*).

Classically, analgesia may be produced by electrical stimulation of or injection of morphine into the periaqueductal gray (76, 77, 92, 108). Further, enkephalin-rich brain extracts and D-ala-met-enkephalin mimic morphine's analgesic actions when injected here (99). Morphine analgesia is reduced if the raphé nucleus is lesioned beforehand (113). Since both the periaqueductal gray and dorsal raphé contain moderate to dense concentrations of opiate receptors and enkephalin, it is conceivable that some opiate-induced analgesic effects take place at enkephalinergic synapses in these two regions.

The association of both enkephalin and its receptor with pretectal nuclear components of the accessory optic system might relate to pupillary constricting effects of morphine in humans (50).

Diencephalon

Opiate receptors and enkephalin are distributed unevenly through the diencephalon, with concentrations in the infundibulum and median eminence of the hypothalamus, the anterior hypothalamus, portions of the medial habenula, and the dorsal, medial aspects of the thalamus (Table 11–2; Fig. 11–9).

Dissected fragments of medial and anterior monkey hypothalamus show moderate to high receptor binding, whereas the mammillary bodies exhibit lower levels (61). In receptor autoradiographic studies in the rat, grain density is generally low over the hypothalamus, although the infundibulum and a thin layer dorsal to the mammillary bodies exhibit moderate grain densities (2) (Fig. 11–9).

Monkey medial thalamus (61) and human dorsomedial, centromedian, and pulvinar thalamic regions (46) show elevated binding in dissection studies, while more lateral regions have considerably lower binding. Autoradiographic studies in the rat demonstrate high receptor densities in the periventricular, lateral geniculate, intralaminar, and medial thalamic regions with lower densities ventrally and laterally (2). Epithalamic regions studied include the zona incerta, displaying moderate grain density, and the habenula, with dense grains over the lateral aspect of its medial nucleus (2).

Enkephalin activity assayed by radioreceptor or radioimmunoassay is high in the hypothalamus, higher in anterior than in posterior regions (118,123; Table 11–2). Initial immunohistofluorescence studies show dense enkephalin fluorescence in the areas of the periventricular, ventromedial, dorsomedial, and medial preoptic nuclei, in the floor of the hypothalamus, and in the infundibulum. Less fluorescence occurs in the supraoptic, arcuate, mammillary, and suprachiasmatic nuclei (31,119) (Fig. 11–9). In the median eminence region, there are enkephalin-containing fibers, at least some of which appear to end on portal capillaries (R. Elde, *personal communication;* G. Uhl, M. J. Kuhar, and S. H. Snyder, *unpublished observations*). Lower fluorescence densities are evident in the suprachiasmatic nuclei (31,119). Colchicine treatment has revealed apparent enkephalinergic cell bodies in several hypothalamic nuclei; more detailed mapping of these aspects of hypothalamic enkephalin fluorescence is in progress. β-Endorphin fluorescence is also seen in the hypothalamus in what appear to be neuronal structures. Although some enrichment of endorphin fluorescence is seen in periventricular regions, detailed elucidation of its localization is incomplete (F. Bloom, *personal communication*).

Thalamic enkephalin activity measured by radioreceptor assay is generally moderate to low; nevertheless, monkey medial thalamus displays higher levels than the lateral thalamus or pulvinar (118). Immunohistofluorescence in the thalamus is densest in medial dorsal regions and in the intralaminar nuclei (119), whereas more ventral and lateral regions display little enkephalin fluorescence. The lateral border of the medial habenula shows elevated fluorescence as does the zona incerta.

Receptor and enkephalin activities in the thalamus are concentrated in dorsomedial and intralaminar areas. Thalamic intralaminar nuclei are thought to be associated with the more affective components of pain appreciation; conceivably, some of opiates' analgesia could be mediated at apparent enkephalinergic synapses here. Dorsomedial thalamic areas are strongly associated with frontal and limbic cortical regions thought to be more generally involved with affect; these thalamocortical systems might be involved in opiates' production of euphoria. Opiate receptor, enkephalin, and endorphin systems noted in the hypothalamus and median eminence might represent loci for opiates' effects on endocrine systems (36). The presence of enkephalin terminals on portal blood vessels suggests that enkephalin might be in a position to affect pituitary function after transmission through these portal capillary beds, in analogy to the well-described effects of the releasing hormones. Alternatively, enkephalin might modify the effective release of these classic releasing hormones into the portal circulation through local axoaxonic synapses.

The high density of opiate receptors and/or enkephalin associated with discrete portions of the habenula, fasciculus retroflexus, and interpeduncular nucleus seems to suggest an association of enkephalin with the habenular-interpeduncular pathway.

Telencephalon

Opiate receptors and enkephalin are present in many forebrain areas, with concentrations in certain amygdaloid nuclei, patches of the striatum, the globus pallidus, and interstitial nuclei of the stria terminalis (Table 11–2; Fig. 11–10).

Amygdaloid fragments show high binding levels in dissection studies of monkey and human tissue (61). In autoradiographic studies in the rat, high receptor grain density is seen in the medial, basal, central, and especially

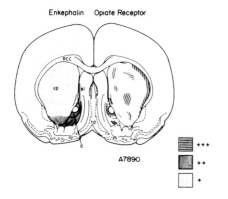

Enkephalin   Opiate Receptor

A7890

+++
++
+

FIG. 11–10. Distribution of enkephalin (*left*) and opiate receptors (*right*) in the anterior telencephalon. Abbreviations are as follows: cp, nucleus caudatus putamen; RCC, radiatio corporis callosi; sl, nucleus septi lateralis; td, nucleus tractus diagnolis (Broca). Derived from (113,119).

cortical amygdaloid nuclei. The lateral amygdala has a contrastingly low grain density (3).

The hippocampus of monkey shows moderate levels of receptor binding in dissection studies, although autoradiography of rat hippocampus reveals moderate grain densities only in the molecular layer, with low densities elsewhere (3,61). Interestingly, presubicular cortex, especially posteriorly, exhibits dense grains.

The monkey caudate nucleus has fairly high binding in dissection studies, while binding to the putamen is considerably lower (61). The rat caudate/putamen shows striking patches of dense grains on autoradiography, with interposed areas of low density (3).

In dissection studies of monkey brain and in rat autoradiographic studies, the globus pallidus exhibits moderate receptor activity (3,61).

Dissection studies of monkey and human cerebral cortex show most binding in the frontal, superior temporal, and parahippocampal gyri, whereas other regions possess lower binding levels (46,61). Autoradiography of the rat cerebral cortex shows that, except for densities over the presubicular cortex, cortical areas have only low densities most concentrated in deeper cortical layers (3).

Receptor autoradiography also reveals high grain densities over patches of the nucleus accumbens, the subfornical organ, the entopeduncular nucleus, and the interstitial nucleus of the stria terminalis. Moderate density occurs in the nucleus triangularis septi; other septal nuclei have lower grain densities (3).

By radioreceptor assay, monkey amygdala possesses moderate levels of enkephalin, while enkephalin immunohistofluorescence is dense in the rat central amygdaloid nucleus and somewhat less dense in corticomedial and basolateral areas (31,118,119). The central amygdaloid nucleus also possesses substantial β-endorphin fluorescence, with apparent fluorescent cell bodies (F. Bloom, *personal communication*).

The hippocampus exhibits little enkephalin in dissection studies or by immunohistofluorescence (118,119). Both rat striatum and monkey caudate possess high levels of enkephalin by radioreceptor and radioimmunoassays, respectively (118,123). Moderate to sparse fluorescence is seen in the rat striatum, with perhaps some of the patchiness seen with the receptor distribution (31,119). The monkey globus pallidus exhibits high levels of enkephalin radioreceptor activity; gray matter areas of the globus display the densest fluorescence in the rat brain (119,149; Fig. 11–7). By contrast, little β-endorphin fluorescence is seen in the globus pallidus, although substantial fluorescence is seen in the caudate (F. Bloom, *personal communication*).

Monkey cerebral cortical regions have generally low levels of enkephalin activity, with temporal gyri somewhat more enriched (61). Immunohistofluorescence in rat cerebral cortex is also sparse, but more concentrated in intermediate to deep cortical layers (119).

The rat nucleus accumbens, lateral septal nucleus, and interstitial nucleus of the stria terminalis all possess fairly dense (119) fluorescence.

Manipulation of certain forebrain structure leads to marked changes in reactivity and apparent affect; "sham rage" following septal lesions (4) and the taming of the Klüver-Bucy syndrome (58) following temporal lesions including the amygdala are among these. The association of opiate receptor and enkephalin concentrations with these areas suggests that they might be loci for opiates' effects on affect.

The patchy distribution of opiate receptor, and to a lesser extent, of enkephalin in the rat striatum may exhibit parallels with a patchiness found by Goldman and Nauta (40) in projections from the monkey frontal cortex to the caudate. Conceivably, some of the receptor-dense areas of the striatum could represent areas of interactions with frontal or limbic cortex. Alternatively, this patchiness could reflect a "mosaic" organization of the striatum.

Pituitary

Opiate receptor binding and nonenkephalin opioid peptides are found in the pituitary gland, with notably high concentrations in the intermediate lobe.

Dissection studies (123,127) of bovine pituitary demonstrate substantial opiate receptor binding in the posterior and intermediate lobes. Binding to anterior lobe membranes, on the other hand, is negligible.

Pituitary and brain opiate receptors have similar affinities for many opiate drugs. Met- and leu-enkephalins, however, are about 20-fold less potent at displacing ^{3}H-naloxone from pituitary than from brain receptors, although morphine has a 10-fold lower affinity in the pituitary than in the brain (127). By contrast, β-endorphin is roughly equipotent at brain and pituitary receptors (127).

Little of the pituitary's content of opiate-receptor-active substances is enkephalin. Gel chromatography shows essentially all activity eluting in fractions containing substances with the apparent molecular weight of β-endorphin (110). This corresponds well with preliminary observations that, in the pituitary proper, only very sparse enkephalin immunofluorescence can be observed (31; G. Uhl, M. J. Kuhar, and S. H. Snyder, *unpublished observations*).

Cells of the intermediate lobe of the pituitary do show α- and β-endorphin fluorescence (8) (Fig. 11–11). This fluorescence appears to be granular and to overlie the nonnuclear portions of virtually all pars intermedia parenchymal cells. The same cells stain with antisera directed against both α- and β-endorphins. The apparent intermediate lobe localization of α- and β-endorphins is interesting in light of the known presence of β-lipotropin in this lobe (27). Unfortunately, this picture is clouded somewhat by the high cross-reactivity of the β-endorphin antiserum used in these studies with β-lipotropin.

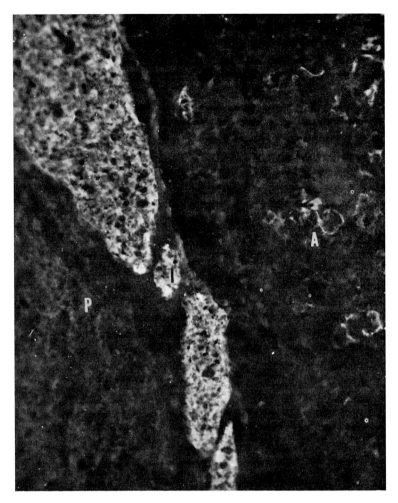

FIG. 11–11. β-Endorphin immunohistofluorescence. A, anterior lobe of pituitary; I, intermediate lobe; P, posterior lobe. Photograph courtesy of F. Bloom.

Granular α- and β-endorphin fluorescence is also seen in certain cells of the anterior pituitary; positive cells are often noted to be in close apposition to blood vessels (8). In light of this localization, it is tempting to speculate about a possible hormonal role for pituitary endorphin.

Opioid peptides other than the well-characterized α- and β-endorphins have been detected in the pituitary (41). The finding that most opiate-receptor-active material in pituitary extracts elutes from gel-filtration columns in fractions corresponding to the molecular weight range of endorphin, however, is consistent with the idea that the endorphins are the predominant pituitary peptides. The greater affinity of β-endorphin relative to the enkephalins for pituitary opiate receptor binding is also consistent with this hypothesis. Opiates have effects on several pituitary hormones. Acute effects of opiate administration may differ from those produced by chronic administration, with apparent tolerance/dependence phenomena (36). Many of these effects are reviewed elsewhere (28,36,37,39,62).

Systemic morphine causes a release of vasopressin, an effect which can be mimicked by microinjection of morphine into the supraoptic nucleus of the hypothalamus (50). This effect is suggestive of a supraoptic hypothalamic locus of the action of morphine; unfortunately, low enkephalin fluorescence and low receptor grain densities seen in this nucleus make this perhaps a less attractive locus to which to assign morphine's effect on vasopressin. The few receptors present could, of course, still account for the action of morphine. Alternatively, the finding of opiate receptors in the posterior pituitary may hint that some of morphine's effect on vasopressin is directly mediated through neurohypophyseal receptors.

Growth hormone (GH) release from the anterior pituitary is thought to be under dual control of somatostatin and growth hormone releasing hormone (75). Morphine stimulates the release of GH (29,59,109). β-Endorphin, met-enkephalin, and D-ala-met-enkephalin also facilitate GH release when injected intracerebroventricularly in rats pretreated with somatostatin antiserum (29). Administered intraventricularly or intravenously, β-endorphin is similarly effective in producing a naloxone-reversible GH release in steroid-primed and normal rats, although the lower doses of met-enkephalin and α-endorphin in this study are ineffective in releasing GH (109). The stimulation of GH release in rats with depleted circulating somatostatin suggests that morphine and opioid peptides exert their effects through release of growth hormone releasing factor from the hypothalamus (29). Failure of morphine, α-endorphin, β-endorphin, or met-enkephalin to affect GH release from pituitaries cultured *in vitro* renders a pituitary site for opiates' actions on GH release less likely. Thus, enkephalin and/or endorphin synapses on hypothalamic cells mediating growth hormone releasing hormone release are likely candidates for the site of action of opiate drugs on GH release.

Naloxone-reversible prolactin release from the pituitary follows the intraventricular or intravenous administration of morphine or β-endorphin (30, 80,109). Met-enkephalin is similarly effective when injected intraventricularly in high doses (30). Although some investigators report that morphine, enkephalin, and α-endorphin are ineffective in causing prolactin release from pituitary cell cultures (109), others find that enkephalin increases prolactin secretion in such cultures (69). The reasons for these differences are not clear. Hypothalamic influences on pituitary prolactin secretion are primarily inhibitory (62). Release of dopamine from dopaminergic terminals in the median eminence is thought to have a physiological role in the inhibition of prolactin secretion (30,74). Conceivably, hypothalamic β-endorphin and enkephalin synapses onto median eminence dopaminergic neurons could inhibit dopamine release, and thereby allow increased prolactin secretion (30).

Morphine stimulates pituitary secretion of ACTH when administered acutely (36). This effect of systemic morphine can be replicated by local injection of morphine into several hypothalamic regions (73). Areas where morphine is effective in causing ACTH release include the anterior, paraventricular, dorsomedial, and ventromedial hypothalamic areas. Electrolytic lesions of the anterior median eminence abolish morphine-elicited ACTH release (36). These findings have been interpreted in support of a hypothalamic localization of morphine's effects, possibly through actions on corticotropin releasing hormone (CRH; 38). Interestingly, many of those hypothalamic regions where locally injected morphine is effective in causing ACTH release have substantial enkephalin immunohistofluorescence. This parallel raises the possibility that opioid peptide synapses on the hypothalamic cells that secrete CRH might be loci for the ACTH effects of morphine.

Secretion of TSH is also stimulated by morphine (37). Systemically injected morphine and morphine microinjected into the preoptic/chiasmatic hypothalamus or the posterior-supramammillary hypothalamus cause TSH release. Although neither enkephalin fluorescence nor opiate receptor density is especially high in either of these areas, morphine's effects could conceivably be mediated by receptor/opioid peptide systems of low density.

Gonadotropin (FSH and LH) release is decreased by morphine (36,39). Conceivably, this effect may be mediated through hypothalamic processes modifying gonadotropin releasing hormone secretion (36).

In most cases, the effects of opiates on endocrine systems are thus thought to be mediated by hypothalamic-level interactions with releasing hormone systems. Although the lack of localized opiate receptor densities in the hypothalamus as detected by *in vivo* autoradiographic studies is not encouraging, substantial receptor binding seen in *in vitro* studies indicates that receptors with densities below those detectable by autoradiographic methods do exist in the hypothalamus.

Opiate receptor binding in the anterior and, especially, intermediate lobes of the pituitary suggests that some opiate actions might be mediated there. However, the function of the mammalian pars intermedia is not clear.

Opioid peptide/receptor systems in extrahypothalamic brain regions might provide loci for some opiate effects on endocrine processes. For example, the central amygdala is rich in enkephalin, β-endorphin, and opiate receptors, and is thought to be intimately involved in the control of the secretion of growth hormone (75) and gonadotropins (33).

CONCLUSION

A series of investigations, triggered by the demonstration of opiate receptor binding in brain membranes, has begun to unravel the details of several apparent brain/pituitary systems that were previously unknown. Increasing morphological, biochemical, and physiological evidence supports the hypothesis that the enkephalins, and perhaps the endorphins, have neurotransmitter-like roles in the brain, interacting with the physiological receptors labeled by tritiated opiate drugs. Differences between the brain and pituitary complements of opiate receptors and opioid peptides suggest the existence of distinct "enkephalinergic" and "endorphinergic" opiate-sensitive subdivisions. β-Endorphin, perhaps formed from β-lipotropin, might act in a neurotransmitter-like role in the brain, and have a hormonal function in the pituitary. The neurotransmitter-like activities of enkephalins seem to take place, at least in part, at axoaxonic synapses. The physiological actions of opiates ought, in general, to be explicable ultimately by their effects on opioid peptide/opiate receptor systems.

ACKNOWLEDGMENTS

Supported by USPHS Grant DA-00266, and by NIMH RSDA Awards MH-33128 to S.H.S. and 5T01 GM01183–13 to G.R.U. We thank Drs. M. Molliver, R. LaMotte, and J. Campbell for their helpful comments on sections of the manuscript, Susan M. Garonski for manuscript preparation, and Pamela D. Morgan and Carl E. Kenyon for their assistance.

REFERENCES

1. Atweh, S., and Kuhar, M. J. (1977): Autoradiographic localization of opiate receptors in rat brain. I. Spinal cord and lower medulla. *Brain Res.,* 124:53–67.
2. Atweh, S., and Kuhar, M. J. (1977): Autoradiographic localization of opiate receptors in rat brain. II. The brainstem. *Brain Res. (in press).*
3. Atweh, S., and Kuhard, M. J. (1977): Autoradiographic localization of opiate receptor in rat brain. III. Forebrain. *Brain Res. (in press).*
4. Bard, P., and Mountcastle, V. B. (1948): Some forebrain mechanisms involved in expression of rage with special reference to expression of angry behavior. *Res. Publ. Assoc. Res. Nerv. Ment. Dis.,* 27:362–404.
5. Belluzzi, J. D., Grant, N., Garsky, V., Sarantakes, D., Wise, C. D., and Stein, L. (1976): Analgesia induced *in vivo* by central administration of enkephalin in rat. *Nature,* 260:625–626.
6. Belluzzi, J. D., and Stein, L. (1977): Enkephalin may mediate euphoria and drive-reduction reward. *Nature,* 266:556–558.
7. Belluzzi, J. D., Wise, C. D., and Stein, L. (1976): Enkephalin: Intraventricular self-administration in the rat. Sixth Annual Meeting of the Society for Neuroscience, *Neurosci. Abstr.,* 564.
8. Bloom, F. E., Battenberg, E., Rossier, J., Ling, N., Leppaluoto, J., Vargo, T., and Guillemin, R. (1977): Endorphins are located in the intermediate and anterior lobes of the pituitary gland, not in the neurohypophysis. *Life Sci.,* 20:43–48.
9. Borison, H. (1971): The Nervous System. In: *Narcotic Drugs: Biochemistry and Pharmacology,* edited by D. Clouet. Plenum Press, New York.
10. Bradbury, A. F., Smyth, D. G., and Snell, C. R. (1976): The peptide hormones: Molecular and cellular aspects. *Ciba Found. Symp.,* 41:61–75.
11. Bradbury, A. F., Smyth, D. G., and Snell, C. R. (1976): Lipotropin: Precursor to two biologically active peptides. *Biochem. Biophys. Res. Commun.,* 69:950–956.
12. Bradbury, A. F., Smyth, D. G., Snell, C. R., Birdsall, N. J. M., and Hulme, E. C.

(1976): C fragment of lipotropin has a high affinity for brain opiate receptors. *Nature,* 260:793–795.

13. Bradley, G. (1976): The effect of CO_2, body temperature, and anesthesia on the response to vagal stimulation. In: *Respirator Centers and Afferent Systems,* edited by B. Duron, INSERM, Paris.

14. Büscher, H. H., Hill, R. C., Römer, D., Cardinaux, F., Closse, A., Hauser, D., and Pless, D., Jr. (1976): Evidence for analgesic activity of enkephalin in the mouse. *Nature,* 261:423–424.

15. Carenzi, A., Guidotti, A., Revuelta, A., and Costa, E. (1975): Molecular mechanisms in the action of morphine and viminol on rat striatum. *J. Pharmacol. Exp. Ther.,* 194:311–318.

16. Chang, J. K., Fong, B. T. W., Pert, A., and Pert, C. B. (1976): Opiate receptor affinities and behavioral effects of enkephalin: Structure-activity relationship of ten synthetic peptide analogues. *Life Sci.,* 18:1473–1482.

17. Cheung, A., and Goldstein, A. (1976): Failure of hypophysectomy to alter brain content of opioid peptides (endorphins). *Life Sci.,* 19:1005–1008.

18. Childers, S., and Snyder, S. (1977): Enkephalin levels in brains of morphine-dependent rats. *Neuropharmacology (in press).*

19. Clendenium, N., Petraitis, M., and Siman, E. (1976): Ontological development of opiate receptors in rodent brain. *Brain Res.,* 118:157–160.

20. Collier, H. O. J., and Roy, A. C. (1974): Morphine-like drugs inhibit stimulation by E prostaglandins of cyclic AMP formation by rat brain homogenate. *Nature,* 248:24–27.

21. Coons, A. H. (1958): Fluorescent antibody methods. In: *General Cytochemical Methods,* edited by J. Daniell. Academic Press, New York.

22. Cox, B. M., Goldstein, A., and Li, C. H. (1976): Opiate activity of a peptide, β-lipotropin-61-91, derived from β-lipotropin. *Proc. Natl. Acad. Sci. USA,* 73:1821–1823.

23. Coyle, J., and Yamamura, H. (1976): Neurochemical aspects of the ontogenesis of cholinergic neurons in the rat brain. *Brain Res.,* 118:429–440.

24. Creese, I., Pasternak, G. W., Pert, C. B., and Snyder, S. H. (1975): Discrimination by temperature of opiate agonist and antagonist receptor binding. *Life Sci.,* 16:1837–1842.

25. Creese, I., and Snyder, S. H. (1975): Receptor binding and pharmacological activity of opiates in the guinea pig intestine. *J. Pharmacol. Exp. Ther.,* 194:205–219.

26. Cuatrecasas, P. (1974): Membrane receptors. *Annu. Rev. Biochem.,* 43:169–214.

27. Dessy, C., Herlant, M., and Cretieu, M. (1973): Immunohistofluorescent detection of lipotropin synthesizing cells. *C. R. Acad. Sci. [D] (Paris),* 276:335–338.

28. DeWied, D., van Ree, J., and De Jong, W. (1974): Narcotic analgesia and the neuroendocrine control of anterior pituitary function. In: *Narcotics and the Hypothalamus,* edited by E. Zimmerman and R. George. Raven Press, New York.

29. Dupont, A., Cusan, L., Garon, M., Labrie, F., and Li, C. H. (1977): β-endorphin: Stimulation of growth hormone release *in vivo*. *Proc. Natl. Acad. Sci. USA,* 74:358–359.

30. Dupont, A., Cusan, L., Labrie, F., Coy, D., and Li, C. H. (1977): Stimulation of prolactin release in rat by intraventricular injection of β-endorphin and methionine-enkephalin. *Biochem. Biophys. Res. Commun.,* 75:76–82.

31. Elde, R., Hökfelt, T., Johannson, O., and Terenius, L. (1976): Immunohistochemical studies using antibodies to leu-enkephalin: Initial observations on the nervous system of the rat. *Neurosci.,* 1:349–355.

32. Enna, S., Yamamura, H., and Snyder, S. (1976): Development of muscarinic cholinergic and GABA receptor binding in chick embryo brain. *Brain Res.,* 101:177–183.

33. Flerkó, B. (1975): Hypothalamic mediation of neuroendocrine regulation of hypophysial gonadotrophic functions. In: *Reproductive Physiology,* edited by R. Greep. University Park Press, Baltimore.

34. Fratta, W., Yang, H., Hang, J., and Costa, E. (1977): Stability of met-enkephalin

content in brain structures of morphine-dependent or foot-shock stressed rats. *Nature (in press)*.

35. Garcin, F., and Coyle, J. (1976): Ontogenetic development of [³H]naloxone binding and endogenous morphine-like factor in rat brain. In: *Opiates and Endogenous Opioid Peptides*, edited by H. W. Kosterlitz. North Holland, Amsterdam.

36. George, R. (1971): Hypothalamus: Anterior pituitary gland. In: *Narcotic Drugs: Biochemical Pharmacology*, edited by D. Clouet. Plenum Press, New York.

37. George, R. (1973): Effects of narcotic analgesics on hypothalamo-pituitary-thyroid function. Drug effects on neuroendocrine regulation. *Prog. Brain Res.*, 30:339–345.

38. George, R., and Way, E. (1959): The role of the hypothalamus in pituitary-adrenal activation and antidiuresis by morphine. *J. Pharmacol. Exp. Ther.*, 125:111–115.

39. Gold, E., and Ganong, W. (1967): Effects of drugs on neuroendocrine processes. In: *Neuroendocrinology, Vol. 2*, edited by L. Martini and W. Ganong. Academic Press, New York.

40. Goldman, P., and Nauta, W. (1977): An intricately patterned prefronto-caudate projection in the rhesus monkey. *J. Comp. Neurol.*, 171:369–386.

41. Goldstein, A. (1976): Opioid peptides (endorphins) in pituitary and brain. *Science*, 193:1081–1083.

42. Goldstein, A., Lowney, L. I., and Pal, B. K. (1971): Stereospecific and nonspecific interactions of the morphine congener levorphanol in subcellular fractions of the mouse brain. *Proc. Natl. Acad. Sci. USA*, 68:1742–1747.

43. Gromysz, H., and Karczewski, W. (1976): Responses of the brain stem respiratory neurons to stimulation of the vagal input. In: *Respiratory Centers and Afferent Systems*, edited by B. Duran. INSERM, Paris.

44. Hambrook, J. M., Morgan, B. A., Rance, M. J., and Smith, C. F. C. (1976): Mode of deactivation of the enkephalins by rat and human plasma and rat brain homogenates. *Nature*, 262:782–783.

45. Herz, A., and Teschemacher, H. (1971): Activities and sites of antinociceptive action of morphine-like analgesics. *Adv. Drug Res.*, 6:29–111.

46. Hiller, J., Pearson, J., and Simon, E. (1973): Distribution of stereospecific binding of the potent narcotic analgesic etorphine in human brain: Predominance in the limbic system. *Res. Commun. Chem. Pathol. Pharmacol.*, 6:1052–1062.

47. Hughes, J. T. (1975): Isolation of an endogenous compound from the brain with the pharmacological properties similar to morphine. *Brain Res.*, 88:295–308.

48. Hughes, J., Smith, T. W., Kosterlitz, H. W., Fothergill, L., Morgan, B. A., and Morris, H. R. (1975): Identification of two related pentapeptides from the brain with potent opiate agonist activity. *Nature*, 258:577–579.

49. Hughes, J., Smith, T., Morgan, B., and Fothergill, L. (1975): Purification and properties of enkephalin-possible endogenous ligand for morphine receptors. *Life Sci.*, 16:1753–1758.

50. Jaffe, J., and Martin, W. (1975): Narcotic analgesics and antagonists. In: *The Pharmacological Basis of Therapeutics*, edited by L. Goodman and A. Gilman, pp. 245–283. Macmillan, New York.

51. Jones, C. R., Gibbons, W. A., and Garsky, V. (1976): Proton magnetic resonance studies of conformation and flexibility of enkephalin peptides. *Nature*, 263:779–782.

52. Kerr, F. (1975): Neuroanatomical substrates of nociception in the spinal cord. *Pain*, 1:325–356.

53. Kitahata, L., Kosaka, Y., Taub, A., Bauikos, K., and Hoffeit, M. (1974): Lamina-specific suppression of dorsal horn unit activity by morphine sulfate. *Anesthesiology*, 41:39–48.

54. Klee, W. A., and Nirenberg, M. (1974): A neuroblastoma × glioma cell line with morphine receptors. *Proc. Natl. Acad. Sci. USA*, 71:3474–3477.

55. Klee, W. A., and Nirenberg, M. (1976): Mode of action of endogenous opiate peptides. *Nature*, 263:609–611.

56. Klee, W. A., Sharma, S. K., and Nirenberg, M. (1975): Opiate receptors as regulators of adenylate cyclase. *Life Sci.*, 16:1869–1874.

57. Klee, W. A., and Streaty, R. A. (1974): Narcotic receptor sites in morphine-dependent rats. *Nature*, 248:61–63.

58. Klüver, H., and Bucy, P. (1938): An analysis of certain effects of bilateral temporal lobectomy in the rhesus monkey with special reference to psychic blindness. *J. Psychol.,* 5:34–54.
59. Kokko, N., Garcia, J., and Elliott, H. (1973): Effects of acute and chronic administration of narcotic analgesics on growth hormone and corticotrophin (ACTH) secretion in rats. Drug effects on neuroendocrine regulation. *Prog. Brain Res.,* 39:347–358.
60. Kosterlitz, H. W., and Waterfield, A. A. (1975): *In vitro* models in study of structure-activity relationships of narcotic agents. *Annu. Rev. Pharmacol.,* 15:29–47.
61. Kuhar, M. J., Pert, C. B., and Snyder, S. H. (1973): Regional distribution of opiate receptor binding in monkey and human brain. *Nature,* 245:447–450.
62. Labrie, F., Bougeat, P., Ferland, L., Lemay, A., Dupont, A., Lemaire, S., Pelletier, G., Borden, N., Drouin, J., De Léan, A., Bélanger, A., and Jolicoeur, (1975): Mechanism of action and modulation of activity of hypothalamic hypophysiotrophic hormones. In: *Hypothalamic Hormones,* edited by M. Motta, P. Crosignani, and L. Martini. Academic Press, New York.
63. Lambertson, C. (1974): Neurogenic factors in control of respiration. In: *Medical Physiology,* edited by V. B. Mountcastle, pp. 1447–1497. C. V. Mosby, St. Louis.
64. Lamotte, C., Pert, C. B., and Snyder, S. H. (1976): Opiate receptor binding in primate spinal cord: Distribution and changes after dorsal root section. *Brain Res.,* 112:407–412.
65. Law, P. Y., Wei, E. T., Lseng, L. F., Loh, H. H., and Way, E. L. (1977): Opioid properties of β-lipotropin fragment 60–65. *Life Sci.,* 20:251–260.
66. Lazarus, L. H., Ling, N., and Guillemin, R. (1976): β-Lipotropin as a prohormone for the morphinomimetic peptides endorphins and enkephalins. *Proc. Natl. Acad. Sci. USA,* 73:2156–2159.
67. Li, C. H. (1964): Lipotropin, a new active peptide from pituitary glands. *Nature,* 201:924.
68. Li, C. H., and Chung, D. (1976): Isolation and structure of an untriakontapeptide with opiate activity from camel pituitary glands. *Proc. Natl. Acad. Sci. USA,* 73: 1145–1148.
69. Lieu, E., Fenichet, R., Garsky, V., Sarantakis, D., and Grant, N. (1976): Enkephalin-stimulated prolactin release. *Life Sci.,* 19:837–840.
70. Ling, N., Burgus, R., and Guillemin, R. (1976): Isolation, primary structure, and synthesis of α-endorphin and γ-endorphin, two peptides of hypothalamic-hypophysial origin with morphinomimetic activity. *Proc. Natl. Acad. Sci. USA,* 73:3942–3946.
71. Ling, N., and Guillemin, R. (1976): Morphino-mimetic activity of synthetic fragments of β-lipotropin and analogs. *Proc. Natl. Acad. Sci. USA,* 73:3308–3310.
72. Loh, H. H., Tsent, L. F., Wei, E., and Li, C. H. (1976): β-Endorphin is a potent analgesic agent. *Proc. Natl. Acad. Sci. USA,* 83:2895–2898.
73. Lotti, U., Kokko, N., and George, R. (1969): Pituitary-adrenal activation following intrahypothalamic microinjection of morphine. *Neuroendocrinology,* 4:326–332.
74. MacLeod, R., and Lehmeyer, J. (1974): Studies on the mechanism of the dopamine-mediated inhibition of prolactin release. *Endocrinology,* 94:1077–1085.
75. Martin, J., Tannerbaum, G., Willoby, J., Renand, L., and Brazeau, P. (1975): Functions of the central nervous system in regulation of pituitary GH secretion. In: *Hypothalamic Hormones,* edited by M. Motta, P. Crosignani, and L. Martini. Academic Press, New York.
76. Mayer, D., and Hayes, R. (1975): Stimulation-produced analgesia: Development of tolerance and cross-tolerance to morphine. *Science,* 188:941–943.
77. Mayer, D., and Liebeskind, J. (1974): Pain reduction by focal electrical stimulation of the brain: An anatomical and behavioral analysis. *Brain Res.,* 68:73–93.
78. Mayer, D., and Price, D. (1976): Central nervous system mechanisms of analgesia. *Pain,* 2:379–404.
79. Meglio, M., Hasobuchi, Y., Loh, H., Adams, J., and Li, C. H. (1977): β-Endorphin: Behavioral and analgesic activity in cats. *Proc. Natl. Acad. Sci. USA,* 74:774–776.
80. Meites, J. (1966): Control of mammary growth and lactation. In: *Neuroendocrinology,* Vol. 2, edited by L. Martini and W. Ganong, pp. 669–707. Academic Press, New York.

81. Minneman, K. P., and Iversen, L. L. (1976): Enkephalin and opiate narcotics increase cycle GMP accumulation in slices of rat neostriatum. *Nature,* 262:313–314.
82. Morin, O., Caron, M. G., DeLean, A., and LaBrie, F. (1976): Binding of opiate-like pentapeptide methionine-enkephalin to a particulate fraction from rat brain. *Biochem. Biophys. Res. Commun.,* 73:940–946.
83. Pasternak, G. W., Goodman, R., and Snyder, S. H. (1975): An endogenous morphine-like factor in mammalian brain. *Life Sci.,* 16:1765–1769.
84. Pasternak, G. W., Simantov, R., and Snyder, S. H. (1975): Characterization of an endogenous morphine-like factor (enkephalin) in mammalian brain. *Mol. Pharmacol.,* 12:504–513.
85. Pasternak, G. W., Snowman, A. M., and Snyder, S. H. (1975): Selective enhancement of ^{3}H-opiate agonist binding by divalent cations. *Mol. Pharmacol.,* 11:735–744.
86. Pasternak, G. W., and Snyder, S. H. (1975): Identification of novel high-affinity opiate receptor binding in rat brain. *Nature,* 253:563–565.
87. Pasternak, G. W., and Snyder, S. H. (1975): Opiate receptor binding: Enzymatic treatments discriminate between agonist and antagonist interactions. *Mol. Pharmacol.,* 11:474–478.
88. Pasternak, G. W., Wilson, H. A., and Snyder, S. H. (1975): Differential effects of protein modifying reagents on receptor binding of opiate agonists and antagonists. *Mol. Pharmacol.,* 11:478–484.
89. Paton, W. D. M. (1957): Action of morphine and related substances on contractions and on acetylcholine output of coaxially-stimulated guinea pig ileum. *Br. J. Pharmacol. Ther.,* 12:119–127.
90. Pearse, A. (1976): Peptides in brain and intestine. *Nature,* 262:92–94.
91. Pert, A. (1976): Behavioral pharmacology of d-alanine^2-methionine enkephalin amide and other long-acting opiate peptides. In: *Opiates and Endogenous Opioid Peptides,* edited by H. W. Kosterlitz, pp. 87–94. North Holland, Amsterdam.
92. Pert, A., and Yaksh, T. (1974): Sites of morphine-induced analgesia in primate brain: Relation to pain pathways. *Brain Res.,* 80:135–140.
93. Pert, C., Aposhian, D., and Snyder, S. (1974): Phylogenetic distribution of opiate receptor binding. *Brain Res.,* 75:356–361.
94. Pert, C. B., Bowie, D. L., Fong, B. T. W., and Change, J. K. (1976): Synthetic analogues of met-enkephalin which resist enzymatic destruction. In: *Opiates and Endogenous Opioid Peptides,* edited by H. W. Kosterlitz, pp. 79–86. North Holland, Amsterdam.
95. Pert, C. B., Kuhar, M. J., and Snyder, S. H. (1975): Autoradiographic localization of opiate receptor in rat brain. *Life Sci.,* 16:1849–1854.
96. Pert, C. B., Kuhar, M. J., and Snyder, S. H. (1976): Opiate receptor: Autoradiographic localization in rat brain. *Proc. Natl. Acad. Sci. USA,* 73:3729–3733.
97. Pert, C. B., Pasternak, G. W., and Snyder, S. H. (1973): Opiate agonists and antagonists discriminated by receptor binding in brain. *Science,* 182:1359–1361.
98. Pert, C. B., Pert, A., and Tallman, J. F. (1976): Isolation of a novel endogenous opiate analgesic from human blood. *Proc. Natl. Acad. Sci. USA,* 73:2226–2230.
99. Pert, A., Simantov, R., and Snyder, S. H. (1977): A morphine-like factor in mammalian brain: Analgesic activity in rats. *Brain Res. (in press).*
100. Pert, C. B., Snowman, A. M., and Snyder, S. H. (1974): Localization of opiate receptor binding in synaptic membranes of rat brain. *Brain Res.,* 70:184–188.
101. Pert, C. B., and Snyder, S. H. (1973): Opiate receptor: demonstration in nervous tissue. *Science,* 179:1011–1014.
102. Pert, C. B., and Snyder, S. H. (1973): Properties of opiate receptor binding in rat brain. *Proc. Natl. Acad. Sci. USA,* 70:2243–2247.
103. Pert, C. B., and Snyder, S. H. (1974): Opiate receptor binding of agonists and antagonists affected differentially by sodium. *Mol. Pharmacol.,* 10:868–879.
104. Queen, G., Pinsky, C., and LaBella, F. (1976): Subcellular localization of endorphine activity in bovine pituitary and brain. *Biochem. Biophys. Res. Commun.,* 72:1021–1027.
105. Ralston, H. (1968): The fine structure of neurons in the dorsal horn of the cat spinal cord. *J. Comp. Neurol.,* 132:275–302.

106. Rethely, M., and Szentagothai, J. (1969): The large synaptic complexes of the substantia gelatinosa. *Exp. Brain Res.,* 7:258–274.
107. Rexed, B. (1954): A cytoarchitectonic atlas of the spinal cord of the cat. *J. Comp. Neurol.,* 100:297–379.
108. Reynolds, D. (1969): Surgery in the rat during electrical analgesia induced by focal brain stimulation. *Science,* 164:444–445.
109. Rivier, C., Vale, W., Ling, N., Brown, M., and Guillemin, R. (1977): Stimulation *in vivo* of the secretion of prolactin and growth hormone by β-endorphin. *Endocrinology (in press).*
110. Ross, M., Divigledine, R., Cox, B., and Goldstein, A. (1977): Distribution of endorphines (peptides with morphine-like pharmacological activity) in pituitary. *Brain Res.,* 124:523–532.
111. Ross, M., Su, T. P., Cox, B. M., and Goldstein, A. (1976): Brain endorphines. In: *Opiates and Endogenous Opioid Peptides,* edited by H. W. Kosterlitz, pp. 35–40. Amsterdam, North Holland.
112. Rouges, B. P., Garbay-Jaurequiberry, C., Oberlin, R., Anteunis, M., and Lala, A. K. (1976): Conformation of met-enkephalin determined by high field PMR spectroscopy. *Nature,* 262:778–779.
113. Samanin, R., Gumulka, W., and Valzalli, L. (1970): Reduced effects of morphine in midbrain raphé lesioned rats. *Eur. J. Pharmacol.,* 10:339–343.
114. Sharma, S. K., Nirenberg, M., and Klee, W. A. (1975): Morphine receptors as regulators of adenylate cyclase activity. *Proc. Natl. Acad. Sci. USA,* 72:590–594.
115. Simantov, R., Childers, S. R., and Snyder, S. H. (1977): ^{3}H-opiate binding: Anomalous properties in kidney and liver membranes. *Mol. Pharmacol. (in press).*
116. Simantov, R., Childers, S. R., and Snyder, S. H. (1977): Opioid peptides; Differentiation by radioimmunoassay and radioreceptor assay. *Brain Res. (in press).*
117. Simantov, R., Goodman, R., Aposhian, D., and Snyder, S. H. (1976): Phylogenetic distribution of a morphine-like peptide, "enkephalin." *Brain Res.,* 14:204–211.
118. Simantov, R., Kuhar, M. J., Pasternak, G. W., and Snyder, S. H. (1976): The regional distribution of morphine-like factor enkephalin in monkey brain. *Brain Res.,* 106:189–197.
119. Simantov, R., Kuhar, M. J., Uhl, G., and Snyder, S. H. (1977): Opioid peptide enkephalin: Immunohistochemical mapping in the rat central nervous system. *Proc. Natl. Acad. Sci. USA (in press).*
120. Simantov, R., Snowman, A., and Snyder, S. H. (1976): A morphine-like factor "enkephalin" in rat brain: Subcellular localization. *Brain Res.,* 107:650–657.
121. Simantov, R., Snowman, A. M., and Snyder, S. H. (1976): A morphine-like factor in rat brain: Subcellular localization. *Brain Res.,* 107:650–657.
122. Simantov, R., Snowman, A. M., and Snyder, S. H. (1976): Temperature and ionic influences on opiate receptor binding. *Mol. Pharmacol.,* 12:977–986.
123. Simantov, R., and Snyder, S. (1976): Brain-pituitary opiate mechanisms: **Pituitary** opiate receptor binding, radioimmunoassays for methionine enkephalin and leucine enkephalin, and ^{3}H-enkephalin interactions with the opiate receptor. In: *Opiates and Endogenous Opioid Peptides,* edited by H. W. Kosterlitz. North Holland, Amsterdam.
124. Simantov, R., and Snyder, S. H. (1976): Elevated levels of enkephalin in morphine-dependent rats. *Nature,* 262:505–507.
125. Simantov, R., and Snyder, S. H. (1976): Morphine-like factors in mammalian brain: Structure elucidation and interactions with opiate receptor. *Proc. Natl. Acad. Sci. USA,* 73:2515–2519.
126. Simantov, R., and Snyder, S. H. (1976): Morphine-like factors, leucine-enkephalin and methionine enkephalin: Interactions with opiate receptor. *Mol. Pharmacol.,* 12:987–988.
127. Simantov, R., and Snyder, S. H. (1977): Opiate receptor binding in the pituitary gland. *Brain Res.,* 124:178–184.
128. Simon, E. J., and Groth, J. (1975): Kinetics of opiate receptor inactivation by sulfhydryl reagents: Evidence for conformational change in presence of sodium ions. *Proc. Natl. Acad. Sci. USA,* 72:2404–2407.

129. Simon, E. J., Hiller, J. M., and Edelman, I. (1973): Stereospecific binding of the potent narcotic analgesic ³H-etorphine to rat brain homogenate. *Proc. Natl. Acad. Sci. USA,* 70:1947–1949.
130. Simon, E. J., Hiller, J. M., Groth, J., and Edelman, I. (1975): Further properties of stereospecific opiate binding sites in rat brain on the nature of the sodium effect. *J. Pharmacol. Exp. Ther.,* 192:531–537.
131. Smith, T. W., Hughes, J., Kosterlitz, H. W., and Sosa, R. P. (1976): Enkephalins: Isolation, distribution and function. In: *Opiates and Endogenous Opioid Peptides,* edited by H. W. Kosterlitz, pp. 57–62. North Holland, Amsterdam.
132. Snyder, S. H., Pasternak, G. W., and Pert, C. B. (1975): Opiate receptor mechanisms. In: *Handbook of Psychopharmacology, Vol. 5,* edited by L. L. Iversen, S. D. Iversen, and S. H. Snyder, pp. 329–360. Plenum Press, New York.
133. Snyder, S. H., and Simantov, R. (1977): The opiate receptor and opioid peptides. *J. Neurochem.,* 29:13–20.
134. Terenius, L. (1973): Characteristics of the "receptor" for narcotic analgesics in synaptic plasma membrane fractions from rat brain. *Acta Pharmacol. Toxicol.,* 33:377–384.
135. Terenius, L., and Wahlstrom, A. (1974): Inhibitor(s) of narcotic receptor binding in brain extracts and in cerebrospinal fluid. *Acta Pharmacol. (Kbh.) [Suppl. 1],* 35:55.
136. Terenius, L., and Wahlstrom A. (1975): Morphine-like ligand for opiate receptor in human CSF. *Life Sci.,* 16:1759–1764.
137. Teschmacher, H., Opheim, K. E., Cox, B. M., and Goldstein, A. (1975): Peptide-like substance from pituitary that acts like morphine. *Life Sci.,* 16:1777–1782.
138. Traber, J., Fischer, K., Latzin, S., and Hamprecht, B. (1975): Morphine antagonizes action of prostaglandin in neuroblastoma and neuroblastoma × glioma hybrid cells. *Nature,* 253:120–122.
139. Uhl, G., Kuhar, M., and Snyder, S. H. (1977): Immunohistochemical localization of neurotensin and enkephalin in rat CNS. *Neurosci. Abstr. (in press).*
140. Ungar, G., Ungar, C. L., and Malin, D. H. (1976): Brain peptides with opiate antagonist activity. In: *Opiates and Endogenous Opioid Peptides,* edited by H. W. Kosterlitz, pp. 121–128. North Holland, Amsterdam.
141. Van Ree, J. M., DeWeid, D., Bradbury, A. F., Hulme, E. C., Smyth, D. G., and Snell, C. R. (1976): Induction of tolerance to the analgesic action of lipotropin C-fragment. *Nature,* 264:792–794.
142. Waterfield, A. A., Hughes, J., and Kosterlitz, H. W. (1976): Cross tolerance between morphine and methionine enkephalin. *Nature,* 260:624–625.
143. Way, E. L., and Adler, T. K. (1962): The biological disposition of morphine and its surrogates. *Bull. WHO,* 27:359–394.
144. Wei, E., and Loh, H. (1976): Chronic, intracerebral infusion of morphine and peptides with osmotic minipumps, and the development of physical dependence. In: *Opiates and Endogenous Opioid Peptides,* edited by H. W. Kosterlitz, pp. 303–310. North Holland, Amsterdam.
145. Weissman, B. A., Gershon, H. and Pert, C. B. (1976): Specific antiserum to leu-enkephalin and its use in a radioimmunoassay. *FEBS Lett.,* 70:245–248.
146. Wilkening, D., Mishra, R. K., and Makman, M. H. (1976): Effects of morphine on dopamine-stimulated adenylate cyclase and on cyclic GMP formation in primate brain amygdaloid nucleus. *Life Sci.,* 19:1129–1138.
147. Wilson, R. S., Rogerts, M. E., Pert, C. B., and Snyder, S. H. (1975): Homologous N-alkylnorketobeminidones. Correlation of receptor binding with analgesic potency. *J. Med. Chem.,* 18:240–242.
148. Wong, D. T., and Horng, J. S. (1973): Stereospecific interactions of opiate narcotics in binding of ³H-dihydromorphine to membranes of rat brain. *Life Sci.,* 13:1543–1556.
149. Yaksh, T., and Rudy, T. (1976): Analgesia mediated by a direct spinal action of narcotics. *Science,* 192:1157–1158.

Frontiers in Neuroendocrinology, Vol. 5,
edited by W. F. Ganong and L. Martini.
Raven Press, New York © 1978.

Chapter 12

Biotransformation and Degradation of Corticotropins, Lipotropins and Hypothalamic Peptides

Neville Marks

*N.Y. Institute for Neurochemistry and Drug Addiction,
Rockland Research Institute,
Wards Island, New York 10035*

INTRODUCTION

Neuropeptides represent some of the most powerful pharmacologically active agents ever described, yet relatively little is known about their biosynthesis and breakdown. Such processes are mediated in many cases by proteolytic enzymes playing dual roles: (a) in the cascade of events linked to the packaging, processing, and conversion from precursors; and (b) in peptide inactivation. The assertion that many neuropeptides have neurotransmitter properties (48), coupled with potential clinical applications, has lent urgency to studies on the role that proteolytic enzymes play in regulating their manifold biological activities.

The present account is focused on brain enzymes available for biotransformation of cortico- and lipotropins and well-characterized hypothalamic peptides such as LRH, TRH, somatostatin, and substance P. Examples are cited for peptides in non-CNS tissues where these illustrate aspects involved in peptide processing that may have general application.

The discovery of multiple molecular forms for many hormones has raised a host of questions related to: (a) the nature of the gene product, (b) the biological roles of the different oligomeric forms, (c) the exact anatomical sites or compartments involved in processing (central versus peripheral sites), (d) mechanisms involved in transport, (e) specificity of the enzymes involved in conversion, (f) potential inhibitors or activators of such enzymes, and (g) the role of N- and C-terminal extensions present in precursor forms. As a general comment, it might be stressed that pathways involved in protein and polypeptide metabolism within tissues are poorly understood (107, 118). As a result, knowledge concerning those related to neuropeptides may help to shed light on this obscure area. Processes of formation, secretion, and transport of neuropeptides can be viewed as part of the general phenomena associated with "neurosecretion" as enunciated by Scharrer and Bargmann (7,175) and as such represents a vital branch of peptidology.

Conversion—Terminology and Methodology

Studies on conversion of pancreatic zymogens, complement formation, and blood clotting have led to the recognition of several principles for the identification of precursors (38,42,76,143). Such processes are all characterized by limited proteolysis of the larger forms which contain inactivating N- or C-terminal sequences. Evidence for the larger forms can be obtained by the use of labeled amino acids in pulse-chase type experiments, followed by their isolation and then conversion into the smaller (active) forms by controlled digestion, utilizing purified extra- or intracellular enzymes. Such studies were helped immeasurably by the presence in tissues in high concentration of zymogens relative to active forms, and by the availability of purified intracellular enzymes that activate the precursor. It is generally assumed that the N- or C-peptide extensions alter polypeptide geometry and thus affect specificity of the converting enzymes. Differentiation of true precursors from simple aggregates is generally provided for by treatment with urea or some other dissociating agent.

Improvement in bioassay techniques, along with introduction of radioimmunoassay, led to the discovery by Steiner et al. (181–183) of proinsulin in pancreatic islets followed shortly thereafter by the discovery of larger forms for parathyroid hormone (PTH), ACTH, glucagon, gastrins, and more recently opioid peptides (118,136). At the present time, there is no consensus concerning the terminology for these larger forms, which are referred to in the literature as: *prepro, pre, pro* or *big big, big, intermediate, small, little,* and *mini*. Studies on pancreatic zymogens may provide a rational basis for restricting the term "pre" to precursors having only N-terminal extensions. It has been argued in the latter case that the inactivating sequence is formed prior to the catalytic center by N-terminal attachment to the nascent chain of the ribosome in order to prevent premature expression of enzyme activity (143). A rational terminology for biologically active peptides, however, must await new knowledge concerning the structure of prohormones with regard to the number and site of peptide extensions (Fig. 12–1).

A number of remarkable analogies exist in conversion processes for ACTH, PTH, β-lipotropin (β-LPH), gastrins, and insulins with the bonds most vulnerable to cleavage being adjacent to paired basic residues such as Lys-Lys, Arg-Arg, and Lys-Arg. This suggests the presence of intracellular proteinases with unique tryptic-like specificities differing from exocrine trypsin, which largely cleaves bonds adjacent to a carboxy group of a single amino acid. Body fluids, however, contain enzymes similar to exocrine trypsin involved in conversion processes such as plasmin (blood clotting), and acrosin (fertilization). A feature about (exocrine) trypsin frequently overlooked is that it acts best on smaller peptic fragments and exists in two ionic forms, one of which (anionic) cleaves slowly the bond between two basic residues (210). The high degree of specificity of intracellular converting enzymes (re-

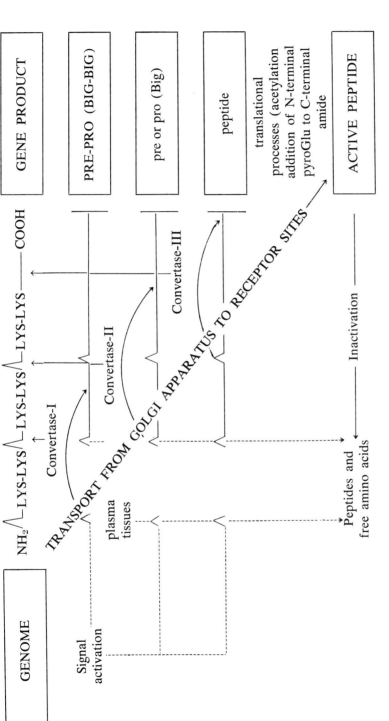

FIG. 12-1. Schematic representation of conversion processes as mediated by a series of converting enzymes (convertases 1-111). In this scheme the intermediate steps of conversion and transport are shown as being regulated by the released peptide extensions according to the proposals of Bloobel and Dobberstein (17). After conversion of precursor to active hormone, the hormonal peptides are inactivated by soluble or membrane bound degradative enzymes to release inactive peptides or amino acids as the final end-products.

ferred to for convenience as convertases) is illustrated by enterokinase, which activates trypsinogen only at 1 of 16 potential lysyl sites, the bond adjacent to the N-extension, Val^1-Asp-Asp-Asp-----Lys^6. This example demonstrates further that studies using exocrine trypsin *in vitro* must be treated with caution since they are unlikely to simulate exactly the remarkable specificities of convertases *in situ*. Purification of intracellular convertases represents one of the major challenges in studies on peptide processing, especially with respect to insulin and cortico- and lipotropins.

All studies on biotransformation and fate of peptides must take into account the problems associated with inadvertent breakdown during extraction and isolation procedures (118,202). Processing generally occurs within specialized compartments which may not be exposed to lysosomal or other enzymes released by fragmentation of tissues. Such changes can be prevented, in part, by the use of specific inhibitors. The use of specific inhibitors may be a critical factor in studies connected with affinity binding or other *in vitro* tests involving the use of tissue membranes. There is a distinction to be made between inhibitors *per se* which interact with the active sites of enzymes, and the role of inactivating peptide extensions which are covalently bound to the active sequence. Other than altering the geometry of polypeptides, the role of peptide extensions has not been defined. It has been speculated by Blobel and Dobberstein (17) that these extensions have informational content and act as signals to activate convertases or specific transport mechanisms involved in peptide processing (Fig. 12–1). These peptide extensions once released may have useful clinical applications for diagnosis of clinical disorders: C-peptide of proinsulin, for example, is considered to be diagnostic of hypoglycemia associated with renal failure (109).

Biosynthesis of neuropeptides frequently involves post-translational changes to introduce blocked N- and C-terminal residues such as pyroGlu, N-acetyl, and C-terminal amides. PyroGlu can also be formed by nonenzymatic cyclization of Gln. The finding of pyroGlu in many peptides raises an interesting question as to the true biological form of such peptides *in situ* and also whether pyroglutamyl peptidases (E.C.3.4.11.8) play a role in their metabolism. Formation of C-terminal amides poses a problem since mechanisms involving formation without chain shortening have not been described. Bradbury et al. (20) have suggested that C-terminal amide could be formed by transamidation involving an enzyme such as cathepsin C (dipeptidyl transferase, E.C.3.4.14.1) acting reversibly in presence of ammonia as indicated:

$$R - R - R - R - NH_2 + NH_3 \rightleftharpoons R - R - NH_2 + R - R - NH_2$$

This hypothesis implies that peptides with C-terminal amides are derived from larger forms having C-terminal extensions and that there might be a regulatory role for ammonia in tissues.

The many structural homologies that exist for zymogens have led to speculation about their phylogenetic origin utilizing a common catalytic sequence
accompanied by evolutionary adaptations favoring a specific function. In this
respect, there exists a remarkable phylogenetic relationship for neurohypophyseal peptides such as vasopressin (1). The preservation of an active
sequence for neuropeptides or zymogens could represent a cellular economy
with modification of function modulated by the presence of N- and C-terminal
extensions. In the case of neuropeptides, more information is required to define evolutionary aspects related to conversion, as, for example, the existence
of a family of related tryptic-like enzymes involving an identical pathway for
activation. Also of particular interest is the finding of similar immunoreactive
peptides in gut and central nervous system (CNS), suggesting that they are
derived from cells of common embryological origin (2,152). The functional
roles of gut peptides in the CNS (gastrins, vasoactive intestinal peptide), or,
conversely, the peptides typical of nerve tissue in the gut (somatostatin, enkephalins), pose questions of considerable significance.

Processing of Non-CNS Peptides

Parathyroid hormone (PTH) has served as a useful model for studying
conversion since it is formed from precursor macromolecules termed pro-
and prepro PTH (73,117). ProPTH is a single polypeptide chain with an
N-terminal (basic) hexapeptide (Lys-Ser-Val-Lys-Arg) and may also possess
additional C-terminal sequences in prohormone from human and bovine
sources (73). ProPTH and PTH are associated with membranous structures,
and present evidence points to transport of newly formed prohormones to the
endoplasmic reticulum of the Golgi region, the predominant site for conversion. Consideration of the structure of the hexapeptide-hormone combination has led to expectation that a "tryptic-like" cleavage can accomplish the
conversion into active PTH. Digestion of bovine PTH with trypsin was reported to yield a peptide comigrating with an intact hormone marker; also,
trypsin cleaved a synthetic analogue consisting of hexapeptide covalently
bound to the N-terminal of an active hormonal fragment (-Arg^8-Ala^7) to
release in high yield the peptide extension before a cleavage of the hormone
occurred (53). MacGregor et al. (117) studied a particulate-bound enzyme
of bovine parathyroid glands tentatively termed "convertase," which converted proPTH to an active hormone but which did not possess "tryptic-like"
properties (no inhibition by benzamidine, transylol) and differed from cathepsin B (no inhibition by chloroquine). Convertase differed also in its properties from a Ca^{2+}-sensitive peptidase acting only on PTH at pH 6.0.

It is of interest that the hexapeptide extension in the case of proPTH is
similar to that attached to proalbumin (169). Such sequence may serve to
act as a signal for activation of tryptic-like enzymes cleaving in paired basic
residues (Fig. 12–1). MacGregor et al. (117) proposed that the hexapeptide

may have additional informational content to facilitate transport of PTH into distinct cell compartments that contain required enzymes for processing.

Extensive studies on proinsulin conversion have provided an excellent model for studies on conversion. These studies show that β-cells of pancreatic islets contain a mixture of proteinases, some having similarities to exocrine pancreatic enzymes. Two enzymes in particular have received attention; one is a tryptic-like intracellular proteinase capable of cleaving the Arg-Gly bonds adjacent to the two sets of double basic residues connecting the C-peptide to insulin (210). There is evidence based on studies *in vitro* with purified enzymes for separate release of these basic amino acids by sequential action of an intracellular carboxypeptidase B. These converting enzymes are not available in purified form for studies on specificity. Conversion appears to be initiated within the Golgi apparatus or in newly secreted granules which contain converting enzymes, as demonstrated *in vitro* by the generation of insulin from prelabeled endogenous precursors. As in the case of ACTH, the ultimate gene product (preproinsulin) has yet to be separated and identified.

In studies using synthetic substrates resembling the activation sites, Zuhlke et al. (210) observed a carboxypeptidase B-like enzyme in islets requiring Zn^{2+} in addition to the tryptic-like enzyme. The possibility exists that these two processing enzymes have similarities to cathepsins B1 and B2 which are of lysosomal origin (181). Studies with specific inhibitors indicate only partial suppression by thiol compounds (iodoacetamide, parachloromercuribenzoate) and site-specific reagents active against serine-like proteins (109). Measurements of circulatory proinsulin and C-peptide have facilitated diagnosis of different disorders including those associated with hypoglycemia and certain malignancies. The half-lives of proinsulin and C-peptide are comparatively short—in the range of 10 min (151). The possibility exists that conversion processes *per se* are involved in pancreatic dysfunction associated with diabetes (95).

Less is known about glucagon conversion although larger forms have been detected in fish, birds, and mammals (180). Limited proteolysis of a precursor from angelfish was shown to generate active hormone. Tager and Steiner (186) in studies on a proglucagon have isolated a 37-residue sequence connected by Lys-Arg to the active hormone which could represent one of the circulating sequences.

Growth Hormone

Graf et al. (55) have observed some sequence homologies between human growth hormone (residues 1 to 23), porcine secretin (residues 5 to 20), and the C-fragment of porcine β-LPH (residues 70 to 91). This underscores a possible common evolutionary origin. The homologies also pose questions as to whether similar enzymatic mechanisms are involved in activation of larger prohormonal forms. In a number of studies on growth hormone labeled with leucine and isolated from pituitaries by gel electrophoresis, three forms ranging from 20,000 to over 100,000 have been observed. Heterogeneity has been observed in plasma forms of GH (112,115). Several explanations have been proposed to account for GH heterogeneity. These include association of nascent peptides attached to its polysome, and aggregation, since some forms are dissociated in guanidine hydrochloride and by urea treatment (115).

Gastrins

The CNS is reported to contain components cross-reacting to antisera against intestinally derived peptides. Gastrins are present in portions of intestinal mucosa and in plasma with high concentrations in the Zollinger-Ellison syndrome and pernicious anemia. Altogether five forms, all biologically active, have been described ranging from a *mini* (13 residues) and a *little* (17 residues) to a *big* (34 residues) and a *big big* gastrin of 20,000 molecular weight. There is also an *intermediate* gastrin which in size is between *big* and *big big* (58). In terms of conversion there are some striking similarities to proinsulin and β-LPH since tryptic digestion *in vitro* of "big" gastrin yields "little" gastrin by cleavage of junctional sequence Lys^{16}-Lys^{17}-Glu^{18} at bonds 17 to 18. The N-terminal glutamine could spontaneously cyclize to form the pyroGlu present in the heptadecapeptide sequence. There is no good explanation for formation of the C-terminal Phe-NH_2 other than by transamidation; however, this would presuppose an even larger prohormonal form with a C-terminal extension. Since removal of Phe-NH_2 inactivates gastrins, a prohormone with C-terminal modification is likely to be biologically inactive. Studies on the characterization of gastric precursors are aided by the fact that prohormonal forms themselves are biologically active in contrast to most other prohormones that are inactive or only weakly active.

Corticotropins

Pituitary extracts contain a variety of corticotropic-related peptides of which ACTH is the most studied because of its manifold biological activities (see reviews, 77,111,159,190). Of particular interest is the finding that some sequences prepared synthetically (notably ACTH 4–10) have potent behavioral effects (94,200) and that this heptapeptide is common to several polypeptides (Fig. 12–2).

The nomenclature adopted for active sequences is arbitrary; ACTH 4–10, for example, could be labeled α-MSH 4–10, β-MSH 7–13, or LPH 47–53. Generally, active sequences are related to ACTH, and this is convenient provided no assumptions are made concerning their existence *per se* in tissues or their production. Since lipotropins do not contain the ACTH 1–39 sequence and thus may be derived by a different biosynthetic pathway, they are described separately below.

Clues concerning possible sites of ACTH conversion into melanotropic or

PROACTH

Ser-Tyr-Ser-*Met-Glu-His-Phe-Arg-Trp-Gly*-Lys-Pro-Val-Gly-Lys-Lys-Arg-Arg-Pro-Val-
Lys-Val-Tyr-Pro-Asn-Gly-Ala-Glu-Asp-Glu-Ser-Ala-Glu-Ala-Phe-Pro-Leu-Glu-Phe

ACTH

ACTH 1–16 followed by carboxypeptidase, acetylation, amination

Ac-Ser-Tyr-Ser-*Met-Glu-His-Phe-Arg-Trp-Gly*-Lys-Pro-Val. NH₂

α-MSH

Asp-Glu-Gly-Pro-Tyr-Lys-*Met-Glu-His-Phe-Arg-Trp-Gly*-Ser-Pro-Lys-Asp

β-MSH

ACTH ⎡ 17–38
aminopeptidase ⎣ 18–38
          (CLIP)

Glu-Leu-Ala-Gly-Ala-Pro-Pro-Glu-Pro-Ala-Arg-Asp-Pro-Glu-Ala-Gly-Ala-Ala-Ala-Arg-
Ala-Glu-Leu-Glu-Tyr-Gly-Leu-Val-Ala-Glu-Ala-Glu-Ala-Ala-Glu-Lys-Lys-Asp-Glu-Gly-Pro-Tyr-
Lys-*Met-Glu-His-Phe-Arg-Trp-Gly*-Ser-Pro-Pro-Lys-Asp-Lys-Arg-Tyr-Gly-Gly-Phe-Met-Thr-Ser-Glu-
Lys-Ser-Gln-Thr-Pro-Leu-Val-Thr-Leu-Phe-Lys-Asn-Ala-Ile-Val-Lys-Asn-Ala-His-Lys-Lys-Gly-Gln

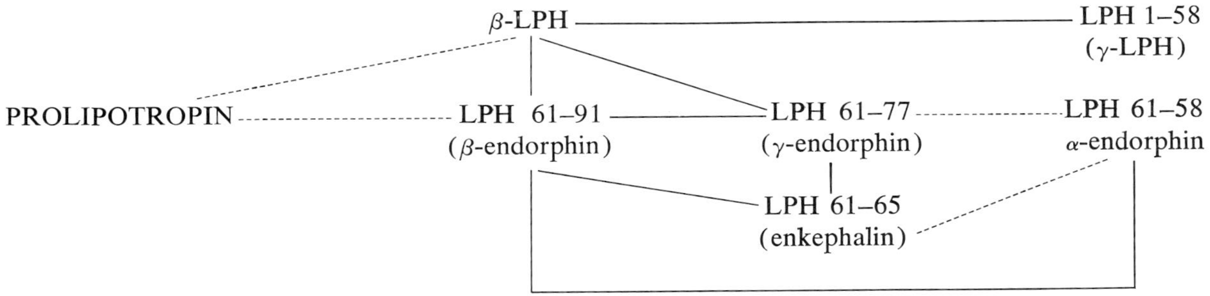

β-LPH —————————— LPH 1–58
(γ-LPH)

PROLIPOTROPIN

LPH 61–91 ————— LPH 61–77 --------- LPH 61–58
(β-endorphin)   (γ-endorphin)   α-endorphin

LPH 61–65
(enkephalin)

FIG. 12–2. Schemata for the conversion and processing of ACTH, melanotropins and lipotropins. The composition or the precursors for ACTH and lipotropin are unknown. Postulated pathways involving conversion of these prohormones is indicated in both cases by the broken lines. Direct conversion of β-lipotropin to form β-MSH has not been demonstrated using tissue extracts; there is indirect evidence that enzymes present in pituitary extracts can cleave one of the bonds close to the C-terminus as described in the text. There is evidence for the conversion of β-endorphin to form γ- and α-endorphin, enkephalin and other peptide fragments when incubated with washed synaptosomal membranes [or striatal slices or rat brain (4b, 179 a).] A heptapeptide sequence common to ACTH, melanotropins and lipotropin in italics. Abbreviations used are: ACTH, adrenocorticotropin; LPH, lipotropin; MSH, melanocyte stimulating hormone; CLIP, corticotropin-like intermediate peptide.

other fragments are supplied from studies on anatomical localization. ACTH 1–39 is present in extracts of the pars distalis and α-MSH is found largely in pars intermedia which may be one of the sites for its conversion (28,177, 179). Early reports that these occur also in the hypothalamus of the dog and pig were confirmed recently by Krieger et al. (72,103,174), who found a concentration that was 1% of the concentration in the pituitary in rats. The occurrence of extrapituitary peptide has given rise to speculation concerning a pituitary source by retrograde flow involving the hypophyseal or systemic circulations, although this notion is offset by persistence of corticotropin levels in the hypothalamus 10 days after hypophysectomy. This implies that the peptide is of diencephalon origin.

Conversion Processes

Sensitive radioimmunoassay procedures enabled Yalow and Berson (207) to detect the presence of a "big ACTH" in tumors associated with ectopic ACTH production, and in plasma of patients with Cushing's syndrome. Big ACTH is present only as a minor component in rat pituitaries, and apparently absent in mice. Among the criteria used for the identification was separation of big ACTH by gel filtration, cross-reaction with antisera to ACTH 1–39, and subsequent conversion into the active form by controlled tryptic digestion. The fact that big ACTH was unaltered following urea treatment provided evidence that it was not a simple aggregate (206,208). Species differences exist since in mouse pituitary and its cultured cell lines an intermediate rather than a big form has been isolated which cannot be converted by tryptic digestion (147). This finding implies the existence of a different biosynthetic pathway and raises a number of questions concerning the ultimate gene product for ACTH in tissues. The biological role of these oligomeric forms of ACTH is unknown but has been linked to the ratio of plasma corticosterone to cortisol in some species (39). Of interest clinically is the finding that levels of big ACTH in plasma appear to be indicative of the presence of lung tumors (206).

Scott et al. (178) observed that pars intermedia tissue of the rat and pig contained substantially more C- than N-terminally immunoreactive ACTH-like material. Subsequently they isolated and characterized a new ACTH-like peptide from pars intermedia. This material resembled ACTH 18–39 and was termed corticotropin-like intermediate peptide (CLIP). They suggested that CLIP and α-MSH are formed by intracellular cleavage mediated by a neutral proteinase, followed by secondary metabolic transformation (Fig. 12–2). This represents an example of an active hormone itself acting as a precursor for smaller (active) fragment. Methodologically it is also of interest, since it illustrates the use of antisera directed toward the N- and C-termini for demonstrating the existence of a possible transformation step. The amounts of α-MSH and CLIP in rat pituitary were approximately equivalent, providing evidence of a common precursor. CLIP has been isolated from whole rat pituitaries, acetone powders of pig posterior lobe, and human bronchial tumors associated with hypersecretion of ACTH. Localization of α-MSH and β-MSH in pars intermedia suggests that cleavage of LPH to β-MSH, and ACTH to α-MSH may occur at similar anatomical sites (177). Cleavage of the paired basic residue of ACTH (Lys-Arg) to release the 17–39 sequence has similarities to proinsulin-insulin conversion.

Degradation

Intensive studies have been conducted on the structure of ACTH and its analogues for the purpose of altering its diverse biological properties to favor one or more of its actions. These include steroidogenesis, release of growth hormone, melanophore stimulation in amphibia, fat mobilizing effects, alterations of glucose and protein metabolism, and behavioral effects (28,159).

It was long suspected that the C-terminal 24–39 portion of ACTH was not essential, as shown by its removal following treatment with pepsin (111). Nevertheless, based on the potency of ACTH 1–39 relative to that of shorter sequences *in vivo,* the C-terminal extension appears to play a role in stability (11,159). Studies with ACTH 1–24 or analogues show that the active steroidogenic site resides in the 6–13 sequence and that 1–5 and 15–18 (the basic core, Fig. 12–2) play roles in attachment to receptors. ACTH is a linear peptide readily susceptible to digestion as demonstrated by its inactivation when incubated with tissue extracts (11,28,159). Modification of the N-terminal (oxidation, N-acetylation, aminopeptidase actions) generally results in loss or reduction of steroidogenesis accompanied by accentuation of extra-adrenal actions (159). Blocking the N-terminal with D-Ser, D-Ala, β-Ala, GABA, or Sar prolongs action *in vivo* by retarding or blocking the action of aminopeptidase. Thus, a commonly used analogue is D-Ser[1], Lys[17,18] ACTH 1–24 (19,43,91). Chemical manipulation is aimed generally at enhancing a desired property with reduction or loss of endocrinological or other unwanted side effects. Such studies must take account of species differences in rates of metabolism. For example, ACTH is lipolytic in the tissue of rats and rabbits, whereas MSH is lipolytic only in the rat. Rudman et al. (168) ascribe these differences to rates of degradation in these species although other explanations have been presented (see reviews, 28,169).

Even small peptide fragments (ACTH 6–9) retain MSH effects when tested by very sensitive bioassay procedures (131,176,207). Elongation by addition of Gly[10], Glu[5], and Met[4] yields fragments with progressive increases in lipolytic activity (28), illustrating the fine relationships between structure and activity. Alteration in activity by substituting with D-amino acids is dependent on the length of the peptide fragment: D-Arg and D-Phe do not alter the pigmenting effects of ACTH 6–10, but these are reduced in D-Phe-ACTH 4–10 (75,101). Complete replacement in the case of ACTH 6–10 by D-amino acids is reported to reverse the MSH action, lightening previously darkened skin (75). Greven and de Wied (59,60), in a series of elegant studies involving stepwise shortening of ACTH 1–10 or ACTH 4–10, showed that the tetrapeptide ACTH 4–7 bears the essential elements required for the behavioral activity associated with ACTH 1–39 and MSH. Selected fragments with behavioral effects can be stabilized by substitution with D-amino acids and other groups as shown strikingly by the 1,000-fold increase in potency for Met $(0)^4$, Arg^8, D-Phe^9 ACTH 4–9. One nanogram of this compound given to rats subcutaneously delayed pole jump avoidance behavior for several hours (192,193,203). Analogues with potencies up to 10^6-fold have been prepared. These contain two D-lysyl residues such as Met (0 or 0_2)-$(Ala)_3$-D-Lys-Phe-Gly-D-Lys-Pro-Val-Gly-$(Lys)_2$. The trialanine can be replaced by Glu-His-Phe or Ala-Ala-Phe (52). Studies by Witter et al. (203) showed that the improved activity of the synthetic hexapeptide (Met-0-Glu-His-Phe-D-Lys-Phe) appeared to be related to its relative resistance to breakdown as shown by studies *in vitro* using rat brain homogenates or plasma. This analogue or ones containing dimethylated derivatives had half-lives of 38 and 74 min in brain homogenates and plasma as compared to 1 and 3 min for Lys^8Phe^9ACTH (192,193). The major end-product of this synthetic hexapeptide was the C-terminal tripeptide Phe-D-Lys-Phe, which by itself possessed only minimal activity. The presence of free Phe in small amounts indicated that the tripeptide was subject to further degradation. In our studies, breakdown of this analogue was evaluated by the release of free amino acids when incubated with brain extracts and rat serum (128). Failure to detect D-Lys but presence of Phe showed that the remaining dipeptides Phe-D-Lys or D-Lys-Phe were not cleaved to any significant extent. Of interest clinically was the finding that this analogue was not degraded significantly when incubated with human serum. In contrast, α-MSH and ACTH 4–10 were degraded rapidly by rat brain extracts and serum. The patterns of release of amino acids indicated probable cleavage of Phe-Arg for α-MSH and ACTH 4–10 by an endopeptidase followed by the secondary action of exopeptidases; in the case of the hexapeptide the primary point of cleavage appeared to be His-Phe. Cleavage of α-MSH at the Phe-Arg bond is in accord with the findings of Lowery and McMartin (116) for intestinal enzymes.

In studies on ACTH degradation in adrenal preparations, Saez et al. (171) indicated that binding and degradation occurred by two independent processes. Degradative activity was associated largely with a crude 20,000 g pellet and split 1–24 more rapidly than the inactive fragment 11–24. This finding points to different affinities of the peptide fragments, some of which can inhibit breakdown; thus 1–10 inhibited breakdown of 11–24, and 11–24 was inhibited by 1–24. Interference with degradation of fragments by competitive inhibition may represent a subtle but little studied mechanism of hormonal regulation. Lowery and McMartin (116) in detailed studies on actual peptide bonds split by intestinal enzymes using corticotropin 1–24 or its D-Ser[1]-Lys[17,18] analogue showed that the -Phe[7]-Arg[8]-bond and the N-terminal were particularly labile. The presence of D-Ser appeared to confer a marked protection to aminopeptidase action. Release of free amino acids indicated other peptide bonds were susceptible to intestinal and membrane-bound mucosal enzymes of everted intestinal sacs. Aminopeptidases associated with the everted sac had properties akin to those of brush border cells.

In studies with isolated adrenal cells, Bennett et al. (11) found a more rapid breakdown of ACTH 1–24 as compared to 1–39, which was not inhibited by trasylol, a known tryptic inhibitor, or by bacitracin. Bacitracin is not a recognized peptidase inhibitor but appears to suppress glucagon breakdown by substrate competition (82) and more recently has been used with success to retard breakdown of enkephalins (134), endorphins (167) and TRH (129).

Lipotropins

Lipotropins are polypeptides with either 1–58 (γ-lipotropin) or 1–91 residues (β-lipotropin, LPH). They were isolated by Li, Chretien, Graf, and collaborators over a decade ago (32,33,35,54). They have lipolytic actions *in vitro* but their biological significance *in vivo* until recently remained an enigma. Since their sequence contains structures with known melanocyte stimulating activity (β-MSH) or opioid functions (Fig. 12–3), studies on biotransformation of lipotropins are now attracting considerable interest. The variety of lipotropic peptides is dependent on the species employed, the specific areas of pituitary or brain extracted, and the procedures used for identification (34,55,71). Identification involves direct extraction followed by chromatography with separation and sequencing of the peptides, or in some studies attempted identification based on the use of radioimmunoassay or radioreceptor assays. The term "endorphin" is generic and refers to all materials with opioid actions but without differentiation between *in vivo* and *in vitro* actions (85). Endorphins are generally considered as peptide fragments derived from LPH 61–91, but larger than LPH 61–65, which is referred to as enkephalin. Enkephalins are described separately below (see also Chapter 11).

In porcine whole pituitary extracts, Bradbury et al. (20–23) found by chromatographic separation evidence for LPH 1–58, 1–91, 1–38, 61–91, 61–87, and 41–58 in addition to CLIP and ACTH (for nomenclature see Fig. 12–2). Guillemin et al. (71) found LPH 61–76, 61–77 in posterior lobes with attached stalk and median eminence. Li and Chung (113) found largely LPH 61–91 in camel pituitaries. La Bella et al. (106), using a radioimmunoassay with N-terminal directed antiserum, found evidence for lipotropins in high concentrations in the intermediate lobe. The concentration was lower in the adenohypophysis. In extracts prepared by gel filtration subjected to radioimmunoassay for lipotropins or receptor assays for opioid fragments, the same β-Lipotropin   GLU ——————————————————— GLN⁹¹

γ-Lipotropin   GLU ——————————— ASP⁵⁸

N-Fragment   GLU ——— LYS³⁸

β-MSH   ASP⁴¹ ——— ASP⁵⁸

Enkephalin   TYR⁶¹ ——— MET⁶⁵

α-endorphin   TYR⁶¹ ——————— THR⁷⁶

γ-endorphin   TYR⁶¹ ——————— LEU⁷⁷

C′-fragment   TYR⁶¹ ——————— LYS⁸⁷

β-endorphin   TYR⁶¹ ——————————— GLN⁹¹

FIG. 12-3. Lipotropic fragments reported present in extracts of brain and neurosecretory regions. Only the first and terminal residues are indicated; for full structures see Fig. 12-2.

group found different profiles in pituitary as compared to brain with LPH 1–39, 1–58, and 2,000 to 3,000 molecular weight units, but not any approaching enkephalin size (mol. wt. 500). In brain LPH 1–91 was detected but not its N-terminal fragments, which was taken as pointing to rapid breakdown of the latter by amino or other peptidases. In terms of C-terminal activity, only an unidentified 2,000 unit was found. The source of CNS lipotropins is currently unknown, although there has been speculation that they may be derived in part from pituitary by mechanisms involving retrograde transport via hypophyseal portal circulation.

Rubenstein et al. (167) recently showed the presence of several opioid fragments in rat adenohypophysis, with the number and quantity present in each chromatographic peak dependent on the conditions selected for extraction. Lipotropins were identified by amino acid analysis and others (α-, β-, γ-endorphins, and enkephalin) by their chromatographic profile on columns and their affinities in receptor binding assays. Evidence that breakdown is a factor affecting yield of β-LPH was provided by the high yield (15 pmoles/ mg) following extraction in the presence of a protease inhibitor. In fresh material, β-endorphin levels were approximately 0.3 pmoles/mg. The finding of a high molecular weight form (approx. 30,000 daltons) capable of yielding opioids upon trypsinization suggests the presence of a prolipotropin.

Immunohistochemical studies have indicated the presence of β-LPH in the intermediate lobe (106,153) along with evidence for β-endorphin (18). In the pituitary and the brain, β-LPH and its larger cleaved fragments are present in particulates and are sedimentable at 12,000 g. These may represent secretory granules involved in the formation of β-MSH and opioid peptides, but studies of their enzymic content are unavailable (158). The antigenic determinants of β-endorphin appear to reside at LPH 6–15, but there appears to be no correspondence between immunoreaction of LPHs and the opioid action *in vivo* of smaller fragments, notably LPH 61–65 and 20–31 (114).

Conversion

Chretien et al. (36), using *in vitro* pulse labeling techniques, demonstrated the transformation of β-LPH to γ-LPH in pituitaries. However, Bretagna et al. (24) failed to show formation of β-MSH from the same precursor. The finding of fragments contiguous with β-MSH led Bradbury et al. (22) to propose that biotransformation is a possibility. They showed that incubation of β-LPH with trypsin led to cleavage of the peptide bond adjacent to the paired basic residues at positions 60 and 61 (C-terminal of β-MSH), and this type of cleavage could be reproduced using the synthetic peptide Lys-Asp-Lys-Arg-Tyr-Gly. In marked contrast, the bond adjacent to the N-terminal of β-MSH was resistant to cleavage, as confirmed also *in vitro* with a synthetic heptapeptide. When incubated with trypsin, this peptide was hydrolyzed at the Lys-Lys bond (Ala-Glu-Lys-Lys-Asp-Glu-Gly), implying that if cleavage of Lys-Asp- were to occur *in vivo,* it must be mediated by a tryptic enzyme with specificity differing from that cleaving Arg-Tyr-. Speculations arising from such findings can be resolved only by purification of the enzymes in question. In addition to tryptic-like enzymes, the overall conversion process for production of β-MSH must involve participation by a carboxypeptidase B-like enzyme capable of removing C-terminal Arg and Lys on the C-terminal of the LPH fragment. There is no explanation currently on why other bonds adjacent to basic residues in β-MSH are resistant (Lys^6-Met^7- and Arg^{11}-Trp^{12}), although this may be explained ultimately by conformational considerations. The slow cleavage of the Lys^{40}-Asp^{41} bond might account for the accumulation of γ-LPH rather than β-MSH within the gland. It might be noted that studies *in vitro* have a number of limitations since short synthetic peptides are unlikely to reproduce the conformational characteristics that often determine the specificity of intracellular proteinases involved in conversion. Earlier reports that human pituitaries, which have only a vestigial pars intermedia, contained a 22 amino acid β-MSH (44) have been discounted (20,25). There have been studies on structure activity relationships of β-MSH, which may be of interest to metabolism and which show differential actions on melanocytes versus lipolysis on alteration of residues 8 and 10 (179,205).

Opioid Peptides

Graf et al. (54–57) in studies on crude extracts of rat adenohypophysis showed the presence of two different classes of convertases operating at high and low pH. The enzyme active at pH 8.0 termed lipotropic activating enzyme (LA) cleaved the Arg^{60}-Tyr^{61} bond and as such may have similarities to the one proposed for the processing of β-MSH (20,55). This enzyme was largely particulate, present in large granules and microsomes, and could be differentiated from that of exocrine trypsin by failure of soybean inhibitor to affect its activity. The major product was LPH 1–60, and there was a low yield of 61–91 (β-endorphin). If loss of β-endorphin occurred as a result of secondary cleavage, this may be of interest since a lipotropic fragment prepared by digestion with plasmin (LPH 52–60) appears to act as an inhibitor of this conversion process. Other plasmin fragments prepared by Graf et al. (55) include sequences 1–46, 1–51, 1–60, 1–79, 52–79, 61–79, and 80–91, some of which retain a weak fat-mobilizing effect and one of which has opiate-like properties *in vitro.* Inhibitors that affect the bioavailability of β-endorphin, a potent analgesic and behavioral peptide *in vivo* (86,189), may be of interest in terms of clinical applications. Graf et al. (55) in preliminary studies observed that an aldehyde of LPH 58–60 had properties in this respect in contrast to LPH 61–65 (Met-enkephalin) and LPH 57–60 amide, which were inactive.

A second enzyme involved in conversion was active at the lower pH of 6.5. It cleaved the Leu^{77}-Phe^{78} bond in the presence of Cleland's reagent and

EDTA (56). Thus, sequential action of pH 8.0 and 6.5 enzymes could lead to the formation of γ-endorphin, or, acting sequentially with a carboxypeptidase, the formation of α-endorphin (Fig. 12–3). Since these two LPH fragments lack activity *in vivo,* the pH 6.5 enzyme can be regarded in terms of an agent more for inactivation rather than for conversion to active compounds. Unfortunately, not all enzymes involved in biotransformation of β-LPH have been sufficiently purified to define their catabolic mechanisms. A distinction may prove necessary on the types of conversion that can occur with the full 91 amino acid sequence as compared to its fragments (LPH 41–58, LPH 61–91) in view of probable differences in their conformation and number of basic charges.

Breakdown of β-Endorphin

In view of the biological actions of β-endorphin, studies have been conducted on mechanisms available for inactivation. Early studies indicated a lower rate of biodegradation relative to that of enkephalins, implying that this would be a factor contributing to its potent *in vivo* actions (86,87). Studies based on the release of amino acids and peptides as detected by microdansylation procedure showed only partial breakdown upon incubation with brain extracts for short periods (122) with evidence for release of 3 to 6% of Tyr, Phe, Ser, Glu, Leu, Lys, Ile, and His. At longer incubation periods all amino acid residues were detected in yields ranging from 37% (Gly) to 100% (Tyr). The low yield of Gly was indicative of a rate-limiting split of Gly-Gly by a slow-acting glycyl glycine dipeptidase in brain extracts (Tables 12–1 and

TABLE 12–1. Cleavage of β-endorphin and a D-alanyl analogue by mouse brain extracts

			Percent breakdown							
		Time (min)	Tyr^{16}	Gly	Phe	Met	Thr	Ser	Glu	Val-
	LPH 61–91	5	6	0	4	0	0	5	7	0
$D-Ala^2$	LPH 61–91		tr	tr	tr	0	0	0	0	0
	LPH 61–91	60	100	37	70	88	62	55	90	67
$D-Ala^2$	LPH 61–91		49	12	22	23	20	22	53	32

		Time (min)	Glu^{91}	Lys	His	Ala	Asn	Ile	Leu-
	LPH 61–91	5	0	3	3	0	0	6	6
$D-Ala^2$	LPH 61–91		0	6	0	tr	0	tr	0
	LPH 61–91	60	40	70	47	50	60	63	85
$D-Ala^2$	LPH 61–91		9	42	tr	23	59	51	53

Residues released upon incubation of 50 nmoles, peptide for 5–60 min with 0.1 ml of mouse brain ultrafiltrate (33 vols of 1% NaCl submitted to double passage through a UM-10 Amicon filter) and 0.1 ml of 50 mM Tris-HCl buffer.

12–2). Peptide products were detected on polyamide plates, but no significant yield of LPH 61–65 was observed.

The paired lysyl residues at the C-terminal of β-endorphin appear to confer stability on the C-terminal Gln and Gly when exposed to carboxypeptidase A or the carboxypeptidase actions of washed rat brain synaptosomes or membranes used for study of opiate receptors (50). The stability may be due in part to the positive charges as shown by studies on model peptides; Ala-Tyr-Lys-Lys-Gly-Gln was resistant to degradation by carboxypeptidase but became susceptible following acetylation and citraconylation, or incubation carried out at higher pH. The synthetic hexapeptide corresponded with part of the C-terminal of human β-endorphin (residues LPH 87–91). A pentapeptide with only one lysine was rapidly degraded by carboxypeptidase A. Previous studies have established that carboxypeptidase A is largely a particulate enzyme and absent in sucrose supernatants (70). Breakdown of β-endorphin by an ultrafiltrate of mouse brain prepared with hypotonic buffers or saline led to the release of Gln and Gly, but release of these two residues does not differentiate release of C-terminal from internal residues (position 62–63,70). In the case of D-Ala²-β-endorphin where N-terminal release was retarded at short incubation periods, there was no evidence at all for Glu or Gly; at longer incubation periods Glu and Gly were less than one-fourth that of unsubstituted peptide (Table 12–2). This evidence favors the view that the C-terminal of β-endorphin is not readily degraded by brain carboxypeptidases. In the case of D-Ala²-α- and γ endorphins, N-terminal release was reduced to trace levels, and only at longer intervals were significant quantities of C-terminal groups released. The anomalous preservation of

TABLE 12–2. Cleavage of α- and γ-endorphins and D-alanyl analogues

N-terminus	Time (min)	Percent breakdown			
		Tyr[61]	Gly	Phe	Met-
D-Ala-α	5	0	0	0	0
	60	3	tr	tr	10
D-Ala-γ	60	tr	0	tr	11

C-terminus	Time (min)	Percent breakdown					
		Leu[77]	Thr[76]	Val	Pro	Glu	Lys-
D-Ala-α	5	—	7	4	0	0	0
	60	—	80[a]	74	41	0	0
D-Ala-γ	60	60	78[a]	44	34	16	48

Release of residue upon incubation with bovine brain extract.

[a] Based on the assumption that this is derived solely from position 76 and not from other positions in the polypeptide chain.

N-terminal on D-Ala^2-substituted α and γ-endorphins as compared to the longer β-endorphin sequence cannot be explained in the absence of data on changes in conformation induced by substitution with D-amino acids. The release of Lys in high yield from γ but not α-D-Ala^2-endorphin implies a conformational effect of the C-terminal Leu on susceptibility to carboxypeptidase-like enzymes. Structure-activity studies on β-endorphin are incomplete, but studies with purified enzymes as related to *in vitro* activities provide some information. Treatment with trypsin and chymotrypsin results in considerable loss of activity (45). The lack of effect observed with carboxypeptidase A by Doneen et al. (45) is understandable in view of the stability of the C-terminal portion His-Lys-Lys-Gly-Glu as noted in studies by Geisow and Smyth (50). Ronai et al. (166) have indicated a proximity between the helical LPH 73–89 region with the nonhelical LPH 61–65 portion when studied in an α-helix-promoting environment. Intramolecular interactions between the N-terminal LPH 61–65 of β-endorphins and other regions might account for its slower breakdown as compared to shorter fragments (79).

Evidence for conversion of β-endorphin into enkephalin and other peptides has been provided by Smyth and co-workers (4a,4b). They showed that ^{125}I labeled peptide undergoes stepwise cleavage when incubated for prolonged periods at pH 7.4 in presence of bacitracin to form γ-endorphin and small amounts of enkephalin, and even more rapidly at pH 5.0 to form α-endorphin, enkephalin and small amounts of hexa- and heptapeptides (for structures see Fig. 12–2). The slow rate of enkephalin production at physiological pH requires some comment. This might indicate only low levels of enzyme in washed synaptosomal preparations or conformational restraints such as to prevent rapid cleavage at sites adjacent to the C-terminus of enkephalin. Studies with purified enzymes show that conformational considerations do apply since the region Thr^{76}-Leu-Phe-Lys-Asn^{80} is vulnerable to a number of proteases when incubated under relatively mild conditions. Thus Leu-Phe is split by renin at pH 4.0 to release γ-endorphin but at higher enzyme concentration and longer periods of incubation it split also Phe^{64}-Met^{65}. Similarly, chymotrypsin at pH 7.4 cleaved Phe-Lys but with protracted incubations cleaved the Phe^{64}-Met^{65}. Trypsin under mild conditions cleaved Lys-Asn and with more vigorous conditions Lys^{69}-Ser^{70}. Proteases from armillaria or staphylococcus split Phe-^{78}-Lys^{79} and Gly^{68}-Lys^{69} respectively. None of these enzymes cleaved Met^{65}-Thr^{66} to liberate enkephalin indicating that brain membranes contain enzymes with different specificities possibly akin to that of neutral endopeptidases (cathepsin M, 120). The possibility exists also that there is endopeptidase cleavage at another site followed by sequential action of exopeptidases. Brain particulates including synaptosomes contain membrane bound carboxypeptidases active at neutral and acid pH (70) which could serve this role. Also, brain is known to contain renin-like enzymes (see 120), that could serve to form γ-endorphin which appears to be the major metabolite at physiological pH. Even in the case of β-LPH the precursor of

β-endorphin the bond Thr[77]-Leu[78] is vulnerable to enzymes present in adenohypophysis (56) and cleavage of this precursor form may precede that of other lipotropic fragments. The chief differences between action of renin and enzymes present in adenohypophysis is the pH optima which may indicate that some or part of the conversion processes are mediated by 'lysosomal' enzymes rather than soluble tissue endopeptidases. Since brain renin has similarities to brain cathepsin D (see 120) it will be of interest to determine if conversion can be mediated by lysosomal enzymes active at pH 3–6 such as the endopeptidases cathepsins D and B1, or exopeptidases such as cathepsins A, B2, and C (70,120). Formation of γ-endorphin at acid pH may account for the finding of this peptide in acid extracts prepared from brain or neurosecretory materials (71) and this explanation may apply to other opiod fragments (80) unless special precautions are taken to prevent breakdown during extraction procedures. Purification of intracellular proteinases together with information on the anatomical sites is necessary in order to propose mechanisms for the conversion of prolipotropin, β-LPH or other lipotropic fragments that may be found in the CNS. Since α- and γ-endorphins do not have any functional properties that they may simply serve as intermediates in the formation of enkephalins which are then rapidly inactivated at their target sites. In further studies Smyth and Snell (179a) showed that striatal slices can degrade β-endorphin to form γ-endorphin, enkephalin, and smaller amounts of other peptides (β-endorphin, hexa, and heptapeptides). Its half-life was 3.2 h without change on addition of bacitracin was considered by the authors to indicate that breakdown is initiated by endo- rather than exopeptidases. The presence, however, of Tyr as one of the products does indicate action by aminopeptidases and is in line with our findings made with soluble brain extracts incubated for shorter periods. The half-life of γ-endorphin was shorter (1.1 hr) with notable increase on addition of bacitracin which could indicate more rapid action of aminopeptidases or other enzymes. Uptake of radiolabeled peptide into slices was not demonstrated suggesting that breakdown was mediated by extra- rather than intracellular enzymes. However, it is likely that some intracellular enzymes may have leaked from the slice or its damaged surfaces. All these results appear to indicate that the conformation of β-endorphin (and probably its precursor forms) favors hydrolysis at the region LPH 76–80 and that there are restraints affecting production of shorter sequences closer to the N-terminus. Conformational aspects therefore supply a critical factor to regulation of intracellular pathways involved in conversion processes. This is demonstrated by the rapid degradation of shorter sequences such as LPH 61–65 by aminopeptidases or LPH 61–67 by chymotrypsin at the Phe-Met bond, and by brain membranes within 1 h at 37°C in presence of bacitracin to yield enkephalin and the dipeptide Thr-Ser. Brain particulates are known to contain a C-terminal dipeptidase capable of removing moieties similar to those of Thr-Ser and may be involved in the conversion process (122a). Alterations in levels of enzymes involved in the conversion processes especially if there is an insufficiency may be linked to phenomena such as those associated with development of tolerance or altered mental states (86).

Enkephalins

The enkephalins, pentapeptide components with opioid properties *in vitro,* were first isolated by Hughes (80) from acetone powders, using acid extraction. Their peptidyl nature was shown by their rapid destruction by leucine aminopeptidase and carboxypeptidase A. Subsequently, Hughes et al. (81) showed that these materials were pentapeptides, one with the composition of LPH 61–65 and the other Leu[65] LPH 61–65. The widespread occurrence of enkephalins as shown by bio- and immunoassay raises a number of questions concerning their source. Clouet and Ratner (37) observed incorporation of labeled glycine given intracisternally into an "enkephalin-like" fragment, but further studies are required to show if this occurred by *de novo* synthesis from precursor amino acids or by breakdown of a larger form. It is known that tissue extracts of liver, kidney, brain, and cerebrospinal fluid contain endorphin-like materials (see Chapter 11). It is unlikely that leu-enkephalin is derived from known lipotropins since none of the latter contain leucine in position 65 (55).

Degradation

Enkephalins are rapidly hydrolyzed when exposed to tissue extracts (87, 122), membrane fractions (132,134), or plasma *in vitro* (74), or if labeled peptide is administered intraventricularly (132) or by intracarotid injection (93). The rapid destruction of this peptide might be regarded as in keeping with suggestions that it has putative neurotransmitter properties (102).

Studies on activity *in vitro* show that a minimum sequence of five amino acids is essential since removal of its N- or C-terminal groups results in loss of activity when tested *in vitro* (138). Tyr is essential but need not be at the N-terminal, since LPH 60–65 (Arg-Tyr-) has activity *in vitro* (108). In the case of the pentapeptide, the Tyr-Gly- bonds are particularly vulnerable to aminopeptidases as shown by studies using brain fractions (87,122), and this could account for failure to detect activity *in vivo* (86). Hambrook et al. (74) using labeled met-enkephalin found evidence for release of Tyr along with the formation of a tetrapeptide LPH 62–65 at short incubation periods. This tetrapeptide is formed also in studies in our laboratories on incubation with analogues bearing D-Phe and D-Met in positions 64 and 65 (Table 12–3).

Further studies with enkephalin analogues show that it is necessary to block N- and C-terminals simultaneously to prevent breakdown and improve potency as evaluated by an analgesic test *in vivo.* Thus, D-Ala in position 62

TABLE 12–3. *Breakdown of enkephalin analogues by mouse brain soluble extracts*

Substrate	Time (min)	Products (percent breakdown)
LPH 61–65	1	Tyr (40), Gly-Gly-Phe-Met
	5	Tyr (90), Gly (10), Gly-Gly (40), Phe (40), Met (50)
D-Ala^{62}	5	Tyr (trace), Met (trace)
	60	Tyr (62), Met (76), Phe (62)
D-Ala^{64}	5	Tyr (100), Gly-Gly (21), Gly-D-Ala-Phe-Met
D-Met^{65}	5	Tyr (82), Gly-Gly (trace), Gly-Gly-D-Phe-Met
Met.NH$_2^{65}$	5	Tyr (50), Phe (4)
	60	Tyr (60), Gly-Gly (20), Phe (44), Met (34), Met.NH$_2$ (18)
D-Ala^{62}, Met.NH$_2^{65}$	5	None
	60	Tyr (3)
D-Met, Pro.NH$_2$	5	None
	60	Tyr (20), D-Met-Gly-Phe-Pro.NH$_2$

For details see Table 1. The doubly substituted analogs that resist digestion by soluble extracts prepared from mouse brain are known to be active as analgesic agents when given in vivo as noted in Table 12–4. Removal of Tyr in the case of LPH 61–65 (enkephalin) is known to result in inactivation. Intermediate formation of Gly-Gly as a product is attributable to a slow acting Gly-Gly dipeptidase of brain which has a requirement for Co^{2+}.

retarded release of N-terminal groups but did not prevent rapid C-terminal cleavages. In contrast, D-Ala in position 63 blocked C-terminal cleavage but not the action of aminopeptidases present in brain extracts. Action of carboxy- but not aminopeptidases was blocked by D-Phe and D-Met in positions 64 and 65 leading to the accumulation in digests of the tetrapeptide LPH 62–65. The presence of methionamide on the C-terminal delayed breakdown, but in combination with D-Ala in position 62 gave a peptide that was relatively nonmetabolizable; only trace levels of Tyr were detectable at 5 min and 3% at 60 min (Table 12–3). These results indicated that these substitutions led to an intramolecular interaction between N- and C-termini so as to induce a conformational change inimical to the action of degradative hydrolases. Detailed studies on the conformation of enkephalin led to the conclusion that there is a secondary structure, characterized by a β-bend with restricted rotation for Tyr but not for Phe and Met (83,135); presence of amide on the C-terminal could thus engender a more stable configuration. The remarkable resistance of D-Ala-enkephalamide to breakdown may be a factor to enhance potency *in vivo,* as demonstrated following its application to periaqueductal gray (154,155) or given intraventricularly (195), and its enhanced affinity to opiate receptors and action on gut and vas deferens (40).

Other analogues also show higher activity as compared to enkephalin, leading to the assumption that reduced susceptibility to degradation is an important factor (Table 12–4). Pert et al. (154) found that substitutions by D-amino acids, L-DOPA, Sar at the N-terminal, or Ala, Pro, Sar in position 63 in combination with methionamide at the C-terminal 63 decreased binding

TABLE 12–4. *Stabilization of enkephalins toward degradation: correlation to biological activity* in vitro *and* in vivo

---

1. Substitutions that lead to loss of activity *in vitro* (guinea pig ileum, mouse vas deferens, or receptor binding assays)
   position 1: D-Tyr (or des-Tyr), O-methyl Tyr, Phe, Sarcosine, L-DOPA, Trp, His
   position 2: Pro, Sar, D-Val, D-Phe
   position 3: D-Ala*
   position 4: Gly, D-Phe*
   position 5: D-Met*
2. Substitutions that lead to an enhancement of activity:
   D-Ala^2.Met.NH$_2$[a],[b]*
   D-Met^2.Pro NH$_2$* (or NH Et)[b],[c]
   D-Ala^2.Pro NH$_2$ (or NH Et)[b]
   N-(methyl) Tyr[1b]
   N-(methyl) Tyr[1b]

Data taken from studies by several groups (6, 23, 40, 134, 154, 155). Analogues with an asterisk are described separately in terms of breakdown in Table 12–3. The small letters refer to activity measured *in vitro* (a), *in vivo* (b), or if active when given intravenously (c).

to opiate receptors *in vitro*, although in the case of some double-substituted analogues weak analgesia activity was detectable *in vivo*. Breakdown was implied as a factor responsible for the enhanced activity of D-Ala-enkephalinamide since exposure of it to washed membranes was without effect on binding capacity as compared to enkephalins. This is in agreement with findings of Miller et al. (134) who found that binding of enkephalin but not D-Ala^2-enkephalinamide was improved at 0° as compared to 25°C, implying that breakdown was involved. Also, binding of enkephalin but not the active analogue was improved in the presence of proteolytic inhibitors, notably soybean inhibitor and bacitracin.

Bradbury et al. (23) observed improved activities of "stabilized" enkephalins such as N-methylated LPH 61–65 and its amide when injected intraventricularly, although these compounds were less active than β-endorphin on a molar basis. In addition to analgesia, they produced catatonic changes. More recently, Bajusz et al. (6) prepared analogues that were equal to or higher in analgesic potency as compared to β-endorphin; these included the (D-Met^{2}Pro^{5}NH$_2$), (D-Met^{2}ProNHEt), and (D-Ala^{2}ProNHEt) analogues of enkephalins. The first analogue had double the activity of β-endorphin and was active when given intravenously. This analog also was resistant to degradation by brain soluble enzymes (Table 12–3). The development of "superactive" analogues having only five residues may indicate that the active sequence of β-endorphins with respect to analgesia is shorter than previously supposed. Furthermore, the use of analogues supports the hypothesis that breakdown is a factor that must be considered in evaluating the activity of opioid fragments. Failure to demonstrate an *in vivo* action for enkephalins does not exclude the possibility for its release close to the active site by an endogenous process followed by rapid breakdown. As noted elsewhere (119,

120) breakdown is one of several factors contributing to an enhanced activity; others include transport across membranes and increased receptor affinity.

Studies on enkephalins using purified exopeptidases confirm the susceptibility of the Tyr-Gly group to N-terminal cleavage as shown by studies with aminopeptidase. Law et al. (108) using the LPH 60–65 indicated that the Arg-Tyr bond is not cleaved by gut enzymes based on qualitative studies of extracted material present in gut bath. The stability of peptides to gut enzymes is of interest but may not be analogous to degradation by CNS hydrolases.

HYPOTHALAMIC PEPTIDES

Biosynthesis of Hypothalamic Hormones

There is only fragmentary evidence for the existence of precursors for hypothalamic releasing factors such as LRH and somatostatin, neurohypophyseal hormones, and neurophysins, all of which are known to be present in hypothalamic areas. In most cases studies on synthesis using labeled amino acids as precursors are handicapped by the rapid destruction of precursor forms and the active peptides, indicating the need for development of specific inhibitors or the use of other strategies. Neurophysins represent an example of polypeptides without hormonal properties that are formed in association with oxytocin and vasopressin (see Chapter 2), and which appear to play a role in their packing and transport (48,170). Based on labeling patterns *in vivo* of neurosecretory granules of the supraoptic and paraventricular regions, there is evidence that neurophysins are formed with neurohypophyseal peptides, possibly from a common precursor. Neurophysins themselves are a group of cysteine-rich polypeptides, occurring in neurosecretory regions (hypothalamus, neurohypophysis, and pineal gland) which have been subjected to intensive study with respect to their primary structure and to their metabolism (1,196). Sachs (170) was the first to demonstrate incorporation of labeled amino acids into neurophysins and associated peptides by infusion of ^{35}S-cysteine and ^{3}H-tyrosine into the third ventricle of dogs. The labeling pattern observed favored the hypothalamus as the primary site of biosynthesis (specific activities higher than in neurohypophysis following pulse labeling). This was confirmed subsequently by sectioning the stalk and preventing the accumulation of labeled materials in the posterior lobe. Biosynthesis could also be demonstrated *in vitro* using the median eminence, but not the posterior lobe (170). Inhibition by puromycin of vasopressin synthesis *in vitro* and *in vivo* supports the view that this component is formed via a classic ribosomal mechanism at sites outside the neurosecretory granules. Since vasopressin and oxytocin contain a C-terminal amide, post-translational changes of these precursor forms are indicated. Although studies imply existence of precursors for neurohypophyseal peptides, these have yet to be isolated and identified. If such active peptides are formed in association with neurophysins, then a number of critical questions remain to be answered: these refer to the biological role of neurophysins *per se;* the anatomical sites involved in biosynthesis and packaging; and the enzymes involved, if any, in processing of the complex at the sites of synthesis or during flow down the axon to the posterior lobe. Gainer et al. (49) have provided the best evidence to date for the existence of a precursor form by isolation of a 20,000 molecular weight complex following placement of ^{35}C-cysteine at sites adjacent to the supraoptic nucleus of rat. This was presumed to be a putative precursor since the larger form disappeared with time with the concomitant increase in a labeled unit with a molecular weight of 12,000. Both larger and smaller forms cross-reacted with a specific antiserum directed toward neurophysin. The synthesis of neurophysin complexes within the supraoptic nucleus coupled with their conversion during axonal transport is a further example of neurosecretion as conceived by the Scharrers (175). Cleavage of neurophysins by intragranular hydrolases at sites of synthesis or by specific hydrolase or cathepsin during transport could account in some cases for presence of smaller neurophysins or their fragments in tissues (41,146); in this respect, neurophysin is a known substrate for brain cathepsin D (156).

Oxytocin itself is regarded as a possible prohormone for MSH-inhibiting factor (MIF), since Pro-Leu-Gly·NH$_2$ is present on the C-terminal of oxytocin and is reported to be released by enzymes present in the hypothalamus (197) but absent in brain (121). The authenticity of MIF as a true hypothalamic inhibitory factor has been questioned, but studies on the metabolic fate of this tripeptide have attracted interest following reports that it has *in vivo* actions on behavior (92,94). The tripeptide is rapidly degraded by brain and serum enzymes, with release of Pro, Leu, and Gly·NH$_2$, but the primacy of enzymes cleaving Pro-Leu versus Leu-Gly·NH$_2$ has yet to be decided; studies with these two dipeptides using brain and serum show cleavage at both bonds by aminopeptidases and arylamidases (198). Since Gly·NH$_2$ and not Gly was detected as an end-product, there is no indication that this tripeptide, in contrast to pyroGlu-His-Pro·NH$_2$ (TRH), is inactivated by deamidation. MIF is remarkably stable when incubated with human serum but not with rat (Table 12–5; 198). In further studies on structure-activity relationships of other oxytocin fragments on MSH release, Celis et al. (31) showed that Cys-Tyr-Ile-Gln-Asn, Ile-Gln-Asn, and Tyr-Ile-Gln-Asn in nanogram concentrations were effective in decreasing pituitary levels of MSH even following lesioning of the median eminence. Thus, they appeared to act directly on the gland.

Previous claims that a number of hypothalamic factors including LRH, TRH, and PIF are formed *de novo* from precursor amino acids by nonribosomal soluble systems have yet to be corroborated. In the case of TRH,

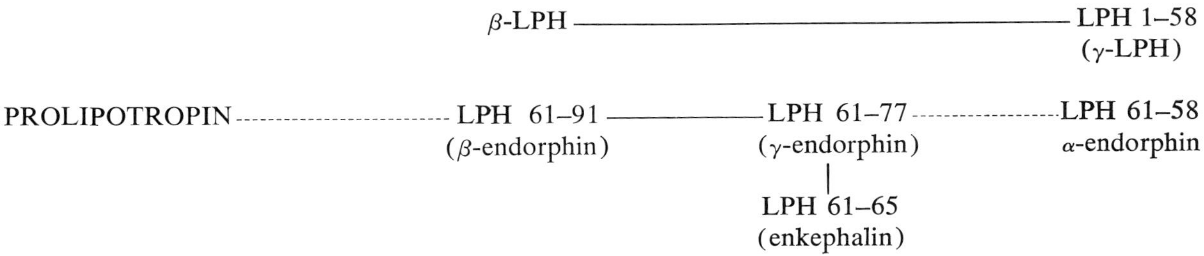

β-LPH ———————————————— LPH 1-58
(γ-LPH)

PROLIPOTROPIN --------- LPH 61-91 --------- LPH 61-77 ------------- LPH 61-58
(β-endorphin)   (γ-endorphin)   α-endorphin
                              |
                        LPH 61-65
                        (enkephalin)

FIG. 12-2. Schemata for the conversion and processing of ACTH, melanotropins and lipotropins. The composition of the precursors for ACTH and lipotropin are unknown. Postulated pathways involving conversion of these prohormones is indicated in both cases by the broken lines. Direct conversion of β-lipotropin to form β-MSH has not been demonstrated using tissue extracts; there is indirect evidence that enzymes present in pituitary extracts can cleave one of the bonds close to the C-terminus as described in the text. There is evidence for the conversion of β-endorphin to form γ- and α-endorphin, enkephalin and other peptide fragments when incubated with washed synaptosomal membranes [or striatal slices of rat brain (4b, 179 a).] A heptapeptide sequence common to ACTH, melanotropins and lipotropin in italics. Abbreviations used are: ACTH, adrenocorticotropin; LPH, lipotropin; MSH, melanocyte stimulating hormone; CLIP, corticotropin-like intermediate peptide.

TABLE 12–5. Cleavage of LRH, somatostatin, TRH MIF, and analogues by serum enzymes

Peptide	Residues	Percent released			
		Human		Rat	
		4 hr	24 hr	4 hr	24 hr
LRH	Leu	14	60	52	100
	Gly·NH₂	0	24	68	82
(des-Gly¹⁰)-LRH ethylamide	Leu	34	60	24	76
(des-Gly¹⁰-D-Ala⁶) LRH-ethylamide	Leu	nd	6	nd	12
H₂-somatostatin	Lys	28	58	58	63
	Phe	10	31	50	50
N-acetyl-des-Ala¹- Gly²-somatostatin	Lys	14	nd	nd	nd
	Phe	5			
(D-Trp⁸)-somatostatin	Lys	nd	nd	5	nd
	Phe			0	
TRH	His	5	30	25	80
(3-Me-His²)-TRH	3-Me-His	80	85	90	100
His-Pro·NH₂	His	nd	nd	23	90
Pro-Leu·Gly·NH₂	Leu	0	trace	100	100

Reaction mixtures consisting of 50 nmoles substrate, or 100 nmoles TRH, were incubated at 37°C with 0.2 ml of serum at pH 7.6. Breakdown of LRH is based on the release of two residues: Leu, indicating endopeptidase activity, and Gly·NH₂, indicating activity of a C-terminal cleaving enzyme. Breakdown of somatostatin is based on the release of Lys and Phe; TRH degradation is based on the release of His; MIF on liberation of Leu. Data based on that of Benuck et al. (13,14) and Walter et al. (198). and, not determined.

Bauer and Lipmann (9,10) found that the labeled moiety isolated by Reichlin (163) using single-dimension chromatography could not be identified as the tripeptidyl hormone if subjected to chromatography in a second dimension. Rapid degradation and identification of hormonal products when present in trace amounts represent formidable problems in tackling questions of biosynthesis. Microprocedures for extraction of peptides and radioimmunoassays have been used by some investigators, who have reported biosynthesis of TRH in tissue fragments retaining cellular structure in the hypothalamus and the placenta (51,130). Despite these observations, it is not known if classic ribosomal mechanisms are involved in the biosynthesis of TRH, or if there are macromolecular forms of larger dimension from which it can be formed by proteolytic cleavage. As in the case of neurohypophyseal enzymes, these would have to be accompanied by post-translational changes.

In the case of LRH, Moguilevsky et al. (137) showed incorporation of ³H-Tyr into two biologically active forms of LRH which could be separated by gel filtration. The observation that incorporation was increased in castrated rats could suggest steroidal interactions on these anabolic processes (89,137). Larger immunoreactive forms of LRH have been observed independently by two groups (46,133). Millar et al. (133) found that the two forms present in extracts of lyophilized sheep hypothalami were unaffected by urea. They found LRH activity following treatment of tissue with a hypothalamic supernatant fraction or with trypsin. These precursor forms were less abundant in the median eminence compared to the optic chiasm and basal hypothalamus. Catabolism of LRH itself was prevented by addition of peptides containing C-terminal amides. These peptides inhibit brain peptidases by competition, and were used in similar studies shown in Table 12–5. There is only scanty evidence for presence of precursor forms for somatostatin in tissues. Immunoreactive forms have been detected in extracts of stomach, duodenum, and hypothalamus but not in ovaries and other body organs (4).

Degradation of LRH

A large number of analogues of LRH have been synthesized in the search for longer acting derivatives with agonist or antagonist properties. As a result, this peptide has been intensively studied with respect to degradation (119,120). The presence of blocked N- and C-terminal groups implies action by novel enzymes, since such groupings are not readily hydrolyzed by the classic peptide hydrolases. In studies on the timed release of residues on peptide incubation with brain and serum enzymes (124,125), two mechanisms appeared to be involved. One was internal cleavage by a neutral endopeptidase followed by secondary cleavage by other peptidases. The other was a slower C-terminal removal of glycinamide by a second enzyme acting specifically on peptyl amides. Evidence for the endopeptidase was obtained by Koch et al. (98) with isolation of the intermediate peptide (Gln^1------Gly^6), pointing toward a Gly^6-Leu^7 cleavage. These findings are supported by studies on analogues containing D-amino acids since such substitutions are known to hinder most tissue enzymes. Thus, D-Ala in position 6 led to a reduced release of adjacent residues at short incubation periods *in vitro* concomitant with an enhanced *in vivo* activity. This substitution failed to block release of the C-terminal glycinamide which can be blocked by substitution of Gly^6 with ethylamide ($C_2H_5 \cdot NH_2$) (Fig. 12–4). The doubly substituted analogue was shown by Fujino and his group (47) to be 80-fold more potent in the intact animal.

There thus appears to be an excellent correlation between relative resistance to biodegradation and potency. Substitution can alter conformation favorable to degradative enzymes or change receptor affinities. Current studies to determine if conformational factors play a role by stabilization of a B-II type bend have not provided a clear explanation of the improved potency of the D-Ala^6 analogues (173). Our original observations on reduced breakdown were confirmed in recent studies by Koch et al. (99), using hypothalamic and anterior pituitary extracts incubated with newer analogues and residual activity measured by radioimmunoassay. They found that D-Ala^6

LH-RH analogue	Degradation rate*	Potency in vivo*
pGlu - His - Trp - Ser - Tyr - Gly - Leu - Arg - Pro - Gly · NH₂	1.0	1.0
pGlu —————— D-ALA[6] ————— Gly · NH₂	0.5	6.0
pGlu —————— D-ALA[6] ————— Et · NH₂	0.01	80
pGlu —————— D-LEU[6] ————— Gly · NH₂	0.5	—
pGlu —————— D-TRP[6] ————— Gly · NH₂	0.2	8
pGlu —————— D-ALA[6](NαMe)LEU[7] —— Gly · NH₂	0	1.0

* Relative to that of LH-RH as 1.0

FIG. 12–4. Cleavage of LRH by extracts of brain and neurosecretory regions (124,125,99). Note that presence of D-amino acids in position 6 blocks or retards action of brain endopeptidases (cathepsin M) and presence of ethylamide blocks the action of C-terminal cleaving enzymes. Substitution by D-Trp[6] and D-Ala[6] (Nα-Me)Leu[7] affects all degradative enzymes (99).

was degraded at two-thirds, D-Leu^6 at half, and D-Trp^6 at 80% the rate of LRH. A double-substituted analogue D-Ala^6, N$^\alpha$-MeLeu^7-LRH was impervious to breakdown implying that there was interference also with C-terminal cleavage (Fig. 12–4.) It is known that some D-amino acids in positions 2 and 6 introduce antagonist properties. Examples include D-Phe^6, D-Phe^2-D-Phe^6, D-Phe^2-D-Leu^6, desHis^2 (D-Ala^6), and its ethylamide D-Phe^3-Phe^3-(D-Phe^6)-des His^2(D-Leu)-LRH. However, the stability and mechanism of action of these analogues are unknown (145,165,173). In the case of the doubly substituted analogue D-Ala^6, N$^\alpha$-MeLeu^7 LRH and its ethylamide, degradation is depressed but action *in vivo* is only moderately enhanced. This would suggest an altered conformation unfavorable to receptor binding as compared to D-Ala^6-LRH-ethylamide and similar analogues.

Inactivation of LRH occurs in all anatomical regions of the CNS, pineal, and pituitary so far investigated, i.e., in hypothalamus, anterior and posterior pituitary, thalamus, spinal cord, and pineal gland (61,100,120). In subcellular fractions, more than 90% of the inactivating activity is associated with the cytosol and less than 5% with synaptosomal, nuclear, and mitochondrial fractions. If contamination is excluded as a factor in such studies, the low levels observed in synaptosomes are of interest because they are the major anatomical location of endogenous peptide (185,199). In addition to nerve tissue, inactivating enzymes are present in serum (13) and organs such as liver and kidney (100). Inactivation in body fluids may contribute to the relatively short half-life of LRH, although rapid distribution into other body compartments *in vivo* must be taken into account. Redding et al. (160) found that labeled LRH given intravenously was degraded with the major products in urine being pyroGlu and pyroGlu-His. This might indicate the presence of a pyroglutamyl peptidase in tissue as one of the degrading enzymes. In our studies, LRH was degraded slowly in blood obtained from the hypophyseal circulation of monkeys (14). Breakdown in portal blood was comparable to that observed in systemic blood of monkeys and humans, and less than breakdown in rat blood (13). Therefore, breakdown is not the factor primarily responsible for the insensitivity of some strains of monkey to LRH and its synthetic analogues (110). Studies on breakdown of D-Ala^6 and D-Ala^6-LRH ethylamide in rat and human serum support the notion that their enhanced activity is attributable in part to their resistance to degradation (Table 12–5).

Little progress has been made on purification of enzymes inactivating LRH, in part because of problems of lability and the absence of a rapid monitoring procedure. On the supposition that a neutral endopeptidase was involved, we succeeded in partial purification of an enzyme, using myelin basic protein as substrate. This substance is a linear peptide with an N-terminal blocked group. Enzyme purified 20- to 30-fold by this procedure was shown to inactivate LRH, as measured by radioimmunoassay (N. Marks and M. Benuck, *unpublished observations*). The enzyme was a neutral endopeptidase that was inhibited by diisopropyl fluorophosphate (DFP) and phenylmethal sulfonyl chloride (PMSF) and had properties akin to cathepsin M (119). Other studies based on the effects of tryptic inhibitors on breakdown by crude tissue extracts are inconclusive (98,100).

Studies on the fate of LRH have received attention with respect to possible feedback regulation by steroids. Higher rates of inactivation have been reported for selected regions of the hypothalamus of male rats as compared to females with alterations of activity in supernatant fractions following gonadectomy. These alterations were reported to be reversed by administration of steroids (estradiol to females and testosterone to males), supporting the view that steroids can affect gonadotrophic secretion by affecting metabolism of LRH (62–64,66). Kuhl and Taubert (104,105) in a series of studies obtained evidence that levels of cysteinyl aminopeptidase in hypothalamus can be regulated by LRH, and that this peptidase in vitro is inhibited by congener substrates with C-terminal amides (LRH itself, oxytocin, TRH, and lysine vasopressin). Griffiths and Hooper (64) found that LRH interfered with the metabolism of oxytocin in supernatant extracts of hypothalami from female rats. All these examples collectively reinforce the notion that there is an interrelationship between metabolism of hormonal peptides and gonadotrophic function. However, further studies are mandatory to establish if these effects are direct or secondary to alterations in electrolyte balance, cAMP levels, or glucose and amine metabolism. The relevance of a cysteinyl aminopeptidase is unclear since LRH does not contain a disulfide bridge. Studies with a cysteinyl aminopeptidase using cysteinyl naphthylamides as substrates shows that purified enzyme from blood and tissues has a broad specificity and acts like a typical aminopeptidase or arylamidase (118,123). As such, cysteinyl aminopeptidase may be involved in secondary cleavage of LRH fragments rather than primary cleavage of LRH itself.

Degradation of TRH

Degradation of TRH by blood and tissue extracts is extensively documented (120). The primary mechanisms involved are removal of the pyroglutamyl moiety by a specific peptidase, or cleavage of pyroGlu-His- or His-ProNH$_2$ bonds by peptidases, or deamination (Fig. 12–5).

An enzyme-degrading TRH is widely distributed in CNS and peripheral tissues (125,157). In the case of brain, the presence of a TRH-degrading system in extrahypothalamic tissue may be related to its neurotropic functions. Levels are reported higher in hypothalamus than cortex and pituitary (157), and higher in male than female rabbit CNS (61,65,67). Taylor and Dixon (187) in a survey of various areas of rat brain found high specific activity in supernatants prepared from hypothalamus. There were lower activities in cerebellum, diencephalon, brainstem, forebrain, and posterior cortex. In subcellular fractions of hamster hypothalami, Prasad and

Neurotensin

PGlu-Leu-Tyr-Glu-Asn-Lys-Pro-Arg-Arg-Pro-Tyr-Ile-Leu

$\longleftarrow$ ——————carboxypeptidases

Thyrotropin (TRH)

pGLU-His-Pro · NH$_2$

↑ ↑ ↑
pyroglutamyl peptidase

peptidase

deamidation

FIG. 12–5. Sites of cleavage of neurotensin and TRH by enzymes present in brain extracts (120,125). The first products upon incubation of TRH with brain extracts is ammonia accompanied by the deamido form of TRH.

Peterkofsky (157) found the highest levels in the past 27,000 g supernatant. Winokur et al. (201) observed inactivation of exogenously added TRH in all particulate fractions but did not observe destruction of TRH native to the tissue and present in organelles. This suggests that TRH is compartmentalized or protected by being present in a bound form. Of potential interest is the finding that some clonal cell lines have a reduced capability for breakdown of added TRH, which could suggest neuronal/glial differences of functional significance. TRH degradation appears to be lower in cell strains that lack TRH receptors. If degradation is intracellular following transport into cells, the strains with reduced capacity may never accumulate sufficient TRH to detect breakdown.

Incubation of TRH by brain extracts leads initially to the production of deamido-TRH along with His and Pro and/or Pro·NH$_2$, depending on the methods used. To some extent, results have depended on the development of suitable analytical procedures for isolation and separation of the split products. In the method adopted by Bauer and Lipmann (10) a supernatant prepared from freeze-dried porcine hypothalamic fragments on incubation at pH 7.4 with ^{3}H-Pro-TRH gave deamido-TRH and Pro·NH$_2$ as the major products and Pro as a minor product. They concluded that Pro was derived from the deamido form, since incubation with Pro·NH$_2$ by itself did not lead to deamidation. In contrast to those results, the ratio of split products was different if supernatant was prepared from fresh tissue, since only the deamido form was detected. Since incubation with homogenates of fresh tissue (in contrast to supernatant) again led to production of Pro·NH$_2$ and Pro, it was concluded that the peptidase responsible for cleavage of the deamido form is particulate-bound but capable of solubilization on freeze drying the tissue. Using a similar chromatographic separation of labeled TRH products, Taylor and Dixon (187) found similar results for extracts of fresh and frozen tissue. This approach suggests that extraction of fresh tissue would be a good source of "deamidating enzymes" free of peptidases capable of releasing Pro·NH$_2$ by cleavage of the His-Pro·NH$_2$ bond. Inactivating enzymes are present also in synaptosomes as shown with uptake studies for H-Pro TRH: these showed uptake of only labeled proline (151a).

There have been some attempts to separate and purify the enzymes inactivating TRH. In one of the earliest attempts, Mudge and Fellows (140) purified 15-fold a pituitary pyroglutamyl peptidase from frozen bovine material by extraction with a phosphate buffer containing EDTA and mercaptoethanol followed by salt precipitation and gel filtration using pyroGlu-Ala as the substrate. Like the bacterial enzyme (E.C.3.4.11.8), it was sulfhydryl dependent and unstable in solution. It stabilized with the inhibitor 2-pyrrolidinone and cleaved TRH with release of His-Pro·NH$_2$. In addition to TRH, it cleaved pyroGlu-His-Pro-O methyl ester and the deamido form without appearance of free Pro and His. The enzyme was sulfhydryl dependent since it was inhibited by iodoacetamide. The pituitary pyroglutamyl peptidase showed similarities to that obtained from other sources; the K_m of 2.3×10^{-4} M was one order of magnitude less than that of rat liver and that obtained from bacterial sources (140). PyroGlu itself is present in tissues with relatively high levels in brain in the range of 0.13 μmoles/g fresh weight (120). The pyroGlu moiety present in peptide form can be formed by nonenzymatic mechanisms resulting from cyclization of N-terminal Glu·NH$_2$. A question often posed is whether pyroGlu found in some peptides is artifactual and whether this grouping exists in the native state. Formation and removal of pyroGlu may represent a regulatory mechanism for a number of biologically active peptides. Prasad and Peterkofsky (157) separated two TRH-degrading enzymes from soluble extracts of hamster hypothalami by gel filtration, one of which possessed pyroglutamyl peptidase activity and the second amidase activity.

Incubation of TRH with serum or plasma leads to a multiplicity of products. Redding and Schally (161,162) concluded from their studies on the fate of injected TRH *in vivo* that several distinct processes contributed to its short half-life of approximately 4 min. These included rapid transport into tissue compartments, breakdown in blood and tissues, and urinary excretion. In their studies with labeled TRH the major end-products found in plasma were deamido-TRH, His-Pro·NH$_2$ and Glu-His-Pro. Visser et al. (194) were unable to detect the deamido form in plasma following injection using a specific antiserum directed against pyroGlu-His-Pro·OH. In studies *in vitro,* incubation of TRH with serum or plasma of different species leads to the release of the deamido form, Pro and pyroGlu-His (141), Pro (9), and Pro and His (13). With the more active analogue, 3-methyl-His-TRH, the end-products included 3-methylhistidine (Table 12–5). There is some evidence for species differences, since the rates of degradation were higher in rat than in human serum (Table 12–5; 13), and degradation was undetected in the blood of carp and terrapin (139). Also, the extent of TRH degradation in serum or plasma appears to be related to developmental and functional changes in some but not all studies (8,161,191). Neary et al. (142) found extensive degradation of TRH in plasma from adult rats but not appreciable breakdown in neonatal blood or plasma from rats aged 4 to 16 months. The failure of neonatal blood to degrade TRH was not attributable to an inhibitor, since there was no without effect on addition of adult plasma. Bauer (9) found that degradation was regulated by thyroid hormones, since breakdown was low in serum from hypothyroid animals (treated with propylthiouracil) but restored on treatment with triiodothyronine (T_3) as judged by the disappearance of labeled TRH using chromatographic separation. These relationships imply a possible feedback mechanism based on relative rates of degradation regulating TRH levels. Attempts to relate degradation to levels of TSH in circulating blood are premature in view of discrepant results on the role of TSH and other hormones as inhibitors. In earlier studies, Redding and Schally (161) found a reduced level of TRH breakdown in blood of hypophysectomized-thyroidectomized rats which was reversed by treatment with T_3. However, breakdown was not reduced in patients suffering from hypothyroidism or hypopituitarism (8). Reasons for discrepant results for TRH degradation are not clear, but one of the major difficulties is the development of sensitive analytical procedures for analysis of the end-products when using low (physiological) levels of hormone.

There has been considerable interest in methods for inhibiting breakdown of TRH for studies attempting to demonstrate biosynthesis *in vitro* by nonribosomal or other pathways (10,88,163). More than one enzyme may be involved, and there have been several approaches. These include addition of nonspecific inhibitors to block all degradative enzymes, and specific inhibitors directed against the pyroglutamyl peptidase, cleavage of the -His-Pro·NH$_2$ bond, or inhibition of the amidase (Table 12–6). In early studies Vale et al. (191) found that the dipeptide pyroGlu-His-OCH[3] effectively inhibited TRH inactivation by serum enzymes. Bauer and Lipmann (10) in studies with this dipeptide in CNS tissue showed that the deamidating enzyme was insensitive, indicating that the degradation of TRH by serum and brain must follow different pathways. Knigge and Schock (97) observed inhibition of the enzyme in rat plasma by substrates with N-terminal pyroGlu (LRH and neurotensin) but not by deamido-TRH, Glu-His-Pro, dipeptide breakdown products, or Pro·NH$_2$. Plasma enzyme was inhibited markedly by Cu^{2+}, BAL, benzamidine, and paramercuribenzoate (pCMB); moderately affected by EDTA and puromycin; and unaffected by mercaptoethanol or TSH.

In studies on enzymes of hamster hypothalamus, Prasad and Peterkofsky (157) found some inhibition in the presence of high concentrations of peptides with C-terminal amides LRH, substance P, tetragastrin, and N-terminal pyroGlu (deamido-TRH, pyroGlu-Ala), pointing to the high

TABLE 12–6. Agents proposed for inhibition of TRH breakdown in vitro

	Deamidation	Peptidase or PyroGlu peptidase
1. Competitive	LRH (-Gly NH₂)	
	Substance P (-Met NH₂)	PyroGlu-His-Pro
		PyroGlu-Ala
	Tetragastrin	Neurotensin
	TSH	
2. Site specific	Tos-Lys-CH₂Cl	Tos-Phe-CH₂Cl
	Iodoacetamide	Benzamidine, pCMB
	N-ethylmaleimide	
3. Other	Angiotensin I, II	Hydrocortisone
	(angiotensinamide)	Tryptic inhibitors
		(soybean, ovomucoid)
	Somatostatin	PyroGlu-His methyl ester
	Heavy metals	Bacitracin
		Co²⁺
		Heavy metals

Data obtained from studies of McKelvy et al. (129), Prasad and Peterkofsky (157), Knigge and Schock (97), Vale et al. (191), Bauer and Lipman (10), and Reichlin (163). In several cases the mechanisms of inhibition and the specific enzyme involved cannot be defined. Bacitracin has been used to suppress breakdown of glucagon (82) but is ineffective in breakdown of ACTH fragments on incubation with isolated adrenal cells (11).

degree of specificity of the TRH-degrading system. Trypsin inhibitors from soybean and ovomucoid, and Tos-Lys CH₂Cl appeared to preferentially inhibit TRH-amidase, whereas Tos-Phe CH₂Cl, benzamidine, and Co²⁺ inhibited the pyroglutamyl peptidase. A variety of heavy metals at high concentration (10 mM), including Ni²⁺, Fe²⁺, Cu²⁺, Zn²⁺, and Ca²⁺, inhibited both activities. Iodoacetamide inhibited both activities suggesting a sulfhydryl requirement. Of hormones tested, TSH inhibited the amidase and cortisol inhibited the pyroGlu peptidase. Inhibition of hypothalamic enzyme by TSH is further indication that the pathways in tissue differ from that in blood. This difference is further reinforced by the finding of McKelvy et al. (129), who showed a noncompetitive inhibition of TRH breakdown in homogenates of guinea pig brain and hypothalami or their subcellular fractions by addition of bacitracin ($K_i = 1.9 \times 10^{-5}$ M). It is noteworthy that there are a number of systems that exhibit minimal or no degradative activity. These include the newt (68) and clonal cell lines (69,188). There would appear also to be considerable potential for examining further analogues of dipeptidyl cleavage products as potential inhibitors of either the pyroglutamyl peptidase or amidase actions.

Substance P

The hypotensive unidecapeptide substance P is a candidate neurotransmitter in primary afferent neurons in spinal cord (148–150). High concentrations of substance P-like peptide occur in the hypothalamus and mesencephalon (see Chapter 1; 26). Release of substance P can be demonstrated from superfused slices of rat hypothalamus or substantia nigra, with the release process dependent on the presence of a normal Ca^{2+}/Mg^{2+} ratio in the external medium (84). Release has also been demonstrated from the isolated spinal cord of newborn rats, with increased release in the presence of high K^+ or upon repetitive stimulation of dorsal roots (150). Substance P was detected only after superfusion of slices; this was attributed to rapid breakdown by soluble enzymes or those associated with the membrane. No reuptake mechanism was demonstrated. Substance P values appear to be stable up to 12 hr post-mortem in brains fixed in a freezing mixture. However, they are unstable in brains obtained by decapitation, an observation that suggests the presence of labile precursors (90).

There is a report that substance P injected intracerebrally or intraperitoneally into mice can induce analgesia that is reversible by naloxone (184). In our own studies, we failed to observe marked analgesia on placement of substance P into the periacqueductal gray of rats, a known analgesic site 85; Y. Jacquet and N. Marks, *unpublished observations*).

Enzymes inactivating substance P are widely distributed in brain regions. They are highest in the pineal gland; lower in posterior pituitary, hypothalamus, pons-medulla, and cortex; and lowest in spinal cord (120). In subcellular fractions, the mitochondrial particulates were characterized by low activity as compared with the cytosol. The soluble enzyme was partially purified by passage through DEAE-cellulose and showed properties akin to a neutral endopeptidase (cathepsin M; 12,119). Internal cleavage was indicated in studies with a bioassay using the guinea pig ileum; inactivation occurred before free amino acids could be detected by a chromatographic procedure. Incubation for longer periods led to the liberation of almost all residues, with the appearance of $Met \cdot NH_2$ at shorter, and free Met at longer periods. The release of breakdown products was consistent with endopeptidase cleavage at -Phe[7]-Phe[8]- and possible -Glu[6]-Phe[7]- bonds in addition to release of N-terminal Arg by an aminopeptidase and release of $Met \cdot NH_2$ by a C-terminal cleaving enzyme (Fig. 12–6). Other amino acids were released by sequential breakdown of intermediate peptides. Studies on model peptides such as $Leu-Met \cdot NH_2$ suggest that the amide is released prior to deamidation when incubated with brain extracts. This contrasts with TRH, where deamidation appears to be a major route for inactivation.

Studies on substance P breakdown using bioassay and immunoassay must take into account the possible reactivity of breakdown products which can elicit contraction of guinea pig gut or depolarize frog spinal motoneurons (150,204). This is illustrated by the work of Yajima et al. (204), who found gut contraction by N-blocked Lys[3]-, Gln[5]-, and Gln[6]----Met-NH₂[II] peptides equal to or exceeding substance P, and by Bergmann et al. (16), who observed good activities for a series of synthetic C-terminal peptides. Niedrich et al. (144) using a large series of synthetic peptides, found that C-terminal pentapeptides of substance P, eledoisins, and physalaemins had potent contracting ability, equal to that found for acylated hexa- and heptapeptides. Similar observations for C-terminal penta- and heptapeptides were found by Bury and Mushford (27). Otsuka et al. (150) have suggested that motor-depolarizing activity is specifically connected with the sequence Phe-X-Gly-Leu-Met·NH$_2$ where X = Ile, Tyr, or Phe. If so, substance P could be a precursor, and be transformed to the real transmitter after removal of some N-terminal amino acids. They found that deca-, nona-, and octapeptides were almost equally as active in the spinal cord preparations,

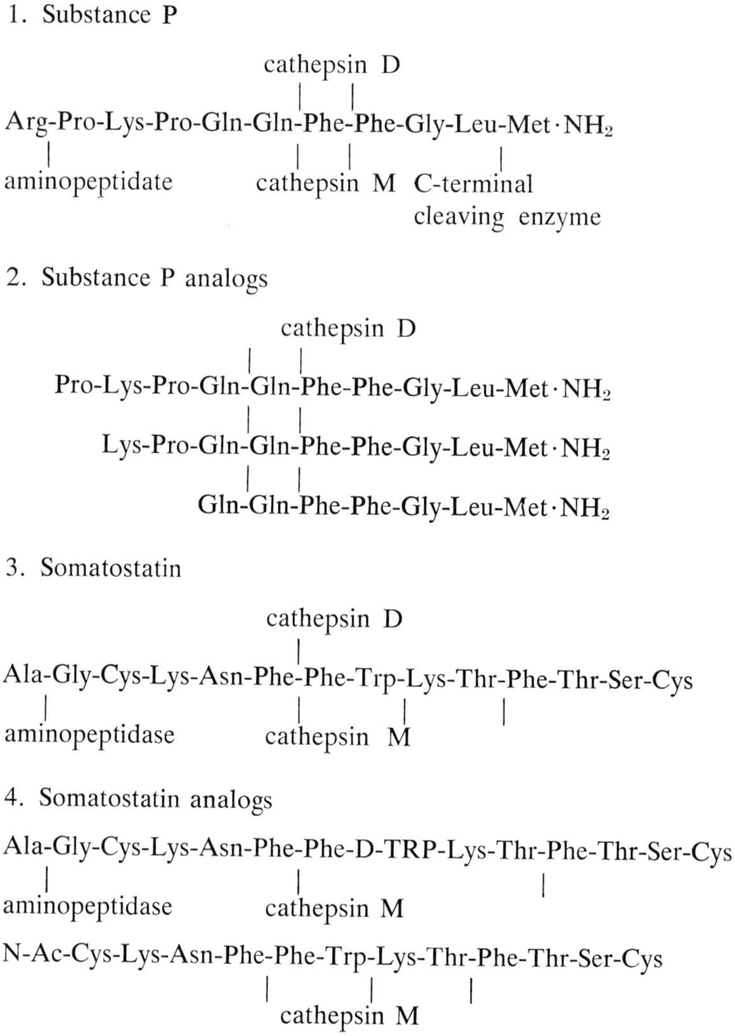

1. Substance P

cathepsin D

Arg-Pro-Lys-Pro-Gln-Gln-Phe-Phe-Gly-Leu-Met·NH$_2$

aminopeptidate   cathepsin M   C-terminal
                                      cleaving enzyme

2. Substance P analogs

cathepsin D

Pro-Lys-Pro-Gln-Gln-Phe-Phe-Gly-Leu-Met·NH$_2$

Lys-Pro-Gln-Gln-Phe-Phe-Gly-Leu-Met·NH$_2$

Gln-Gln-Phe-Phe-Gly-Leu-Met·NH$_2$

3. Somatostatin

cathepsin D

Ala-Gly-Cys-Lys-Asn-Phe-Phe-Trp-Lys-Thr-Phe-Thr-Ser-Cys

aminopeptidase   cathepsin M

4. Somatostatin analogs

Ala-Gly-Cys-Lys-Asn-Phe-Phe-D-TRP-Lys-Thr-Phe-Thr-Ser-Cys

aminopeptidase   cathepsin M

N-Ac-Cys-Lys-Asn-Phe-Phe-Trp-Lys-Thr-Phe-Thr-Ser-Cys

cathepsin M

FIG. 12–6. Sites of cleavage of somatostatin and substance P or analogs by brain enzymes (3,14,15,127).

whereas penta-, tetra-, and tripeptides were practically inactive. These studies emphasize the possible importance of N-terminal peptidases in metabolic studies on the fate of substance P. An unresolved question is the possible heterogeneity of substance P observed in older studies (209).

In addition to inactivation by cytoplasmic enzymes, breakdown of substance P and selected analogues occurs on treatment with lysosomal cathepsin derived from calf brain (15) or bovine hypothalami (3). Brain enzyme cleaved largely at the Phe^7-Phe^8 bond, and in addition hypothalamic enzyme cleaved one of the bonds to yield N-terminal Glu. The cleavage by brain enzyme was completely inhibited on addition of pepstatin, a pentapeptide inhibitor of the lysosomal enzyme. Studies with pepsin showed a similar specificity with cleavage of the Phe-Phe bond. The active heptapeptide Glu^5------Met·NH_2 also was cleaved by cathepsin D of brain with production of N-terminal Phe. Evidence for lysosomal degradation indicates that more than one mechanism exists for breakdown of neuropeptides such as substance P. Regulation by breakdown will therefore be dependent on the anatomical localization of peptide with respect to the degradative system involved. In addition to cathepsin D, brain lysosomes contain cathepsin A, B1, B2, and C. These may play additional roles (70). The large spectrum of enzymes presents a problem in deciding on a relevant system involved in regulation, and it is premature to label any particular enzyme as a leading candidate in the case of substance P.

Neurotensin

Neurotensin is a vasoactive tridecapeptide isolated from hypothalamus that has kinin-like properties. Specific antisera have been developed and studies on its localization show a wide distribution in CNS tissues and the gastrointestinal tract (30). In brain tissue, neurotensin-like substances are present in high concentration in the hypothalamus and brainstem, and in lower concentration in cortex, thalamus, cerebellum, and pituitary. In subcellular fractions, activity is associated with synaptosomes. Studies on breakdown in rat brain homogenates show a C-terminal release of amino acids pointing toward a role for carboxypeptidases as a major route for inactivation (Fig. 12–6). The presence of pyroGlu, as in the case of LRH, probably prevents metabolism by aminopeptidases. An inactive dodecapeptidyl form lacking C-terminal Leu has been isolated from bovine gut. It may have been formed by action of carboxypeptidases (29,30,96). No significant degradation occurred on exposure of neurotensin to washed synaptosomes (96a).

Somatostatin

Somatostatin is the tetradecapeptide first isolated from bovine hypothalamus, and since shown to be of wide occurrence in CNS and gastrointestinal tissue. It inhibits the release of growth hormone and thyrotropin from the pituitary. Its very short half-life has limited its clinical applications, and there has been a search for longer acting derivatives. In studies on inactivation *in vitro* we found a preferential release of internal residues involving the -Trp[8]-Lys[9]- linkage and to a lesser extent bonds adjacent to the Phe residues (Fig. 12–6). The slower release of Ala and Cys suggest that peptide hydrolases are not the primary mechanism for inactivation, especially since Ala and Gly do not appear to be essential for activity (126,127). Further evidence for cleavages was provided by the use of N-blocked analogues that prohibit the action of an aminopeptidase. Incubation of des-Ala-Gly (Ac-Cys[3])-somatostatin or its dicarbo derivative still led to release of internal residues, confirming the action of an endopeptidase which could be partially blocked by substitution of Trp by the D-isomer. Rivier et al. (164,165) have shown that the D-analogue is eightfold more potent *in vivo*. The improved biological activity correlates well with its decreased breakdown, which could be one of several factors affecting its hormonal action. The enzyme inactivating somatostatin was partially purified and showed properties akin to that of the endopeptidase (cathepsin M) inactivating LRH and substance P. In a systematic study on the effects of substitution of each individual residue by Ala, no major change in biological activity was noted except in the case of positions 2 and 8 (127). Such results may reflect changes in receptor occupancy rather than metabolism, since L-amino acids are known to affect breakdown less than the D-isomers. Studies on the tertiary structure of somatostatin indicate that residues adjacent to vulnerable bonds are involved in stabilization of β-type conformation.

Studies on rat and human serum indicate involvement of a similar endopeptidase with partial blockade by insertion of a D-Trp in position 8 (13). Breakdown was significantly greater in rat.

Very little difference in biological activity and rate of degradation has been observed for linear and cyclic forms of somatostatin (164,165). The possibility exists that rapid oxidation occurs in tissues and the active form is cyclic. There have been several attempts to prepare analogues with stabilized ring structures to improve biological stability and potencies (78,172). Studies with purified lysosomal cathepsin D from brain (15) and hypothalamus (3) indicate that the -Phe-Phe bond in positions 6 and 7 of dihydro and cyclic somatostatin is vulnerable to breakdown with production of a new Phe end-group. There is also a slower cleavage of the Trp-Lys bond with release of trace amounts of Lys (Fig. 12–6). Cleavage of the Trp-Lys bond is blocked by the presence of a D-Trp in position 8, and this could be a contributory factor to its enhanced activity *in vivo* (127,165). Since more than one enzyme system is available for inactivation of somatostatin, the same considerations apply to inactivation as apply to substance P. Cleavage at the Phe-Phe bond of dihydrosomatostatin was observed upon incubation with pepsin. Activity of both cathepsin D and pepsin was blocked by pepstatin (15).

ACKNOWLEDGMENTS

I would like to accord my gratitude to the following persons for provision of peptide substrates and for many helpful discussions: Wilfred F. White (Abbott Laboratories, Chicago, Ill.); Jean Rivier (The Salk Institute, San Diego, Ca.); Abba Kastin (V. A. Hospital, New Orleans, La.); Ralph F. Hirschmann (Merck, Sharp and Dohme, West Point, Penn.); and Yasuko Jacquet (Institute for Neurochemistry, Wards Island, N.Y.C.). Also I am indebted to the following persons who have assisted in the research efforts: Myron Benuck, Frederick Stern, and Alice Grynbaum of this Institute. The investigations in this review were supported in part by USPHS grants NB-03226 and NS-12578.

REFERENCES

1. Acher, R. (1976): Molecular evolution of the polypeptide hormones. The peptide hormones: Molecular and cellular aspects. *Ciba Found. Symp.*, 41:31–59.
2. Adelson, J. W. (1971): Enterosecretory proteins. *Nature*, 229:321–325.
3. Akopan, T. N., Arutynyan, A. A., Lajtha, A., and Galoyan, A. A. (1977): Hypothalamus acid proteinase purification, some properties, action on somatostatin, substance P and analogs of substance P. *Neurochem. Res. (in press)*.
4. Arimura, A., Sato, H., Dupont, A., Nishi, N., and Schally, A. V. (1975): Somatostatin: Abundance of immunoreactive hormone in rat stomach and pancreas. *Science*, 189:1007–1008.
4a. Austen, B. M., and Snell, C. R. (1977): The NH_2-terminus of C-fragment is resistant to the action of aminopeptidases. *Biochem. Biophys. Res. Commun.*, 77: 477–482.
4b. Austen, B. M., and Smyth, D. G. (1977): Specific cleavage of lipotropic C-fragment by endopeptidases evidence for a preferred conformation. *Biochem. Biophys. Res. Commun.*, 77:86–94.
5. Bajusz, S., Barabás, E., Széll, E., and Bagdy, D. (1975): Peptide aldehyde inhibitors of the fibrinogen-thrombin reaction. In *Peptides: Chemistry, Structure and Biology*, edited by R. Walter and J. Meienhofer, pp. 603–608. Ann Arbor Science, Ann Arbor, Mich.
6. Bajusz, S., Ronai, A. Z., Szekely, J. I., Graf, L., Dumas-Koracs, Z., and Berzetei, I. (1976): Superactive aminociceptive pentapeptide, D-Met², Pro⁵-encephalinamide. *FEBS Lett.*, 76:91–92.
7. Bargmann, W. (1949): Uber die neurosecretorishe Verknupferung von hypothalamus und Neurohypophyse. *Z. Zellforsh.*, 34:610–634.
8. Bassiri, R., and Utiger, R. D. (1972): Serum inactivation of the immunological and biological activity of TRH. *Endocrinology*, 91:657–667.
9. Bauer, K. (1976): Regulation of degradation of TRH by thyroid hormones. *Nature*, 259:591–593.
10. Bauer, K., and Lipmann, F. (1976): Attempts toward biosynthesis of the thyrotropin-releasing hormone and studies on its breakdown in hypothalamic tissue preparations. *Endocrinology*, 90:230–242.
11. Bennett, H. P. J., Bullock, G., Lower, P. J., McMartin, C., and Peter, J. (1974): Fate of corticotrophins in an isolated adrenal-cell bioassay and decrease of peptide breakdown by cell purification. *Biochem. J.*, 138:185–194.
12. Benuck, M., and Marks, N. (1975): Enzymatic inactivation of substance P by a partially purified enzyme from rat brain. *Biochem. Biophys. Res. Commun.*, 65: 153–160.
13. Benuck, M., and Marks, N. (1976): Differences in the degradation of hypothalamic releasing factors by rat and human serum. *Life Sci.*, 19:1271–1276.

14. Benuck, M., Ferin, M., and Marks, N. (1976): Inactivation of Luliberin (LII-RF) by hypophyseal portal blood of primates. *Neurosci. Abstr.,* 2:848.
15. Benuck, M., Grynbaum, A., and Marks, N. (1977): Cleavage of substance P and somatostatin by lysosomal cathepsin D purified by affinity chromatography. *Brain Res. (in press).*
16. Bergmann, J., Oehme, P., Bienert, M., and Niedrich, H. (1975): Action mechanism of peptides attacking smooth muscles II. *Acta Biol. Med. Ger.,* 34:475–481.
17. Blobel, G., and Dobberstein, B. (1975): Transfer of proteins across membranes. *J. Cell Biol.,* 67:831–835.
18. Bloom, F., Cattenberg, E., Rossier, T., Ling, N., Leppaluolo, T., Varyo, T. M., and Guillemin, R. (1977): Endorphins are located in the intermediate and anterior lobes of the pituitary gland, not in the neurohypophysis. *Life Sci.,* 20:43–48.
19. Boissonas, R. A., Guttman, S., and Pless, T. (1966): Synthesis of D-Ser-Nle⁴-(Val-NH₂)²⁵-β-corticotropin (1–25), a highly potent analogue of ACTH. *Experientia,* 22:526.
20. Bradbury, A. F., Smyth, D. G., and Snell, C. R. (1976): Polypeptide hormone: Molecular and cellular aspects. *Ciba Found. Symp.,* 41:61–75.
21. Bradbury, A. F., Smyth, D. G., and Snell, C. R. (1976): Lipotropin: Precursor to two biologically active peptides. *Biochem. Biophys. Res. Commun.,* 69:950–956.
22. Bradbury, A. F., Smyth, D. G., Snell, C. R., Birdsall, N. J. M., and Hulme, E. C. (1976): C-fragment of lipotropin has a high affinity for brain opiate receptors. *Nature,* 260:793–795.
23. Bradbury, A. F., Smyth, D. G., Snell, C. R., Deakin, J. F. W., and Wendlundt, S. (1977): Comparison of the analgesic properties of lipotropin C-fragment and stabilized enkephalins in the rat. *Biochem. Biophys. Res. Commun.,* 74:748–754.
24. Bretangna, M., Lis, M., and Gilardeau, C. (1974): Biosynthesis in vitro of beef β-lipotropin. *Can. J. Biochem.,* 52:349–358.
25. Broomfield, G. A., Scott, A. P., Lowery, P. T., Gilkes, T. T. H., and Rees, L. H. (1974): A reappraisal of human β-MSH. *Nature,* 252:492–493.
26. Brownstein, M. J., Mroz, E. A., Kizer, J. S., Palkovits, M., and Leeman, S. (1976): Regional distribution of substance P in the brain of the rat. *Brain Res.,* 116:299–305.
27. Bury, W. R., and Mushford, M. L. (1976): Biological activity of C-terminal partial sequences of substance P. *J. Med. Chem.,* 19:854–856.
28. Butt, W. R. (1976): *Hormone Chemistry,* Ed. 2, pp. 96–114. John Wiley & Sons, New York.
29. Carraway, R., and Leeman, S. E. (1975): Structural requirements for the biological activity of neurotensin; a new vasoactive peptide. In: *Peptides: Chemistry, Structure and Biology,* edited by R. Walter and J. Meienhofer, pp. 679–685. Ann Arbor Science, Ann Arbor, Mich.
30. Carraway, R., and Leeman, S. E. (1976): Characterization of radio-immuno-assayable neurotensin in the rat. *J. Biol. Chem.,* 251:7052–7075.
31. Celis, M. E., Nakagawa, S. H., and Walter, R. (1975): Release of melanocyte-stimulating hormone by neurohypophyseal hormone fragments. In: *Peptides: Chemistry, Structure and Biology,* edited by R. Walter and J. Meienhofer, pp. 771–776. Ann Arbor Science, Ann Arbor, Mich.
32. Chretien, M. (1973): Lipotropins LPH. In: *Methods in Investigative and Diagnostic Endocrinology, Vol. 2A,* edited by S. A. Berson and R. S. Yalow, pp. 617–632. North Holland, New York.
33. Chretien, M., Benjannet, S., Dragon, N., Seidah, N. G., and Lis, M. (1976): Isolation of peptides with opiate activity from sheep and human pituitaries: Relationship to β-LPH, *Biochem. Biophys. Res. Commun.,* 72:472–478.
34. Chretien, M., Gilardeau, C., Seidah, N., and Lis, M. (1976): Purification and partial chemical characterization of human pituitary lipolytic hormone. *Can. J. Biochem.,* 54:778–782.
35. Chretien, M., and Li, C. H. (1967): Isolation, purification and characterization of γ-LPH from sheep pituitary glands. *Can. J. Biochem.,* 45:1163–1174.
36. Chretien, M., Lis, M., Gilardeau, C., and Benjannet, S. (1976): In vitro biosynthesis of γ-lipotropic hormone. *Can. J. Biochem.,* 54:566–570.

37. Clouet, D. H., and Ratner, M. (1976): The incorporation of H³-glycine into enkephalin in the brains of morphine treated rats. In: *Opiates and Endogenous Opioid Peptides,* edited by H. W. Kosterlitz, pp. 71–83. Elsevier, Amsterdam.
38. Cooper, N. R., and Ziccardi, R. J. (1976): The nature and reactions of complement enzymes. In: *Proteolysis and Physiological Regulation,* edited by D. W. Ribbons and K. Braw, pp. 167–187. Academic Press, New York.
39. Coslovsky, R., and Yalow, R. S. (1974): Inference of the hormonal forms of ACTH on the pattern of corticosteroid secretions. *Biochem. Biophys. Res. Commun.,* 60:1351–1356.
40. Coy, D. H., Kastin, A. J., Schally, A. V., Morrin, G., Caron, N. G., Latbrie, F., Walter, J. M., Fertel, R., Berntson, G. G., and Sandman, C. A. (1976): Synthesis and opioid activities of stereoisomers and other D-amino acid analogs of methionine enkephalin. *Biochem. Biophys. Res. Commun.,* 73:632–638.
41. Cross, B. A., Dybal, R. E., Dyer, R. G., Jones, C. W., Lincoln, D. W., Morris, J. F., and Pickering, R. T. (1975): Endocrine neurones. *Recent Prog. Horm. Res.,* 31:243–293.
42. Davie, E. W., Fujikawa, K., Legaz, M. E., and Kato Hisao (1975): Role of proteases in blood coagulation. *Proteases and Biological Control. Cold Spring Harbor Conference on Cell Proliferation, Vol. 2,* pp. 65–77. Cold Spring Harbor Laboratory, Cold Spring Harbor, N.Y.
43. Desaulles, P. A., Riniker, B., and Rittel, W. (1969): In: *Protein and Polypeptide Hormones,* edited by M. Margolis, pp. 104–110. Int. Congr. Ser. No. 161, Excerpta Medica, Amsterdam.
44. Dixon, H. B. (1960): Chromatographic isolation of pig and human melanocyte-stimulating hormone. *Biochem. Biophys. Acta,* 37:38–42.
45. Doneen, B. A., Chung, D., Yamashiro, D., Law, P. Y., Loh, H. H., and Li, C. H. (1977): β-Endorphin: Structure-activity relationships in the guinea pig ileum and opiate receptor binding assays. *Biochem. Biophys. Res. Commun.,* 74:656–662.
46. Fawcett, C. P., and Shin, S. H. (1975): Generation of hypophysiotropic activity in hypothalamus extracts *in vitro. Endocrinol Res.,* 2:151–158.
47. Fujino, M., Yamazak, I., Kobayashi, S., Fukuda, T., Shinagawa, S., Nakayama, R., White, W. F., and Rippel, R. H. (1974): Some analogs of LH-RF having intense ovulation-inducing activity. *Biochem. Biophys. Res. Commun.,* 57:1248–1256.
48. Gainer, H. (1976): Peptides and neuronal function. *Adv. Biochem. Psychopharmacol.,* 15:193–210.
49. Gainer, H., Sarne, Y., and Brownstein, M. T. (1977): Neurophysin biosynthesis: Conversion of a putative precursor during axonal transport. *Science,* 195:1354–1356.
50. Geisow, M. T., and Smyth, D. G. (1977): Lipotropin C fragment has a C-terminal sequence with high intrinsic resistance to the action of exopeptidase. *Biochem. Biophys. Res. Commun.,* 75:625–629.
51. Gibbons, J. M., Mitnick, M., and Chiefto, V. (1975): In vitro biosynthesis of TSH and LH-releasing factors by the human placenta. *Am. J. Obstet. Gynecol.,* 121:127–132.
52. Gispen, W. H., van Ree, T. M., and de Wied, D. (1977): Lipotropin and the CNS. *Neuroscience Res. Prog. Bull. (in press).*
53. Goltzman, D. (1976): Conversion of proparathyroid hormone to parathyroid hormone studies *in vitro* with trypsin. *Biochemistry,* 15:5076–5082.
54. Graf, L. (1976): Chemistry of lipotropins. In: *Pharmaceutical Therapeutics,* pp. 753–769. Pergamon Press, Oxford.
55. Graf, L., Cseh, G., Barit, E., Ronai, A. T., Szekely, T. I., Kenessey, A., and Bajusz, S. (1977): Structure formation relationships in lipotropins. *Ann. N.Y. Acad. Sci. (in press).*
56. Graf, L., and Kenessey, A. (1976): Specific cleavage of a single peptide bond (residues 77–78) in β-LPH by a pituitary endopeptidase. *FEBS Lett.,* 69:255–260.
57. Graf, L., Ronai, A. Z., Bajusz, S., Cseh, G., and Szekely, T. I. (1976): Opioid agonist of β-LPH fragments: A possible biological source of morphine-like substances in the pituitary. *FEBS Lett.,* 64:181–184.
58. Gregory, R. A. (1976): Heterogeneity of the gastrins in blood and tissue. Poly-

peptide hormones: Molecular and cellular aspects. *Ciba Found. Symp.*, 41:251–265.

59. Greven, H. M., and de Wied, D. (1967): The active sequence in the ACTH molecule responsible for inhibition of the extraction of conditional behavior in rats. *Eur. J. Pharmacol.*, 2:14–18.

60. Greven, H. M., and de Wied, D. (1973): The influence of peptide derived from ACTH on performance, structure-activity studies. *Prog. Brain Res.*, 39:429–442.

61. Griffiths, E. C. (1976): Peptidase inactivation of hypothalamic releasing hormones. *Horm. Res.*, 7:179–191.

62. Griffiths, E. C., and Hooper, K. C. (1973): The effects of orchidectomy and testosterone propionate injection on peptidase activity in the male rat hypothalamus. *Acta Endocrinol. (Kbh.)*, 72:1–8.

63. Griffiths, E. C., and Hooper, K. C. (1973): Peptidase activity in the hypothalamus of rats treated neonatally with estrogen. *Acta Endocrinol. (Kbh.)*, 72:9–17.

64. Griffiths, E. C., and Hooper, K. C. (1974): Competitive inhibition between oxytocin and LH-RH for the same enzyme system in the rat hypothalamus. *Acta Endocrinol. (Kbh.)*, 75:435–442.

65. Griffiths, E. C., Hooper, K. C., Hubon, D., Jeffcoate, S. L., and White, N. (1977): Hypothalamic inactivation of TRH. *Mol. Cell. Endocrinol.*, 4:215–222.

66. Griffiths, E. C., Hooper, K. C., Jeffcoate, S. L., and Holland, D. T. (1975): The effects of gonadectomy and gonal steroids on the activity of hypothalamic peptidases inactivating LH-RH. *Brain Res.*, 88:384–388.

67. Griffiths, E. C., Hooper, K. C., Jeffcoate, S. L., and White, N. (1976): Inactivation of TRF by peptidases in different areas of rat brain. *Brain Res.*, 105:376–380.

68. Grim-Jorgensen, Y., and McKelvy, J. F. (1974): Biosynthesis of TRH by newt brain *in vitro*. Isolation and characterization of TRH. *J. Neurochem.*, 23:471–478.

69. Grim-Jorgensen, Y., Pieffer, S. E., and McKelvy, J. F. (1976): Metabolism of thyrotropin releasing factor in two clonal cell lines of nervous system origin. *Biochem. Biophys. Res. Commun.*, 70:167–173.

70. Grynbaum, A., and Marks, N. (1976): Characterization of rat brain catheptic carboxypeptidase (cathepsin A) inactivating angiotensin II. *J. Neurochem.*, 26:313–318.

71. Guillemin, R., Ling, N., and Buryas, R. (1976): Endorphins: Hypothalamic and neurohypophysial peptides with morphinomimetric activity. Isolation and primary structure of α-endorphin. *C. R. Acad. Sci. [D] (Paris)*, 282:783–786.

72. Guillemin, R., Schally, A. V., Lipscomb, H. S., Anderson, R. N., and Long, C. N. H. (1962): On the presence in hog hypothalamus of β-corticotropin releasing factor, α and β-MSH, ACTH, lysine vasopressin and oxytocins. *Endocrinology*, 70:471–477.

73. Habener, T. F. (1976): New concepts in the formation regulation of release and metabolism of parathyroid hormone. The peptide hormones: Molecular and cellular aspects. *Ciba Found. Symp.*, 41:197–223.

74. Hambrook, T. M., Morgan, B. A., Rance, M. T., and Smith, C. F. C. (1976): Mode of deactivation of the enkephalins by rat and human plasma and rat brain homogenates. *Nature*, 262:782–783.

75. Hano, K., Koida, M., Kubo, K., and Yajiwa, H. (1964): Evaluation of physiological properties of D-His-D-Phe-D-Arg-D-Trp-Gly in frog melanocyte. *Biochim. Biophys. Acta*, 90:201–210.

76. Hew, C. L., and Yip, C. C. (1976): Biosynthesis of polypeptide hormones. *Can. J. Biochem.*, 54:591–599.

77. Hofman, K. (1974): Relations between chemical structure and function of ACTH and MSH. In: *Handbook of Physiology, Section 7*, edited by K. Krobil and W. H. Sawyer, pp. 29–58. American Physiological Society, Washington, D.C.

78. Holladay, L. A., and Puett, D. (1975): Physiochemical characteristics and a proposed conformation of somatostatin limited β-structure. In: *Peptides: Chemistry, Structure and Biology*, edited by R. Walter and J. Meienhofer, pp. 175–179. Ann Arbor Science, Ann Arbor, Mich.

79. Hollosi, M., Kajtar, M., and Graf, L. (1977): Studies on the conformation of

β-endorphin and its constituent fragments in water and trifluorethanol by CD spectroscopy. *FEBS Lett.*, 74:185–189.

80. Hughes, J. (1975): Isolation of an endogenous compound from the brain with pharmacological properties similar to morphine. *Brain Res.*, 88:295–308.

81. Hughes, J., Smith, T. W., Kosterlitz, H. W., Fothergill, L. A., Morgan, B. A., and Morris, H. R. (1975): Identification of two related pentapeptides from the brain with potent opiate agonist activity. *Nature*, 258:577–579.

82. Iliano, G., and Cuatrecasus, P. (1972): Modulation of adenylate cyclase activity in liver and fat cell membrane by insulin. *Science*, 175:906–908.

83. Isogai, Y., Nemethy, G., and Scheraya, H. A. (1977): Enkephalin: Conformational analysis by means of empirical energy catentations. *Proc. Natl. Acad. Sci. USA*, 74:414–418.

84. Iversen, L. L., Jessel, T., and Kamazawa, I. (1976): Release and metabolism of Substance P in rat hypothalamus. *Nature*, 264:81–83.

85. Jacquet, Y. F., and Lajtha, A. (1973): Morphine action at CNS sites in rat: Analgesia or hyperalgesia depending on site and dose. *Science*, 182:490–492.

86. Jacquet, Y., and Marks, N. (1976): The C-fragment of β-lipotropin: An endogenous neuroleptic or antipsychotogen. *Science*, 194:632–635.

87. Jacquet, Y., Marks, N., and Li, C. H. (1976): Behavioural and biochemical properties of opioid peptides. In: *Opiates and Endogenous Opioid Peptides*, pp. 411–414. Elsevier, Amsterdam.

88. Jeffcoate, S. L., and White, N. (1974): Use of benzamidine to prevent the destruction of TRH by blood. *J. Clin. Endocrinol. Metab.*, 38:135–137.

89. Johannson, N. G., Hooper, F., Sievertison, H., Currie, B. L., and Rolken, K. (1973): Biosynthesis in vitro of LH-RH by hypothalamic tissue. *Biochem. Biophys. Res. Commun.*, 49:650–660.

90. Kanazawa, I., and Jessell, T. (1976): Post mortem changes and regional distribution of Substance P in the rat and mouse nervous system. *Brain Res.*, 117:362–367.

91. Kappler, H., Riniker, B., Rittel, W., Desaulles, P. A., Maier, R., Schar, B., and Stoeblin, N. (1967): In: *The Peptides*, edited by H. C. Beyerman, A. Van de Linde, and W. Maassen van den Brink, pp. 214–221. North Holland, Amsterdam.

92. Kastin, A. J. (1977): Behavioral effects of peptides. *Neurosci. Res. Prog. Bull.* (*in press*).

93. Kastin, A. J., Nissen, C., Schally, A. V., and Coy, D. H. (1976): Blood brain barrier, half-time disappearance and brain distribution for labeled enkephalin and a potent analog. *Brain Res. Bull.*, 1:383–389.

94. Kastin, A. J., Sandman, C. A., Stratton, L. O., Schally, A. V., and Miller, L. H. (1975): Behavioral and electrographic changes in rat and man after MSH. *Progr. Brain Res.*, 42:143–150.

95. Kemmler, W. (1975): Conversion of proinsulin. *Handbk. Exp. Pharmacol.*, 32: 17–56.

96. Kitabyl, P., Carraway, R., and Leeman, S. E. (1976): Isolation of a tridecapeptide from bovine intestinal tissue and its partial characterization as a neurotensin. *J. Biol. Chem.*, 251:7053–7058.

96a. Kitabyl, P., Carraway, P., van Rietschoten, J., Granier, C., Morgat, J. L., Menez, A., Leeman, S., and Frechet, P. (1977): Neurotensin: specific binding to synaptic membranes from rat brain. *Proc. Natl. Acad. Sci. USA*, 74:1846–1850.

97. Knigge, K. M., and Schock, D. (1975): Characteristics of the plasma TRH degrading enzyme. *Neuroendocrinology*, 19:277–287.

98. Koch, Y., Baram, T., Chobsieng, P., and Fridkin, M. (1974): Enzymic degradation of LH-RH by hypothalamic tissue. *Biochem. Biophys. Res. Commun.*, 61:95–103.

99. Koch, Y., Baram, T., Hazum, E., and Fridkin, M. (1977): Resistance to enzyme degradation of LH-RH analogues possessing increased biological activity. *Biochem. Biophys. Res. Commun.*, 74:488–491.

100. Kochman, K., Kendelhue, B., Zog, U., and Jutisz, M. (1975): Studies of enzymatic degradation of luteinizing hormone-releasing hormone by different tissues. *FEBS Lett.*, 50:190–194.

101. Kolda, M., Homo, K., and Iso, T. (1966): Evaluation of in vitro melanocyte-

darkening activities of His-Phe-Arg-Trp-Gly and its nine stereoisomers in Roma nigromaculata. *Jpn. J. Pharmacol.,* 14:243–244.

102. Kosterlitz, H. W., Hughes, T., Lord, T. A. H., and Waterfield, A. A. (1977): Enkephalin, endorphin, and opiate receptors. In: *Neuroscience Symposia,* II, pp. 291–307. Soc. for Neuroscience. Washington. D.C.

103. Krieger, D. T., Liotta, A., and Brownstein, M. T. (1977): Presence of corticotropin in brain of normal and hypophysectomized rats. *Proc. Natl. Acad. Sci. USA,* 74:648–652.

104. Kuhl, H., and Taubert, H. D. (1975): Short-loop feedback mechanism of luteinizing hormone. *Acta Endocrinol. (Kbh.),* 78:649–663.

105. Kuhl, H., and Taubert, H. D. (1975): Inactivation of LH-RF by rat hypothalamic L-crystine arylamidase. *Acta Endocrinol. (Kbh.),* 78:634–648.

106. LaBella, F., Queen, G., Senyshyn, T., Lis, M., and Chretien, M. (1973: Lipotropin: Localization by radioimmunoassay of endorphin precursor in pituitary and brain. *Biochem. Biophys. Res. Commun.,* 75:350–357.

107. Lajtha, A., and Marks, N. (1971): Protein turnover. In: *Handbook of Neurochemistry, Vol. 5,* edited by A. Lajtha, pp. 551–629. Plenum Press, New York.

108. Law, P. Y., Wei, E. T., Tsay, L. F., Loh, H. H., and Way, E. L. (1977): Opioid properties of β-lipotropin fragment 60–65·H-Arg-Try-Gly-Gly-Phe-Met·OH. *Life Sci.,* 20:251–260.

109. Lernmark, A., Chan, J. S., Choy, R., Nathans, A., Carroll, R., Tager, H. S., Rubenstein, A. H., Swift, H. H., and Steiner, D. F. (1976): Biosynthesis of insulin and glucagon: A view of the current state of the art. The peptide hormones: Molecular and cellular aspects. *Ciba Found. Symp.,* 41:7–28.

110. Levitan, D., Beitins, I. Z., Barnes, M. A., and McArthur, T. W. (1976): Insensitivity of Bonnet monkeys to D-Ala^6, des Gly^{10} LH-RH ethylamide, a potent LH-RH analogue in rats and mice. *Endocrinology,* 100:918–922.

111. Li, C. H. (1956): Hormones of the anterior pituitary gland. Growth and adrenocorticotropic hormones. *Adv. Protein Chem.,* 11:101–170.

112. Li, C. H. (1975): The chemistry of human pituitary growth hormone. *Horm. Proteins Peptides,* 3:1–38.

113. Li, C. H., and Chung, C. (1976): Isolation and structure of an untriakontapeptide with opiate activity from camel pituitary glands. *Proc. Natl. Acad. Sci. USA,* 73:1145–1148.

114. Li, C. H., Rao, J., Doneen, B. A., and Yamashiro, D. (1977): β-Endorphin: Lack of correlation between opiate activity and immunosensitivity by radioimmunoassay. *Biochem. Biophys. Res. Commun.,* 75:576–580.

115. Livesey, J. T., Rubenstein, D., and Beck, T. C. (1976): The nature of pituitary large growth hormone as studied by immunoabsorption. The polypeptide hormones: Molecular and cellular aspects. *Ciba Found. Symp.,* 41:77–95.

116. Lowery, P. J., and McMartin, C. (1974): Metabolism of two adrenocorticotropin analogues in the intestine of the rat. *Biochem. J.,* 133:87–95.

117. MacGregor, R. R., Chu, L. L. H., and Cohn, D. V. (1976): Conversion of proparathyroid hormone to PTH by a particulate enzyme of the parathyroid gland. *J. Biol. Chem.,* 251:6711–6716.

118. Marks, N. (1970): Peptide hydrolases. In: *Handbook of Neurochemistry, Vol. 3,* edited by A. Lajtha, pp. 133–171. Plenum Press, New York.

119. Marks, N. (1977): Specificity of breakdown based on the inactivation of active proteins and peptides by brain proteolytic enzymes. In: *Intracellular Protein Catabolism, Vol. II,* edited by V. Turk and N. Marks, pp. 85–102. Plenum Press, New York.

120. Marks, N. (1977): Conversion and inactivation of neuropeptides. In: *Neurobiology of Peptides,* edited by H. Gainer, pp. 221–258. Plenum Press, New York.

121. Marks, N., Abrash, L., and Walter, R. (1973): Degradation of neurohypophyseal hormones by brain extracts and purified brain enzymes. *Proc. Soc. Exp. Biol. Med.,* 142:455–460.

122. Marks, N., Grynbaum, A., and Neidle, A. (1977): On the degradation of enkephalin and endorphins by rat and mouse brain extracts. *Biochem. Biophys. Res. Commun.,* 74:1552–1559.

122a. Marks, N., Benuck, M., and Grynbaum, A. (1978): Conversion and inactivation of brain oligopeptides. In: Mechanism, Regulation and Special Functions of Protein Synthesis in the Brain, edited by S. Roberts, A. Lajtha, and W. H. Gispen. Elsevier, Amsterdam (In press).

123. Marks, N., and Lajtha, A. (1971): Protein and polypeptide breakdown. In: Handbook of Neurochemistry, Vol. 5, edited by A. Lajtha, pp. 49–139. Plenum Press, New York.

124. Marks, N., and Stern, F. (1974): Enzymatic mechanisms for the inactivation of luteinizing hormone-releasing hormone (LH-RH). Biochem. Biophys. Res. Commun., 61:1458–1463.

125. Marks, N., and Stern, F. (1974): Novel enzymes involved in the inactivation of hypothalamo-hypophyseal hormones. In: Psychoneuroendocrinology, edited by N. Hatotani, pp. 153–162. S. Karger, Basel.

126. Marks, N., and Stern, F. (1975): Inactivation of somatostatin (GH-RIH) and its analogs by crude and partially purified rat brain extracts. FEBS Lett., 55:220–224.

127. Marks, N., Stern, F., and Benuck, M. (1976): Correlation between biological potency and biodegradation of a somatostatin analogue. Nature, 261:511–512.

128. Marks, N., Stern, F., and Kastin, A. J. (1976): Biodegradation of α-MSH and derived peptides by rat brain extracts, and by rat and human serum. Brain Res. Bull., 1:591–593.

129. McKelvy, J. F., LeBlanc, F., Landes, C., Perrie, S., Grim-Jorgensen, Y., and Kordon, C. (1976): The use of bacitracin as an inhibitor of the degradation of TRH and LH-RH. Biochem. Biophys. Res. Commun., 71:507–515.

130. McKelvy, J. F., Sheridan, M., Joseph, S., Philips, C. H., and Pirrie, S. (1975): Biosynthesis of TRF in organ culture of the guinea pig median eminence. Endocrinology, 97:908–918.

131. Medzihradszky, K., and Medzihradszky-Schweiger, H. (1976): Small peptides with melanocyte-stimulating activity. FEBS Lett., 67:45–47.

132. Meek, T. L., Yang, H. Y. T., and Costa, E. (1977): Enkephalin catabolism in vitro and in vivo. Neuropharmacology, 16:151–154.

133. Millar, R. P., Achnelt, C., and Rossier, G. (1977): Higher molecular weight immunoreactive species of LH-RH: Possible precursors of the hormone. Biochem. Biophys. Res. Commun., 74:720–731.

134. Miller, R., Chang, K. T., and Cuatrescasas, L. (1977): The metabolic stability of the enkephalins. Biochem. Biophys. Res. Commun., 74:1311–1317.

135. Momany, F. A. (1977): Conformational analysis of methionine-enkephalin and some analogs. Biochem. Biophys. Res. Commun., 75:1098–1103.

136. Monograph (1976): Polypeptide hormones: Molecular and cellular aspects. Ciba Found. Symp., 41:1–400.

137. Moguilevsky, T. A., Enero, M. A., and Szwarcfarb, B. (1974): LH-RH biosynthesis by rat hypothalamus in vitro. Influence of castration. Proc. Soc. Exp. Biol. Med., 147:434–437.

138. Morgan, B. A., Smith, C. F. C., Waterfield, A. A., Hughes, J., and Kosterlitz, A. W. (1976): Structure activity relationship of methionine enkephalin. J. Pharm. Pharmacol., 280:660–661.

139. Mori, M., and Takemori, Y. (1976): Evolutionary aspects of TRH inactivation in serum. Igaku No Ayami, 97:67–68 (Chem. Abstr., 85:58318, 1976).

140. Mudge, A. W., and Fellows, R. E. (1973): Bovine pituitary pyrrolidone-carboxyl peptidase. Endocrinology, 93:1428–1434.

141. Nair, R. M. G., Redding, T. W., and Schally, A. V. (1971): Site of inactivation of TRH by human plasma. Biochemistry, 10:3621–3624.

142. Neary, J. T., Kieffer, D. J., Federico, P., Mover, H., Maloof, F., and Soodak, M. (1976): Thyrotropin releasing hormone development of inactivation system during maturation of the rat. Science, 193:403–405.

143. Neurath, H., and Walsh, K. A. (1976): Role of proteolytic enzymes in biological regulation (a review). Proc. Natl. Acad. Sci. USA, 73:3825–3832.

144. Niedrich, H., Bienert, M., Mehlis, B., Bergmann, J., and Oehme, P. (1975): Studies on the action mechanisms of peptides attacking smooth muscle. III. Effect of N-acylation upon effectiveness of C-terminal partial sequences of eledosin,

physalemin, and substance P on guinea pig ileum. *Acta Biol. Med. Ger.,* 34:483–489.

145. Nishi, N., Coy, D. H., Coy, E. J., Ansimura, A., and Schally, A. V. (1976): Suppression of LH-RH-induced ovulation in hamsters and rats by synthetic analogs of LH-RH. *J. Reprod. Fertil.,* 48:1119–1124.

146. North, W. G., Valtin, H., Morris, J. E., and LaRochella, F. T. (1977): Evidence for metabolic conversions of rat neurophysins within neurosecretory granules of the hypothalamos-neurohypophyseal system. *Endocrinology,* 101:110–117.

147. Orth, D. N., Nicholson, W. E., Mitchell, W. M., Island, D. P., Shapiro, M., and Byging, R. L. (1973): ACTH and MSH production by a single cloned mouse pituitary tumor cell line. *Endocrinology,* 92:385–395.

148. Otsuka, M., and Konishi, S. (1976): Substance P and excitatory transmitter of primary sensory neurons. *Cold Spring Harbor Symp. Cell. Biol.,* XL:135–143.

149. Otsuka, M., and Konishi, S. (1976): Release of substance P-like immunoreactivity from isolated spinal cord of newborn rat. *Nature,* 264:83–84.

150. Otsuka, M., Konishi, S., and Takahashi, T. (1975): Hypothalamic substance P as a candidate for transmitter of primary afferent neurons. *Fed. Proc.,* 34:1922–1928.

151. Oyama, H., Horima, M., Matsummara, S., Kobayashi, K., and Suetsugu, N. (1975): Immunological half-life of porcine proinsulin. *Horm. Metab. Res.,* 7:520–521.

151a. Parker, R. C., Neaves, W. B., Barnea, A., and Porter, J. C. (1977): Studies on the uptake of (^{3}H)thyrotropin-releasing hormone and its metabolites by synaptosomes preparation of the rat brain. *Endocrinology,* 101:66–75.

152. Pearse, A. G. E. (1976): Peptides in brain and intestine. *Nature,* 262:92–94.

153. Pelletier, G., Leclerc, R., Labne, F., Cole, T., Chretien, M., and Lis, M. (1977): Immunohistochemical localization of β-LPH in the pituitary gland. *Endocrinology,* 100:770–781.

154. Pert, C. B., Bowie, D. L., Fong, B. T. W., and Chang, J. K. (1976): Synthetic analogues of Met-enkephalin and other long-acting opiate peptides. In: *Opiates and Endogenous Opioid Peptides,* pp. 79–102. Elsevier, Amsterdam.

155. Pert, C. B., Pert, A., Chang, J. K., and Fong, B. T. W. (1976): D-Ala²-Met-enkephalinamide, a potent, long lasting synthetic pentapeptide analgesic. *Science,* 194:330–332.

156. Pickup, J. C., and Hope, D. B. (1972): The limited proteolysis of bovine neurophysin by cathepsin D. *J. Neurochem.,* 19:1049–1064.

157. Prasad, C., and Peterkofsky, A. (1976): Demonstrations of pyroglutamyl peptidase and amidase activities toward thyrotropin-releasing hormone in hamster hypothalamus extracts. *J. Biol. Chem.,* 251:3229–3234.

158. Queen, G., Pinsky, C., and LaBella, F. (1976): Subcellular localization of endorphine activity in bovine pituitary and brain. *Biochem. Biophys. Res. Commun.,* 72:1021–1027.

159. Ramachandran, T. (1973): The structure and function of adrenocorticotropin. *Horm. Proteins Peptides,* 2:1–25.

160. Redding, T. W., Kastin, A. J., Gonzalez-Barcena, D., Coy, D. H., Coy, E. J., Schalch, D. S., and Schally, A. V. (1973): The half-life, metabolism and excretion of tritiated LH-RH in man. *J. Clin. Endocrinol. Metab.,* 37:626–663.

161. Redding, T. W., and Schally, A. V. (1969): Studies on the thyrotropin-releasing hormone (TRH). Activity in peripheral blood. *Proc. Soc. Exp. Biol. Med.,* 131:420–425.

162. Redding, T. W., and Schally, A. V. (1972): On the half-life of TRH in rats. *Neuroendocrinology,* 9:250–256.

163. Reichlin, S. (1976): Biosynthesis and degradation of hypothalamic-hypophysiotropic factors. In: *Subcellular Mechanisms in Reproductive Neuroendocrinology,* edited by F. Naftolin, K. T. Ryan, and I. J. Davies, pp. 109–127. Elsevier, Amsterdam.

164. Rivier, J., Brown, M., and Vale, W. (1975): D-Trp-somatostatin: An analog of somatostatin more potent than the native molecule. *Biochem. Biophys. Res. Commun.,* 65:746–751.

165. Rivier, J., Ling, N., Monahan, M., Rivier, C., Brown, M., and Vale, W. (1975): LH-RH and somatostatin analogs. In: *Peptides: Chemistry, Structure and Biology,* edited by R. Walter and J. Meienhofer, pp. 863–870. Ann Arbor Science, Ann Arbor, Mich.
166. Ronai, A. Z., Graf, L., Szehely, J. I., Dumas-Kovacs, Z., and Bajusz, S. (1977): Differential behavior of LPH (61–91)-peptide in different model systems: Comparison of the opioid activities of LPH-(61–91) peptide and its fragments. *FEBS Lett.,* 74:182–184.
167. Rubenstein, M., Stein, S., Gerber, L., and Udenfriend, S. (1977): Isolation and characterization of the opioid peptides from rat pituitary. I. β-Lipotropin. *Proc. Natl. Acad. Sci. USA (in press).*
168. Rudman, D., DiGirolamo, M., Malkin, M. F., and Garcia, L. A. (1965): The adipokinetic property of hypophyseal peptides and catecholamines: A problem in comparative endocrinology. In: *Handbook of Physiology, Section 5,* edited by A. E. Renold and G. Cabrill, pp. 533–540. American Physiological Society, Washington, D.C.
169. Russell, J. H., and Geller, D. M. (1975): The structure of rat proalbumin. *J. Biol. Chem.,* 250:3409–3413.
170. Sachs, H. (1970): Neurosecretion. In: *Handbook of Neurochemistry, Vol. 4,* edited by A. Lajtha, pp. 373–428. Plenum Press, New York.
171. Saez, J. M., Dazoni, A., Morera, A. M., and Bataille, P. (1975): Interactions of adrenocorticotropic hormone with its adrenal receptors. *J. Biol. Chem.,* 250: 1683–1689.
172. Sarantakis, D., Teichman, J., Clark, D. E., and Lien, E. L. (1977): A bicyclosomatostatin analog, highly specific for the inhibition of growth hormone release. *Biochem. Biophys. Res. Commun.,* 75:143–148.
173. Schally, A. V., Kastin, A. J., and Coy, D. H. (1976): LH-releasing hormone and its analogs: Recent basic and clinical investigations. *Int. J. Fertil.,* 21:1–30.
174. Schally, A. V., Lipscomb, H. S., Long, J. H., Dear, W. E., and Guillemin, R. (1962): Chromatography and hormonal activities of dog hypothalamus. *Endocrinology,* 70:478–480.
175. Scharrer, E., and Scharrer, B. (1954): Neurosekretion. In: *Hand. Mikr. Anatomie VI, Pt. 5,* edited by W. von Möllendorf and W. Bargmann, pp. 953–1066. Springer, Berlin.
176. Schwyzer, R., Schiller, P., Seelig, S., and Sayers, G. (1971): Isolated adrenal cell: Log close response curves for steroidogenesis induced by ACTH 1–24, 1–10, 4–10, and 5–10. *FEBS Lett.,* 19:229–230.
177. Scott, A. P., Bloomfield, G. A., Lowery, P. J., Gilke, T. J., Landon, J., and Rees, L. H. (1976): Pituitary adrenocorticotrophin and melanocyte stimulating hormones. In: *Peptide Hormones,* edited by J. A. Parsons, pp. 247–271. University Park Press, Baltimore.
178. Scott, A. P., Ratcliffe, J. G., Rees, H., London, T., Bennett, H. P. T., Lowery, P. J., and McMartin, C. (1973): Pituitary peptide. *Nature [New Biol.],* 244:65–67.
179. Simon, L., Yamashiro, D., Hao, A. J., and Li, C. H. (1976): Synthesis and biological activity of β-melanotropins and analogs. *J. Med. Chem.,* 20:155–158.
179a. Smyth, D. G., and Snell, C. R. (1977): Metabolism of the analgesic peptide lipotropin C-fragment in rat striatal slices. *FEBS Lett.,* 78:225–228.
180. Srikant, C. B., McCorkle, K., and Unger, R. H. (1971): Properties of immunoreactive glucagon fractions of canine stomach and pancreas. *J. Biol. Chem.,* 252: 1847–1851.
181. Steiner, D. F., Kemmler, W., Tager, H. S., and Rubenstein, A. H. (1974): Molecular events taking place during intracellular transport of exportable proteins. The conversion of peptide hormone precursors. *Adv. Cytopharmacol.,* 2: 195–205.
182. Steiner, D. F., Kemmler, W., Tager, H. S., Rubenstein, A. H., Lernmark, A., and Zuhlke, H. (1975): Proteolytic mechanisms in the biosynthesis of polypeptide hormones. In: *Proteases and Biological Control, Cold Spring Harbor Conference on Cell Proliferation, Vol. 2,* pp. 531–549. Cold Spring Harbor Laboratory, Cold Spring Harbor, N.Y.

183. Steiner, D. F., and Oyer, P. E. (1967): The biosynthesis of insulin and a probable precursor of insulin by a human islet cell adenoma. *Proc. Natl. Acad. Sci. USA*, 57:473–480.

184. Stewart, T. M., Gelto, C. T., Neldner, K., Reeve, E. B., Krivog, W. A., and Zimmermann, E. (1976): Substance P and analgesia. *Nature*, 262:784–785.

185. Taber, C. A., and Karavolas, H. J. (1975): Subcellular localization of LH releasing activity in the rat hypothalamus. *Endocrinology*, 96:446–452.

186. Tager, H. S., and Steiner, D. F. (1973): Isolation of a glucagon in containing peptide: Primary structure of a possible fragment of proglucagon. *Proc. Natl. Acad. Sci. USA*, 76:2321.

187. Taylor, W. L., and Dixon, T. E. (1976): The inhibition of thyrotropin-releasing hormone deamidation in porcine hypothalamic tissue. *Biochim. Biophys. Acta*, 444:428–434.

188. Tixier-Vidal, A., Levine, P. H., Pradelles, P., Morgat, T. L., and Fromageot, P. (1976): Fate of TRF after binding and stimulation of prolactin release by GHB cells: Evidence for release of immodified (3H-TRH). *Neuroendocrinology*, 20: 201–211.

189. Tseng, L. F., Loh, H. H., and Li, C. H. (1976): β-Endorphin as a potent analgesia by intravenous injection. *Nature*, 263:234–240.

190. Urquhart, T. (1974): Physiological actions of ACTH. In: *Handbook of Physiology, Section 7*, edited by E. Knobil and W. H. Sawyer, pp. 133–157. American Physiological Society, Washington, D.C.

191. Vale, W., Burgus, R., Dunn, T. F., and Guillemin, R. (1971): In vitro plasma inactivation of thyrotropin-releasing factor (TRF) and related peptides. Its inhibition by various agents and by the synthetic peptide PCA-His-OME. *Hormones*, 2:143–203.

192. Verhoeff, T., Palkovits, M., and Witter, A. (1977): Distribution of a behaviorally highly potent ACTH 4–9 analog in rat brain after intraventricular administration. *Brain Res.*, 126:89–104.

193. Verhoeff, T., and Witter, A. (1976): The *in vivo* fate of a behaviorally active ACTH 4–9 analog in rats after systemic administration. *Pharmacol. Biochem. Behav.*, 4:583–590.

194. Visser, J. T., Kuotwijk, W., Doctor, R., and Henneman, G. (1975): RIA for the measurement of pryGlu-His-Pro, a proposed TRF metabolite. *J. Clin. Endocrinol. Metab.*, 40:742–745.

195. Walker, T. M., Berntson, G. G., Sandman, C. A., Coy, D. H., Schally, A. V., and Kastin, A. J. (1977): An analog of encephalin having prolonged opiate-like effects *in vivo. Science*, 196:85–87.

196. Walter, R., and Breslow, E. (1974): Methods of isolation and identification of neurophysin proteins. *Res. Meth. Neurochem.*, 2:279–297.

197. Walter, R., Griffiths, E. C., and Hooper, K. C. (1973): Production of MIF by a particulate preparation of hypothalamus: Mechanism of oxytocin inactivation. *Brain Res.*, 60:449–508.

198. Walter, R., Neidle, A., and Marks, N. (1975): Significant difference in the degradation of Pro-Leu-Gly·NH$_2$ by human serum, and that of other species. *Proc. Soc. Exp. Biol. Med.*, 148:98–103.

199. Warberg, T., Eskay, A., Barnea, A., Reynolds, R. C., and Porter, T. C. (1977): Release of LH-RH and TRH from a synaptosomic enriched fraction of hypothalamic homogenates. *Endocrinology*, 100:814–825.

200. deWied, D., and Gispen, W. H. (1977). Behavioral effects of peptides. In: *Neurobiology of Peptides*, edited by H. Gainer, pp. 391–441. Plenum Press, New York.

201. Winokur, A., Davis, R., and Utiger, R. D. (1977): Subcellular distribution of TRH in rat brain and hypothalamus. *Brain Res.*, 120:423–434.

202. Witter, A. (1975): Commentary: The in vivo fate of brain oligopeptides. *Biochem. Pharmacol.*, 34:2025–2030.

203. Witter, A., Greven, H. M., and deWied, D. (1975): Correlations between structure, behavioral activity and rate of biotransformation of some ACTH 4–9 analogs. *J. Pharmacol. Exp. Ther.*, 143:853–860.

204. Yajima, H., Kitagawa, K., and Segawa, T. (1973): Studies on peptides XXXVIII. Structure-activity correlations of substance P. *Chem. Pharm. Bull. (Tokyo)*, 21: 2500–2506.
205. Yajima, H., Kueho, V., Kinsmura, Y., and Lande, S. (1966): Studies on peptides XI. The effect of melanotropic activity of altering the Arg residue of His-Phe-Arg-Trp-Gly. *Biochim. Biophys. Acta,* 127:545–549.
206. Yalow, R. S. (1976): Multiple forms of corticotropin (adrenocorticotropic hormone, ACTH) and their significance. The peptide hormones: Molecular and cellular aspects. *Ciba Found. Symp.,* 41:159–181.
207. Yalow, R. S., and Berson, S. A. (1971): Size heterogeneity of immunoreactive human ACTH in plasma and in extracts of pituitary glands and ACTH producing thymoma. *Biochem. Biophys. Res. Commun.,* 44:439–445.
208. Yalow, R. S., and Berson, S. A. (1973): Characteristics of 'Big ACTH' in human plasma and pituitary abstracts. *J. Clin. Endocrinol. Metab.,* 36:415–423.
209. Zetler, G. (1970): Biologically active peptides (substance P). In: *Handbook of Neurochemistry, Vol. 4,* edited by A. Lajtha, pp. 135–146. Plenum Press, New York.
210. Zuhlke, H., Steiner, D. F., Lernmark, A., and Lipsey, C. (1970): Carboxypeptidase β-like and trypsin-like activities in isolated rat pancreatic islets. The peptide hormones: Molecular and cellular aspects. *Ciba Found. Symp.,* 41:183–195.

Author Index

Numbers in parentheses before page of citation are reference numbers.

Abdellal, A. E. (1) 113
Abraham, S. F. (1) 73, (2) 107, (3) 115
Archer, R. (1) 36, (2) 36, (1) 329, 333, 352
Adelson, J. W. (2) 333
Ader, R. (1) 167, 179
Adler, R. A. (1) 215
Adolph, E. F. (4) 102
Aghajanian, G. K. (1) 195
Aguilar Parada, E. (1) 279
Ahern, G. (5) 124
Ahlquist, R. (2) 271
Akert, K. (6) 110
Akopan, T. N. (3) 364, 365, 366
Alford, F. P. (2) 233
Alleva, J. J. (2) 185
Alpert, L. C. (1) 13, (1) 137
Althoff, P. H. (3) 231
Amin, A. H. (2) 16
Amoss, M. (3) 3, 12, (2) 136
Anand, B. (3) 276, (4) 273, 275, (5) 273, 275
Andersson, B. (2) 72, (7) 101, (8) 117, (9) 117, (10) 102, (11) 101
Anson, M. L. (3) 64
Antunes, J. L. (4) 8, 21, (3) 42, (3) 139
Arimura, A. (1) 261, (2) 253
Arnauld, E. (4) 135
Arimura, A. (4) 355
Aschoff, J. (3) 187, 202
Aspelagh, M.-R. (5) 4, 23
Asscher, A. W. (12) 104
Atkins, T. (6) 272
Atkinson, L. E. (3) 249
Atweh, S. F. (6) 17, (7) 17, (1) 308, 312, (2) 313, 315, (3) 317
Aubert, M. L. (4) 208
Austen, B. M. (4a) 347, (4b) 337, 347
Axelrod, J. (4) 40, (2) 177
Ayalon, D. (5) 217

Bajusz, S. (5) 350, (6) 351
Baker, B. L. (8) 12, (9) 12, (10) 13
Balestrery, F. G. (4) 200
Ban, T. (7) 268, 275, 277, (8) 265, 275, 276
Bangham, R. (4) 64
Bard, P. (4) 318
Barden, N. (9) 267
Bargmann, W. (5) 35, (6) 35, 36, 41, 42, (7) 329
Barker, J. L. (11) 23, (5) 152, (6) 138, 141
Barnea, A. (12) 10, (7) 136
Barry, J. (13) 12, 21, (14) 12, (15) 1, (16) 12, (17) 12, (18) 12, (19) 12, (20) 12, (21) 12, (22) 12, (8) 137, (9) 137, (4) 253, 259
Bass, A. (10) 265
Bassi, F. (6) 219
Bassiri, R. (8) 361
Bauer, K. (9) 354, 360, 361, (10) 344, 354, 359, 361, 362
Baumann, G. (7) 215, (8) 215
Baxter, C. R. (5) 64, 69
Beck-Peccoz, P. (9) 210
Beilharz, S. (13) 123
Belluzzi, J. D. (5) 304, (6) 304, (7) 304
Ben-Jonathan, N. (10) 136
Benker, G. (10) 231, 235, (11) 231
Bennet, J. B. (6) 71
Bennett, J. P., Jr. (14) 116, 121
Bennett, H. P. (11) 339, 341, 362
Benscome, S. (11) 269, 279
Benuck, M. (12) 363, (13) 354, 357, 360, 361, 366, (14) 354, 357, 364, (15) 364, 365, 366
Bergman, R. (12) 273
Bergmann, J. (16) 363
Bern, H. A. (25) 1

Bernard, C. (13) 276
Besser, G. M. (12) 232, 233, 234, (13) 218, (14) 231, 232, 233
Bhathena, S. (14) 267
Bhattacharya, A. N. (23) 8, 21, (24) 8, (5) 254
Bing, J. (7) 61
Birge, C. A. (15) 235
Bivens, C. H. (16) 228
Björklund, A. (11) 136, 140, (12) 136, 140, (13) 136, 140
Black, I. B. (3) 164
Black, S. J. (15) 115
Blackard, W. G. (17) 225, (18) 225, 226
Blake, C. A. (15) 145, (19) 212
Blakemore, M. A. (16) 144
Blackwell, R. E. (14) 135
Blair-West, J. R. (16) 106
Blake, C. A. (6) 254, (7) 254
Blass, E. M. (17) 103, (18) 119, (19) 117, (20) 117, (21) 117
Blobel, G. (17) 331, 332
Block, M. (5) 200
Bloom, F. (8) 85, (18) 343
Bloom, F. E. (8) 308, 318, 319
Bloom, S. (15) 279, (16) 279, (17) 279, (18) 274, (19) 273, 274, (20) 269, 273, 274, 279
Boer, K. T. (23) 123, 125
Bohnet, H. G. (20) 215, (21) 215, 218, (22) 213
Boissonas, R. A. (19) 339
Booth, D. A. (22) 107
Borison, H. (9) 313
Bott, E. (24) 124
Böttger, I. (21) 279
Boyar, R. M. (23) 215
Boyd, A. E. III (24) 225
Bradbury, A. F. (10) 301, (11) 301, (12) 301, 314, (20) 332, 341, 344, (21) 341, (22) 341, 343, (23) 341, 351
Bradley, G. (13) 313

Subject Index